CHALLENGES IN RHEUMATOLOGY

Edited by **Miroslav Harjacek**

Challenges in Rheumatology
Edited by Miroslav Harjacek

Published by InTech
Janeza Trdine 9, 51000 Rijeka, Croatia

Publishing Process Manager Adriana Pecar

Technical Editor Teodora Smiljanic

Cover Designer InTech Design Team

Additional hard copies can be obtained from orders@intechopen.com

Challenges in Rheumatology, Edited by Miroslav Harjacek
p. cm.
ISBN 978-953-307-848-9

For EU product safety concerns:
IN TECH d.o.o., Prolaz Marije Krucifikse Kozulić 3, 51000 Rijeka, Croatia,
info@intechopen.com or visit our website at intechopen.com.

Meet the editor

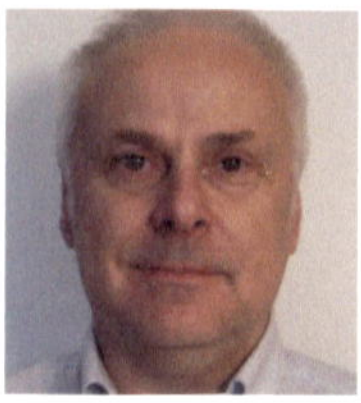

Dr. Miroslav Harjaček is the Head of Division of Pediatric and Adolescent Rheumatology at the Children's Hospital Srebrnjak, Zagreb, Croatia. He graduated in Pediatrics in 1992 (Children's Hospital, Buffalo, NY, USA) and in Pediatric Rheumatology 1996 (Floating Hospital for Children at NEMC, Boston, MA, USA). In 1998, he obtained his PhD in Medical Sciences at the University of Zagreb. He became an Associate Professor of Pediatrics in 2009 at the Medical School Zagreb, Croatia. He is a Fellow of American College of Rheumatology (ACR), member of Pediatric Rheumatology European Society (PRES), and national coordinator of PRINTO (Pediatric International Trial Organization). In 2009 he joined the Children's Hospital Srebrnjak, Zagreb, Croatia, and for the last seven years he has served as co-chairman for the International Summer School in Dubrovnik organized by IUC. Professor Miroslav Harjaček has published numerous papers and given a notable number of invited lectures on Pediatric Rheumatology. He is a reviewer for several international rheumatologic journals.

Contents

Preface

Challenges in Rheumatology aims to provide a general review for those who need quick up-to-date information on various aspects and impacts of rheumatic diseases. Rheumatology is a subspecialty of medicine that focuses on the biology, cause, diagnosis and treatment of a variety of musculoskeletal and other systemic diseases. Rheumatic diseases can present themselves in a number of familiar ways but sometimes are atypical and occasionally puzzling. Patients may appear insidiously or acutely ill and the impact of the disease can range from a temporary irritation, to a condition that is persistent and increasingly disabling, and sometimes a severe, even life-threatening illness. Most clinicians have a basic understanding of common disorders, yet they are often challenged by specific questions regarding the optimal diagnosis and care for patients with rheumatic diseases. More than ever, the care for patients with rheumatic diseases requires a multidisciplinary approach. In addition, the magic of the Internet has allowed our patients to be far better informed about their own health issues. They are demanding, and have the right to be active participants and decision-makers in their own care. If we are to act as their educators and advisors, we must continually strive to expand our own knowledge base.

The field of rheumatology is expanding rapidly and several very exciting developments have occurred in recent years. Firstly, there has been a dramatic shift in our understanding of the nature of inflammation and the possibility of specifically regulating the aberrant immune inflammatory response. Secondly, an understanding of the pathogenesis has lead to the development of new, more targeted therapies. As a practicing pediatric rheumatologist, I have always enjoyed treating the broad range of conditions that challenge my diagnostic skills and treatment abilities on a daily basis. Early in my career, treatment options were far more limited than today, but with the development of biologic therapies, primarily anti-tumor necrosis factor alpha (TNF-α), and others as well, therapeutic success has consequently increased significantly. That development has clearly changed the lives of many of our patients and revitalized an entire generation of rheumatologists.

Challenges in Rheumatology has assembled an impressive group of international experts who have studied specific aspects of certain rheumatic diseases and have extensive experience either in pathophysiology or an in-depth diagnosis and/or management of rheumatic patients. They communicate their knowledge and experience to the reader in chapters that are conveniently organized as pathophysiology, clinical manifestations and diagnosis of selected rheumatic diseases, medical and perioperative orthopedic management, and the economic impact of rheumatic diseases.

I am extremely grateful to the many authors who contributed to this book. I too, have learned a lot on various aspects of experimental and clinical rheumatology form editing the text. My hope is that this book will help our trainees become better physicians and scientists, and practicing rheumatologists to provide better care, and ultimately, improve the quality of life of our patients.

Prof. Dr. Miroslav Harjacek MD, PhD,
Children's Hospital Srebrnjak,
Department of Pediatric and Adolescent Rheumatology,
University of Zagreb, School of Medicine,
Croatia

Part 1

Economic Impact of Rheumatic Diseases

1

Economic Impact of Rheumatic Diseases

Gerardo Quintana L.[1,2] and Paola Coral-Alvarado[2]
[1]*Universidad de los Andes, Fundacion Santa Fe de Bogota*
[2]*Universidad Nacional de Colombia*
Colombia

1. Introduction

The prevalence and incidence of rheumatic diseases (RD) have been growing over the last two decades, related to the timely and accurate diagnosis, affecting in two ways the Health Systems (HS) and society, on one hand to early detection can prevent further functional compromise and sequels; and second, a greater cost in detection, approach, monitoring and treatment that ultimately impact on the prevention of functional decline of patients who suffer it.

The substantial increase in costs of health care service, the growing demand of these services, the increase of users without contributing to its financing and the latest technological advances in medical science have strong implications for the maintenance and provision of services, as well as increase the costs in this sector, creating changes in demand; it makes imperative the economic evaluation of interventions carried out in this social service.

Moreover, the approach to health has evolved significantly and nowadays, not only is essential to consider the evaluation of the patient to describe their evolution but also analyze which health technologies have the best cost/effect in order to achieve that decision makers to choose the most optimal according to the HS and typical econometric conditions of each nation.

In this chapter, will be presented a current view of how to measure the economic and functional impact of RD, the main results in the field and how these concepts are applied from Colombian perspective. Obviously given the relevance of these health technologies, we will approach very much to biological therapies and diseases in which are often used, predominantly Rheumatoid Arthritis (RA)

2. Basic concepts of economic evaluation

The pharmacoeconomics is defined as the description and analysis of how much the drug therapy costs to healthcare systems and society (1). It covers all areas considered like aspects of drugs such as the impact on society, the pharmaceutical industry, pharmacies, national budgets, and so on. It starts with the economic evaluation of health technologies, whose aim is the selection of options with a more positive health impact for appropriate decision-making. This evaluation process is done through comparisons of different alternatives to determine which of them offer the best cost-effect relation; but sometimes this comparison is

not necessarily performed against other drugs, but rather against alternative therapies (surgical or prophylactic).
Additionally, the ethical component is a factor to consider when making decisions, because frequently, the fact of paying more for more effective therapy is not necessary, since in the future, these resources will be able to used for the benefit of many patients and perhaps, more favourable conditions that guarantee the success of treatment (fair distribution of scant resources). In this respect, the physician's role is critical because it must balance between the effectiveness of treatment and its cost associated, to decide the best treatment option that is given to the patient, without neglecting the economic concepts that derive from their decision.
Health authorities are also actors, they have to guarantee a standard approach in the economic evaluation process; an unified evaluation ensures reliable outcomes and therefore their proper utilization and optimal use of resources, always based on the ratio of total healthcare costs (not just the drug itself). Likewise, it should develop a critical and systematic evaluation of these research results to ensure transparency and comparability (audit system).
The pharmaceutical industry also plays a important role, it discovers new products also carries out maintenance or exit of drugs already known, but new drugs must ensure at least a better effectiveness in terms of variables more objective, that truly justifying its use and additional payment; likewise, it has to be interested in promote standard strategies for economic evaluations of drug and integrate them into their research processes, a situation that would help the results of the other components (governments, insurance companies and health authorities).

3. Methods of drug evaluation

This method follows the footsteps of any clinical research in the medical field that is to create a strategic plan for attaining the goals of the study, the proper patient selection, the patients' assessment which they will be submitted, and obviously the objects of measurement.
Measuring the effects of compared options should be clearly established and to it should be led ideally by research with the aim of getting a suitable and clear conclusion, as well as obtaining a high-quality research.
The measurement and identification of costs is made through prospective and / or retrospective studies. The most frequently used are the direct costs (medical and non medical), and indirect costs, which are related to disabilities generated by illness itself, and the intangible costs given by sensations in the patients, it derivated from disease and that are hardly measurable, mainly chronic diseases and psychiatric disorders.
The types of economic evaluation depend on the manner how to measure the effects of a particular drug: cost-benefit; where costs and effects are measured by monetary units and they are compared between different alternatives. In cost-effectiveness, the effects are measured by typical clinical units: (deaths prevented, reduced levels, etc). In cost-utility, the effects are measured through a component that integrates life quality and quantity of life years (quality-adjusted life year -QUALYs). Finally, the cost-minimization compares directly the costs, and it prefers the lower value, but care must be taken when interpreting its results.
The QALY is an indicator that combines survival with quality of life. The measure of quality of life is not standardized and often varies from study to study depending on the disease

and the author preferences about treatment and evaluation. To calculate a QALY, it has to multiply the length of the state of health (in years) by a factor representing the quality ("utility") of this condition. The value of quality (utility) for the economic evaluation usually derived from an index of health, whose scale value 1 equals perfect health and a value of 0 to death (it is also possible to quantify health states with a negative value ("worse than death").

The analysis of results is the last step before making conclusions. There are two types of them: the incremental analysis, where the costs of alternatives (difference) are divided by the differences in effectiveness; and sensitivity analysis, which speculates some assumptions on the values of the most relevant variables, hoping that it does not change the results strikingly.

4. Evaluation of rheumatic diseases

In a series of research from the 1960s, Dorothy Rice et al (2-5) have provided estimates of the economic impact of musculoskeletal diseases, including all forms of arthritis. These estimates were made using constant methods based on the system of national health accounts. The economic burden of musculoskeletal disorders has increased slightly more than half of 1% of Gross Domestic Product (GDP) in the 1960s to just under 3% in 1995 (3% corresponds to $ 215.000). The national data Arthritis Working Group has concluded that about half of this increase was result of an increase in the prevalence of musculoskeletal diseases, due to aging population and higher costs per case, while the other half is due to better accounting methods in each data sources used by Rice and colleagues in their studies.

5. Costs of specific conditions

There have been made many studies on the costs of RA and the results are highly consistent in showing that the direct costs in the U.S. are between $ 4,000 and $ 6,000 a year (average: $5,425), but with the use of biological therapy increases these costs up to $ 19,000 and $ 25,000 / year, while the indirect costs associated with lost wages in the U.S. are between $ 9,000 and $ 24,000 one year (average U.S. $ 9,744) (6.7). In Colombia was made recently a case assessment to calculate the direct costs of early RA during attention first-year and categorized by the severity of the disease, being the average of $1,689, $ 1,805 and $ 23,441 to mild, moderate and severe forms of this disease respectively, and with well differential ranges, especially in the severe form, which allowed the use of anti-TNF therapy (costs in U.S. dollars for 2007) (8).

Hospital admissions represent between 40 and 60% of total direct costs in one year, although only 10% of hospital admissions for people with RA reported their hospital status (9).

Under similar conditions of other variables, the indirect costs of RA are likely to increase in coming decades as women continue to make progress in achieving equality in the labour market. Nowadays, women still have the lowest labour force participation, work fewer hours and lower wages per hour, even after better training and work experience. Moreover, the introduction of biological agents and cyclooxygenase-2 inhibitors has resulted in a dramatic increase of RA direct cost.

Therefore, increasing equality between genders is likely to result in an increase of RA indirect costs, while the development of new agents has led to this increase in direct cost side. On the other hand, while indirect costs are likely to increase in the short term, the advent of biological agents can reduce both direct and indirect costs in the longer term. Randomized clinical trials provide evidence that these agents reduce functional decline (10-13).

The evidence regarding the costs of specific rheumatic diseases is limited. Sutcliffe et al (14) reviewed the literature on the costs of Systemic Lupus Erythematosus (SLE) and reported that the direct costs of this disease were £ 2,613, while indirect costs were £ 5,299, roughly the same proportion as in the AR, it would not surprise, considering that both conditions exist in similar age.

For Colombia, Quintana et al (15) conducted a research to determine the health care costs for the first year of treatment for lupus nephritis (LN). They found a cost of U.S. $ 1,160 for the LN type I and II, the type III and V share the same costs of U.S. $ 3,498 using EURO-LUPUS protocol for induction and maintenance with azathioprine (AZA). In case of use of mycophenolate (MMF), the costs rise to U.S. $ 13,646 for LN type III and U.S. $ 14,161 for the LN type V. In type IV, the cost is U.S. $ 3,499 when using EURO-LUPUS protocol and maintenance with AZA; if it uses MMF for induction and maintenance, the costs amount to U.S. $ 14,163.

In studies of the costs of Ankylosing Spondylitis (AS), the direct costs range from € 1,309 and € 2,686, while indirect costs ranged from € 2,517 up to € 8,862. Maetzel et al (16) summarized the literature on the costs of back pain and they concluded that the costs of this disease were comparable to those associated with heart disease, depression, diabetes, and headaches; most them due to indirect costs. By contrast, in studies of osteoarthritis (OA), this usually affects those who are near or beyond retirement age. Gabriel et al (17, 18) reported that direct costs in USA are $ 1,388, and were 3 times higher than indirect costs ($ 824). Similarly, despite juvenile rheumatoid arthritis has a much higher cost because it affects the population that is not in working age, the direct costs in USA are $ 7,905, nearly 4 times higher than other costs of the same disease (primarily lost wages for parents) (19).

6. Economic evaluations of the rheumatic diseases

As it was mentioned at the beginning of the chapter, it will examine practical aspects of economic evaluations related to RD; therefore it reviews Cost-Effectiveness Analysis (CEA) associated with these diseases, in order to know what the current position and parallel, the situation in our environment.

Independently of the disease, comparing the results of the CEA is difficult due to differences in lifetime horizons, outcomes measurement, treatment sequences, and the perspective taken in estimating costs. Another limitation is that any of the clinical trials used in the CEA included an instrument based on utility to calculate the QALY. Thus, it is necessary new standards to make disease-specific functional scales or measures of Health-Related Quality of life (HRQL), with the purpose of obtaining utility scales. In addition, each CEA uses different utility scores, which has shown an influence on outcomes RA studies from CEA (20). Regardless of this, when is used the monotherapy with Infliximab (INF), Etanercept (ETN) and Adalimumab (ADA), even when some of these are used together with Metotrexate (MTX), they are well tolerated and lead to improvements in HRQL. However, caution is needed because the treatment with biologics can result in adverse effects such as

infections (especially tuberculosis reactivation, although a proper examination can reduce this risk).
For synthetic DMARDs in early RA, it is assumed they are profitable because of its low cost, although published data are limited. There are some CEA that have been carried out to Methotrexate (MTX) (21, 22), Sulfasalazine (SSZ) (21) and Leflunomide (LEF) (23). LEF appears to be cost-effective compared to SSZ (24).
Comparing the efficacy of LEF and MTX, the results of randomized controlled trials (RCTs) (25, 26) are not consistent, which consequently is reflected in the models of this CEA (24). For biological therapy in early RA as the first line of treatment has not been proven to be cost-effectiveness (22).
For ETN monotherapy, during an Indefinite Time Horizon (ITH), Brennan (27) reported an improvement of 1.66 QALY; Jobanputra et al (28) reported an improvement in 0.214; and Tanno et al (29) reported a gain of 2.56 QALY. For combined therapy, ETN + MTX results in a greater increase of 0.37 QALY (5 years) (30). The INF plus MTX increased QALY in 0.34 (ITH) (31), 0.26 (ITH) (32) and 2.98 (10 years) (33). The ADA plus MTX resulted in 2.3 QALY gained (ITH) (34). In terms of incremental cost-effectiveness ratio (ICER), Kobelt (35) found that ETN or INF produced a ratio of $ 96,166 per QALY gained. Studies with long time horizons provide better results. The ICER for the ETN monotherapy ranged between $ 21,000 to $ 32,000 for ITH per QALY (27, 29). Combined therapy with INF plus MTX resulted in an ICER of $ 30,500 to $ 46,000 (31, 33). From the Canadian perspective, Coyle et al (36), reported an ICER of $ 99,305 per QALY (5 years, in a directly way) acquired for therapy with INF combined.
In a recent Colombian study, Quintana et al (37) conducted a CEA where they found that in a time horizon of 2 years, the effectiveness of ETN, ADA and INF is 1.4689, 1.4627 and 1.4340 QALY respectively, versus net costs in Colombian Pesos (COP) of $ 77'938.000, $ 81'975.000 and $ 89'598.000, respectively. ETN dominates over ADA or INF with a cost-effectiveness rate of $ 53'056.723/QALY versus ADA: $ 56'042.654/QALY and INF: $ 62'479.625/QALY. The univariate sensitivity analysis, showed sensitivity of outcomes, mainly to the reduction in the cost / month for the drugs tested.
The Abatacept (ABA) has recently been investigated, this results suggested that is cost-effective for moderate to severe RA after failure to MTX; based on data from the AIM study (38), resulting in $ 47,910 per QALY gained over 10 years and $ 43,041 to ITH.
When failures after one or more anti-TNF are analyzed, Rituximab (RTX) has been profitable (39), this based on data modeling of the REFLEX study. The RTX resulted in QALY gained of 0.526 years. The ICER based on total direct medical cost was £ 11,601, and the addition of RTX, without sequential use of biologics, it generates an ICER of £ 14,690. In this onset, the ABA has also been profitable (40) (the models were based on data from ATTAIN trials); although initially have been rejected by the National Institute for Clinical Excellence (NICE), because it exceeded the threshold of £ 30,000. So far, there are not comparative randomized data head to head of RTX and ABA available. In a summary report, ABA is postulated to be more profitable than RTX (40) in a model derived from AIM and REFLEX.
The cost-effectiveness of anti-TNF therapy on health resources depends on two factors. First, research reviewed, (only those with long time horizons (ITH)) they found that treatments have ICER lower than $ 50,000. However, by definition, a long-term analysis is based on hypotheses for extrapolating the effect of treatment, making it less reliable and

uncertain. Second, reimbursement for treatment with an ICER less than $ 50,000 is only economically viable as long as financial resources do not be diverted into more effectiveness treatments.

A limiting factor common to all CEA of TNF antagonists in RA is the lack of data from long-term randomized studies. As such, researchers must combine data from short-term efficacy with the cohort of long-term observation. This raises many problems such as how to combine data from different sources, to predict the long-term results and alteration of the model after discontinuation of treatment in a biological DMARD. This also influences the lack of standardization of schemes for the use of biologics in relation to the start time and its indications at certain stages of the natural history of disease. It is accepted that treatment for RA is likely to be a sequence of treatments. However, treatment may vary among individuals, clinicians and countries.

Despite of most studies have found that ETN and INF have clinical effects on AS, the study of Boonen et al (41) suggests that high costs from these biological therapies may limit their use in patients who have a BASDAI greater than 4. In fact, an ICER of € 118,022 and 189,564 for ETN and INF provides preliminary evidence that biologics will not be a cost-effectiveness option for individuals with AS, unless a longer-term perspective is adopted. The long-term outcome by Kobelt et al (42) (£ 9,600 per QALY; 30 years) and Kobelt et al (43) ($ 37,491 per QALY, 30 years) it would be a poor indicator, since the clinical outcomes short-term of this trial were extrapolated using epidemiological modeling techniques. The update of the results with data records of longitudinal databases will be needed to verify these findings.

The analysis of TNF antagonists in Psoriatic Arthritis found that the ETN in patients who have previously failed other treatments DMARD was encouraging; but limitations in available data make it difficult to draw definitive conclusions (44). The results on short-term cost-effectiveness of ETN compared with cyclosporine or LEF are not worthwhile. It showed an improvement in the ICER after the first year, but this hypothesis was based on the disease progression founded from poor quality databases. Moreover, the estimations of HRQL from the analysis may not reflect true benefits, since these estimates were based single on HAQ-DI and the EQ-5D (function and quality of life scores).

7. Conclusions

Economic evidence suggests that biologics are not cost-effective compared with DMARDs for RA in adults, with a threshold of cost-effectiveness $ 50,000 per QALY. There is mixed evidence of effectiveness in selected populations about their willingness to pay $ 100,000 per QALY. Definitive conclusions are difficult to make, because there is a lack of consistent studies and high quality. Economic evaluations of biological products are hampered by the lack of data on long-term responses and consequences of responses on health in relation to their utilization and productivity of people.

Likewise, economic analyses support the concept of an early onset with traditional DMARD and rapid progress to the next step when there is an inadequate response. In these specific circumstances, the strategy of incorporating biological treatment, considerably more expensive, seems to provide enough effectiveness. Most current guidelines related to the treatment of RA are consistent with the careful use of social and financial resources.

8. References

[1] Towsend JR. Postmarketing drug research and development. Drug Intell Clin Pharm 1987; 21: 134-36.

[2] Rice D. Estimating the cost of illness. Hyattsville, MD: National Center for Health Statistics, Health Economic Series; 1966: No. 6.

[3] Cooper B, Rice D. The economic cost of illness revisited. Social Security Bulletin 1979;39: 21-35.

[4] Rice D, Hodgson T, Kopstein A. The economic costs of illness: A replication and update. Health Care Finance Rev 1985;7:61-80.

[5] Rice D. The economic burden of musculoskeletal conditions. Praemer A, Furner S, Rice D, editors. Rosemont, IL: American Academy of Orthopaedic Surgeons; 1999.

[6] Yelin E. The worldwide economic and functional impact of rheumatic disease. In: Hochberg M, Silman A, Smolen J, Weinblatt M, Weisman M, editors. Rheumatology. 3rd ed. London: Mosby;2003. p. 31-35.

[7] Pugner K, Scott D, Holmes J, Hieke K. The costs of rheumatoid arthritis: an international long-term view. Semin Arthritis Rheum 2000;29: 305-20.

[8] Mora C, González A, Díaz J, Quintana G. Financial cost of early rheumatoid arthritis in the first year of medical attention: three clinical scenarios in a third-tier university hospital in Colombia. Biomédica 2009;29(1): 43-50.

[9] Yelin E, Wanke L. An assessment of the annual and long-term direct costs of rheumatoid arthritis: the impact of poor function and functional decline. Arthritis Rheum 1999;42: 1209-18.

[10] Cohen S, Wooley J, Chan W. Interleukin-1 receptor antagonist anakinra improves functional status in patients with rheumatoid arthritis. J Rheumatol 2003;30:225-31.

[11] Lipsky PE, van der Heijde DM, St Clair EW, Furst DE, Breedveld FC, Kalden JR, et al. Infliximab and methotrexate in the treatment of rheumatoid arthritis: Anti-Tumor Necrosis Factor Trial in Rheumatoid Arthritis with Concomitant Therapy Study Group. N Engl J Med 2000;343:1594-602.

[12] Bresnihan B, Alvaro-Gracia JM, Cobby M, Doherty M, Domljan Z, Emery P, et al. Treatment of rheumatoid arthritis with recombinant human interleukin-1 receptor antagonist. Arthritis Rheum 1998;41:2196-204.

[13] Mathias S, Colwell H, Miller D, Moreland L, Buatti M, Wanke L. Health-related quality of life and functional status of patients with rheumatoid arthritis randomly assigned to receive etanercept or placebo. Clin Ther 2000;22:129-39.

[14] Sutcliffe N, Clarke A, Taylor R, Frost C, Isenberg D. Total costs and predictors of costs in patients with systemic lupus erythematosus. Rheumatology Oxford 2001;40: 37-47.

[15] Quintana G, Coral-Alvarado P, Díaz J. Direct costs of health care of lupus nephritis in Colombia. Ann Rheum Dis 2011;70(Suppl3):694

[16] Maetzel A, Li L. The economic burden of low back pain: a review of studies published between 1996 and 2001. Best Pract Res Clin Rheumatol 2002;16:23-30.

[17] Gabriel S, Crowson C, Campion M, O'Fallon W. Direct medical costs unique to people with arthritis. J Rheumatol 1997;24:719-25.

[18] Gabriel S, Crowson C, Campion M, O'Fallon W. Indirect and nonmedical costs among people with rheumatoid arthritis and osteoarthritis compared with nonarthritic controls. J Rheumatol 1997;24:43-8.

[19] Allaire SH, DeNardo BS, Szer IS, Meenan RF, Schaller JG. The economic impacts of juvenile rheumatoid arthritis. J Rheumatol 1992;19:952-5.

[20] Marra CA, Marion SA, Guh DP, Najafzadeh M, Wolfe F, Esdaile JM, et al. Not all "quality-adjusted life years" are equal. J Clin Epidemiol 2007 Jun;60(6):616-24.

[21] Choi HK, Seeger JD, Kuntz KM. A cost effectiveness analysis of treatment options for methotrexate-naive rheumatoid arthritis. J Rheumatol 2002;29:1156–65.

[22] Finckh A, Bansback N, Marra CA, Anis AH, Michaud K, Lubin S, et al. Treatment of very early rheumatoid arthritis with symptomatic therapy, disease-modifying antirheumatic drugs, or biologic agents: a cost-effectiveness analysis. Ann Intern Med 2009;151:612–21.

[23] Schädlich PK, Zeidler H, Zink A, Gromnica-Ihle E, Schneider M, Straub C, et al. Modelling cost effectiveness and cost utility of sequential DMARD therapy including leflunomide for rheumatoid arthritis in Germany: II. The contribution of leflunomide to efficiency. Pharmacoeconomics 2005;23:395–420.

[24] Kobelt G, Lindgren P, Young A. Modelling the costs and effects of lefl unomide in rheumatoid arthritis. Eur J Health Econ 2002;3:180–7.

[25] Emery P, Breedveld FC, Lemmel EM, Kaltwasser JP, Dawes PT, Gömör B, et al. A comparison of the efficacy and safety of leflunomide and methotrexate for the treatment of rheumatoid arthritis. Rheumatology (Oxford) 2000;39:655–65. 24.

[26] Strand V, Tugwell P, Bombardier C, Maetzel A, Crawford B, Dorrier C, et al. Function and health-related quality of life: results from a randomized controlled trial of leflunomide versus methotrexate or placebo in patients with active rheumatoid arthritis. Leflunomide Rheumatoid Arthritis Investigators Group. Arthritis Rheum 1999;42:1870–8.

[27] Brennan A, Bansback N, Reynolds A, Conway P. Modelling the cost-effectiveness of etanercept in adults with rheumatoid arthritis in the UK. Rheumatology (Oxford) 2004;43(1): 62-72.

[28] Jobanputra P, Barton P, Bryan S, Burls A. The effectiveness of infliximab and etanercept for the treatment of rheumatoid arthritis: a systematic review and economic evaluation. Health Technol Assess 2002;6(21): 1-110.

[29] Tanno M, Nakamura I, Ito K, Tanaka H, Ohta H, Kobayashi M, et al. Modeling and cost-effectiveness analysis of etanercept in adults with rheumatoid arthritis in Japan: a preliminary analysis. Mod Rheumatol 2006;16(2): 77-84.

[30] Kobelt G, Lindgren P, Singh A, Klareskog L. Cost-effectiveness of etanercept (Enbrel) in combination with methotrexate in the treatment of active rheumatoid arthritis based on the TEMPO trial. Ann Rheum Dis 2005;64(8): 1174-1179.

[31] Wong JB, Singh G, Kavanaugh A. Estimating the cost-effectiveness of 54 weeks of infliximab for rheumatoid arthritis. Am J Med 2002;113(5): 400-408.

[32] Barbieri M, Wong JB, Drummond M. The cost-effectiveness of infliximab for severe treatment-resistant rheumatoid arthritis in the UK. Pharmacoeconomics 2005;23(6): 607-618.

[33] Kobelt G, Jonsson L, Young A, Eberhardt K. The cost-effectiveness of infliximab (Remicade) in the treatment of rheumatoid arthritis in Sweden and the United Kingdom based on the ATTRACT study. Rheumatology (Oxford) 2003;42(2): 326-335.

[34] Bansback NJ, Brennan A, Ghatnekar O. Cost-effectiveness of adalimumab in the treatment of patients with moderate to severe rheumatoid arthritis in Sweden. Ann Rheum Dis 2005; 64(7): 995-1002.

[35] Kobelt G, Eberhardt K, Geborek P. TNF inhibitors in the treatment of rheumatoid arthritis in clinical practice: costs and outcomes in a follow up study of patients with RA treated with etanercept or infliximab in southern Sweden. Ann Rheum Dis 2004;63(1): 4-10.

[36] Coyle D, Judd M, Blumenauer B, Cranney A, Maetzel A, Tugwell P, Wells GA. Infliximab and etanercept in patients with rheumatoid arthritis: a systematic review and economic evaluation [Technology report no 64]. Ottawa: Canadian Coordinating Office for Health Technology Assessment; 2006.

[37] Quintana G, Restrepo JP, Caceres HA, Rueda JD, Rosselli D. Economic evaluation of the treatment of rheumatoid arthritis with anti-TNF biological therapies in Colombia. Acta Med Colomb 2011; 36(1): 24-29.

[38] Vera-Llonch M, Massarotti E, Wolfe F, Shadick N, Westhovens R, Sofrygin O, et al. Cost-effectiveness of abatacept in patients with moderately to severely active rheumatoid arthritis and inadequate response to methotrexate. Rheumatology (Oxford) 2008;47:535–41.

[39] Kielhorn A, Porter D, Diamantopoulos A, Lewis G. UK cost-utility analysis of Rituximab in patients with rheumatoid arthritis that failed to respond adequately to a biologic disease-modifying antirheumatic drug. Curr Med Res Opin 2008;24:2639–50.

[40] Yuan Y, Trivedi D, Maclean R, Rosenblatt L. The cost-effectiveness of abatacept versus rituximab in patients with rheumatoid arthritis in the United States [abstract]. Ann Rheum Dis 2008;67(Suppl II):P582.

[41] Boonen A, van der Heijde D, Severens JL, Boendermaker A, Landewé R, Braun J, et al. Markov model into the cost-utility over five years of etanercept and infliximab compared with usual care in patients with active ankylosing spondylitis. Ann Rheum Dis 2006;65(2): 201-208.

[42] Kobelt G, Andlin-Sobocki P, Brophy S, Jönsson L, Calin A, Braun J. The burden of ankylosing spondylitis and the cost-effectiveness of treatment with infliximab (Remicade). Rheumatology (Oxford) 2004;43(9): 1158-1166.

[43] Kobelt G, Andlin-Sobocki P, Maksymowych WP. The cost-effectiveness of infliximab (Remicade) in the treatment of ankylosing spondylitis in Canada. J Rheumatol 2006;33(4): 732-740.

[44] Bansback NJ, Ara R, Barkham N, Brennan A, Fraser AD, Conway P, et al. Estimating the cost and health status consequences of treatment with TNF antagonists in patients with psoriatic arthritis. Rheumatology (Oxford) 2006;45(8): 1029-1038.

2

Economic Evaluations in Systemic Lupus Erythematosus

Gerardo Quintana[1,2,4,5], Helena Avella Bolivar[3] and Paola Coral-Alvarado[1,2]
[1]*Fundación Santa Fe de Bogotá, Bogotá*
[2]*School of Medicine, Universidad de los Andes, Bogotá*
[3]*School of Nursing, Universidad Nacional de Colombia, Bogotá*
[4]*School of Medicine, Universidad Nacional de Colombia, Bogotá*
[5]*Section of Rheumatology, Faculty of Medicine, Universidad de los Andes, Bogotá*
Colombia

1. Introduction

Systemic lupus erythematosus (SLE) is a prototype of autoimmune diseases with a wide range of clinical and laboratory features that involves almost every organ system. The prevalence is 52 x 100000 inhabitants in U.S, 21 x 100000 in Canada and 25-91 x 100000 in European countries (1). There is an early-onset SLE disease in young women after teenager years and a late-onset before the beginning of fifth decade. Women are affected 9 times more frequently than men.

SLE is a complex disease characterized by recurrent relapses and remissions subsequent. Nowadays, there is no cure for SLE and this disease can be threatening when major organs are affected.

Unfortunately, SLE can be considered as a disease with a high implication in terms of morbi-mortality and also, the patients undergoing a great impairment of quality of life, considering their potential systemic compromise and/or organ-specific. The patients show decline on physical activity as a result of arthritis, undesirable changes in appearance or damage produced by long-term use of steroids (often used therapy to treat patients with SLE) such as osteoporosis, cataracts, or angina, making it one of diseases with major implications at the individual, family, social and economic levels. It affects public health in relation to the increase of resources health consumption.

A better awareness among physicians and patients about this disease, the advent of more effective therapies but also more expensive and longer survival of patients with SLE, it has led toward an important and better perception of the disease in recent years. The socioeconomic data are important as well, since patient survival improves, the accumulation of disease and complications treatment-related are crucial in order to appraisal the financial burden on both individuals and society. In countries where chronic diseases are prevalent, with a growing population and limited economic resources, it is critical a suitable decision-making on resources to health care. Our current knowledge about the economic impact of SLE is very limited and there are only few cost studies conducted by North America and Europe, unfortunately.

This chapter shows a historical description of approaches to economic evaluation in SLE, both at national and international framework and highlighting the main elements that must be considered in clinical practice and decisions to avoid increasing the economic burden of health care. A non-systematic review of all published literature in English, French and Spanish from 1990 to April 2011 was performed using Medline, Pubmed, Cochrane, Lilacs and Scielo in peer-reviewed articles, including the Mesh-terms of systemic lupus erythematosus, direct costs, indirect and intangible cost, economic impact, disease burden, Cost-of-illness (COI) studies, pharmacoeconomics analysis, cost-effectiveness and cost-utility. It will have three types of approaches: the economic impact of the disease, COI studies and finally, a complete pharmacoeconomic assessment.

2. Overview

As previously mentioned, the economic evaluations on autoimmune diseases are lack and most of them have been carried out on Rheumatoid Arthritis (RA). In the case of SLE has virtually been restricted to studies of disease burden and cost-of-illness (COI). The COI studies measures the monetary burden that disease entails on society caused by morbidity and premature mortality in terms of consumption of health resources and lost of productivity.

In 1967, Rice was the first to outline a methodological framework for calculating single-year cost of illness, disability, and death by major category of illness (2). In 1982, Hodgson and Meiners created the first guide to study COI (3). The studies' results are crucial to provide informative data to emphasize the extent of the disease problem and highlight the profile of patients with SLE. They also have the potential to serve as the basis to a major component in economic evaluations such as COI. A valuable COI study included direct, indirect, and intangible cost associated with the disease.

Direct costs represent the opportunity costs of all kind of resources used to treat a disease (3). They usually include direct medical costs and direct non-medical costs. The first refer to the costs involved to provide treatment, including costs associated with the diagnosis, treatment, monitoring, emergency and rehabilitation, while non-medical costs refer to those which patients and their families spend on disease but are not medical in nature, including transportation costs, cost for household expenditures, and informal care.

Indirect costs represent lost productivity associated with morbidity, which may be related to work or non-work activities. Indirect costs usually represent a large proportion of total costs in most of the COI. Indirect costs are usually measured by two methods: Human Capital Approach (HCA) and Friction Cost Method (FCT). The results obtained with one and another are not comparable and the first estimates tend to be lower than the second. The HCA estimates the indirect costs associated with illness and premature death in terms of lost productivity (lost wages), thus excluding the costs of pain and suffering, leisure time and work on a voluntary. The FCT, which considers the amount people would pay to reduce their risk of injury, illness or death, this is subjective and can be difficult to use in children and the elderly, due to the complexity of the questions (4).

Intangible costs refer to patients' psychological pain of, discomfort, anxiety, depression, and stress related to disease or its treatment (5). These are difficult to quantify in monetary terms, therefore, they are usually omitted in COI studies or presented as quality of life.

3. Economic impact of disease

The first assessment about economic impact of SLE was published in 1994 and it was undertaken to assess both the cyclophosphamide (CYC) in intravenous cycles and prednisone PO impact for the treatment of severe lupus nephritis (6). The authors conducted a hypothetical cohort of patients considering the incidence of severe lupus nephritis for U.S. in 1988 (1130 patients). They calculated and compared the costs of prednisone as monotherapy vs. prednisone with intravenous CYC, the rate of renal failure with each comparative option was also considered, as well as age, gender, and economic value of working years gained. The results found that although the costs of combination therapy are greater, the analysis shows an overall savings due to reduced need for dialysis or kidney transplantation, and the economic value of work capacity won. The savings attributable to the costs of patient care were $ 50.8 million and $ 42.3 million earned by working capacity. Finally, they conclude that for a period of 10 years, about $ 93.1 million to year-cohort is saved with the use of combination therapy for treatment of severe lupus nephritis.

Clarke et al (7) presented a study to compare the costs of health care and health status of patients with SLE in three countries (Canada, U.S. and UK), which have different health systems and financing. 708 patients with SLE were involved in 2 centers for each country (Canada 229, UK 268 and U.S. 211), they were evaluated about activity and damage of the disease and information on physical and psychological well-being, satisfaction, social support, and utilization of health resource. All of the costs were calculated using Canadian dollars for 1997. After adjusting for covariate representatives, the Canadian patients, compared with the British and Americans, reported a significantly higher health status in 3 of 8 sub-scales of the SF-36. In general, the annual use of health resources was not significantly different, with an average annual cost per patient of CAD $ 4,853, $ 5,285 and $ 4,760 for Canada, USA and UK, respectively. However, it was found some differences within each resource category. Canadians visited more specialists than British, British visited more general physician. Canadians and Americans used more emergency services, Canadians had higher hospital costs than Americans, and Americans required more paraclinical tests and imaging services.

Zink et al, in 2004, in a comparative study of the disease burden in SLE and rheumatoid arthritis (RA), analyzed retrospectively data of 1,248 patients with SLE and 10,068 patients with RA, who were seen by rheumatologists in 2001. Significant differences were observed in patients who were treated by the rheumatologist; patients with SLE were treated mainly with antimalarials (37%), azathioprine (29%), 61% of patients received at least one immunosuppressive medication plus steroids. In AR, Methotrexate was the drug most used in 63% of patients. A matched analysis showed that SLE patients with a short duration of the disease had pain, functional limitations and general deterioration of health, as well as patients with RA; however, in patients with disease duration of more than ten years, deterioration in health status, was greater in patients with RA. The authors report that in the early stages of both diseases, related costs of health care and burden of disease are similar, but in chronic disease, RA significantly increased costs in relation to pain, poor overall health state and disease activity, as well as greater severity classified by the specialist, suggesting a better long-term prognosis in SLE in the areas observed. Regarding the current treatment, showed an impact when the two diseases are treated by rheumatologists since onset-disease (8).

The same author Clarke et al in 2004, published an interesting study which sought to determine whether the consumption of health resources are correlated with outcome in the health status of SLE patients in three developed countries: USA, UK and Canada. 715 patients were surveyed semi-annually (Canada 231, U.S. 269, and UK 215) to determine the utilization of health resources and outcomes in health status. In 2002, the average cumulative costs per patient over 4 years were CAD $ 15,845, $ 20,244 and $ 17,647 for Canada, USA, and UK respectively, they experimented similar outcomes in health. After adjusting differences in input data, on average, Canadian and British patients utilized 20% and 13% less resources than American patients, respectively. The authors comment that despite incurring higher health expenditure, American patients did not experiment great results in health (9).

Grootscholten C et al in 2007 (10) developed a prospective randomized controlled study to measure the effect of treatment with CYC pulses or azathioprine (AZA) plus methylprednisolone (MP) for a period of 24 months, evaluating health-related quality of life (HRQOL) of patients with Proliferative Lupus Nephritis (PLN). This study measured HRQOL and disease activity at the beginning and after at 12 and 24 months. It was applied the Visual Analog Scale (VAS), SF-36, and a questionnaire to measure activity disease (SLEDAI). The impact of treatment was measured 24 months later and disease activity was measured with the SLEDAI and physician's VAS. They included 87 patients, and only 47 of them completed the questionnaires. HRQOL improved significantly with treatment, particularly during the first year; however, there were no significant differences between the group treated with CYC and AZA/MP; on the other hand, there was a strong favorability in the group treated with AZA/MP when SF-36 was applied. The average reported in the impact on treatment within 24 months was significantly higher in the group treated with CYC. HRQOL was not correlated neither with the SLEDAI nor the physician's VAD. This study concluded that treatment of PLN patients with immunosuppressive drugs and corticosteroid improve QOL, particularly in the first year and this effect was sustained in the second year of treatment. But because such a small sample and lack of differences in HRQOL between CYC and AZA/MP groups, these results should be interpreted with caution. The CYC-treated group showed a high impact on the budget. Data from this study do not support the use of AZA/MP as first line treatment for PLN, but this could be an alternative for women who wish to become pregnant. They propose future studies with Mycophenolate Mofetil and low-dose CYC as therapeutic alternatives in these patients.

An interesting evaluation performed by Campbell et al (11), involved the impact of SLE on working capacity. This study evaluated the status of work (such as job loss, changes in the amount worked) and predictors of job-loss in patients with SLE. The patients with onset-disease recently diagnosed were included, followed-up at least two years and matched by sex and age. Patients were followed-up for an average of 4 years from diagnosis. Work history was obtained through a personal interview during the recruitment and through telephone interviews to follow-up. The authors highlight an important difference for working withdrawals during follow-up between SLE patients and controls (26 vs. 9%, $p < 0.0001$). 92 of SLE patients showed that the cause of abandonment was related to their health status. Patients with SLE who had arthritis were three times more likely to quit their jobs due to changes in health compared with those who did not have arthritis (adjusted OR 3.3 IC95% 1.1 to 8.8). Finally, an association with the presence of pleuritis was founded (adjusted OR 2.3 95% 1.1 to 4.6).

4. Cost-of-illness studies in SLE

Until the last century the most studies in SLE tended to ignore the evaluations that included both loss of productivity in work activities and diary live activities and they focus only on direct costs such as number of hospitalizations and health status measures.

In 1993, Clarke et al (12) published the first assessment which identified the direct and indirect costs of 164 patients with SLE who entered to the Lupus register of Montreal General Hospital between January 1977 and January 1990; they compared the costs with the general population of Quebec and also determined the predictors of costs. The estimated cost was $ 13,094 CAD in 1990, of which 54% represent indirect costs ($ 7,071). In average, SLE hospitalizations were 4 times more frequent than general population of Quebec (matched by gender and age), and the number of outpatient visits were twice than which represented by the general population. The best predictors of direct costs were high levels of creatinine and poor level of physical performance. A poor level of well-being, a combination of education level and employment status, and poor social support were the best predictors for indirect costs.

Clarke et al, in 2000, carried out an indirect costs analysis and it was calculated as a result of decreased productivity in women with SLE. Indirect costs incurred by women with SLE were calculated obtaining the costs from labour and non-labour activities decreased. Six hundred forty-eight women with SLE reported their employment status and time lost for themselves and their employers as well as non-labour activities over a period of 6 months. The average annual indirect costs ranged from $ 1,424 to $ 22,604 CAD to 1997, and they depended on the value assigned to the labour market and non-labour activities (13).

Sutcliffe et al, in 2001, determined the direct costs, indirect costs and predictors in patients with SLE. 105 patients with SLE completed the questionnaires about using of health services and employment history. A multiple regression analysis determined predictors of costs. Direct, indirect and total costs were the depending variables, and demographic data, health status, disease activity, target organ damage, social support and satisfaction with care were used as predictors. The average total annual cost per patient was £7,913. Direct costs were a third of the total costs and indirect costs represented 2/3 of total cost. A good level of education, greater disease activity and reduced physical function were associated with increased direct, indirect and total costs. The major direct costs are also associated with greater impairment and younger age of onset-disease. The authors conclude that SLE has a considerable impact on the health system and society. Improving disease activity and physical health, as well as the prevention of organ damage can significantly reduce costs in SLE (14).

In 2001, Clarke et al compared the direct and indirect costs of care for SLE patients in Canada, USA and UK. In general, the cost of care of patients with SLE is cheaper in UK, because of fewer resources used and number of hospitalizations reduced; however, a significant statistical difference were not found. Additionally, indirect costs of SLE increased dramatically the cost of the disease was another finding. When indirect costs included only job loss, the cost per patient was $ 10,000 a year and if it is considered household task, the cost increased to $ 22,000 (4 times the annual direct costs) (15).

A comparative assessment of costs of rheumatic diseases was made in Germany. In this study, Li et al, in 2006 (16) estimated and compared direct and indirect costs of illness in Rheumatoid Arthritis (RA), Ankylosing Spondylitis (AS), Psoriatic Artritits (PA) and SLE; they evaluated the gender, disease duration and functional status effect on various costs domains. Data were extracted from the German national data set from 1993. The costs were calculated for each patient for the last twelve months prior to recruitment date. The direct costs were € 4,737 per year in RA, € 3,676 in EA, € 3,156 in PA and € 3,191 SLE. Costs increased with duration of disease and they were heavily dependent on functional status. Compared with RA, drug costs in SLE were less than half; patients with AS and PA had less treatment costs in hospitalized patients for acute complications than those with RA and SLE. Calculating the indirect costs were higher in SLE (€ 11.220), followed by AR (€ 10,901).

Panopalis et al in 2007 compared cumulative indirect costs over 4 years in the care of patients with SLE in the U.S., Canada and UK. They surveyed a total of 715 patients with SLE (269 U.S., 231 in Canada and 215 in UK) at baseline and semi-annually, during four years (May 1999-October 2001). Participants completed questionnaires about the use of health resources, employment status, lost work days and lost time spent by caregivers on administrative procedures to access health services and / or daily household tasks. Annually, the patients reported surveys about quality of life, social support, and satisfaction with care. This study is a cross-national comparison of indirect costs in SLE, this is valuable information due to the difficulty of measuring indirect costs and the importance they represent because they contribute to a high percentage of total costs in SLE. The authors found that indirect costs accounted for 74% of total costs, being significantly higher in American patients, and this increase corresponded to the additional labour hours that patients would have worked, if they had not been ill. The authors concluded that indirect costs represent a significant proportion of total costs in the care of patients with SLE and they suggest that among SLE economic evaluations should include indirect costs attributed to productivity lost (17).

Clarke et al in 2008 compared the costs and quality of life among patients with SLE with and without kidney damage; the authors evaluated 715 patients through a semi-annualized interview during four years, in order to determine the use of medical services, loss of productivity and annually the quality of life. The accumulated direct and indirect costs and quality of life (analyzed through the SF-36) were compared between SLE patients with and without renal damage, through of Damage Index for SLE from System Lupus International Collaborating Clinics/ACR. On this scale was considered 0, one patient without renal impairment; 1, with a glomerular filtration rate or creatinine clearance less than 50%; 2, proteinuria greater than 3.5 g; or 3, end-stage kidney disease. Each criterion should be present in at least six months to be considered as kidney damage. Cumulative average direct costs per patient in 2006 were CAD $ 20,337, $ 27,869, $ 51,191 and $ 99,544 for stages 0-3 respectively. For every increased unit on renal damage, it was associated with an increase on average of 24% on direct costs through regression analysis. In addition, patients with end-stage renal disease incurred 103 % more than those without kidney damage. Cumulative indirect costs, lost productivity and the annual change in SF-36 did not show difference between patients (18).

Panopolis et al estimated health care costs and costs associated with changes in labour productivity among people with SLE in the U.S. The data were derived from the University of California. Participants provided information on the use of health resources and employment. Estimations about costs were derived for both of health care costs and costs related to changes in labour productivity. Direct health care costs included hospitalization costs, emergency service use, doctor visits, ambulatory surgery, dialysis and drugs. Productivity costs were calculated by measuring the decrease of productive working hours since onset SLE disease, although these estimates were also compared with general data from U.S. population. For all participants, the average annual direct costs were $ 12,643 (2004, U.S. dollars). The average annual costs of the productivity in working-age people (> or = 18 and <65 years) were $ 8,659. The average total annual costs for working-age were $ 20,924. The increase of disease activity, a longer duration of illness, and mental and physical health impairment were significant predictors of increase in direct costs, because to changes in labour productivity. The authors concluded that the direct costs and costs associated with changes in labour productivity are important and they represent an important contribution to the total costs associated with SLE (19).

Carls et al in 2009 estimated the medical costs related to the productivity of SLE and Lupus Nephritis (LN) in a population of employees between 2000 and 2004. These costs were compared with other chronic diseases costs. The average annual medical expenses and the short-term costs given by disabilities for patients with SLE were US (2005) $ 12,238 and $ 1,184 respectively, in comparison to control diseases. The average medical expenses in LN patients were $ 46,862 higher than the controls. Compared with other chronic health conditions that occurred in this group of employees, SLE / LN was the most expensive condition. The authors conclude that SLE, particularly with LN, is associated with significant costs. The treatment that lead to manage earlier and effective to the patients with SLE, it can result in an important decrease of costs, if they are started on time in order to reduce complications that generate more costs of care (20).

In another study, Zhu T, et al in 2009 determined the direct and indirect costs for patients with SLE in a rheumatology center in Hong Kong. They determined the relationship between Neuropsychiatric SLE (NP-SLE) and costs of the disease through a retrospective cross-sectional, non-randomized study. All participants completed questionnaires on demographic data, employment status and personal expenses. The consumption of health resources was registered in a file.

The onset of NP-SLE since the beginning of SLE was determined using the 1999 ACR criteria. Costs of the disease among patients with and without NP-SLE were compared by the Mann-Whitney test and the predictors of costs were obtained by a multiple linear regression analysis. 306 Chinese patients were recruited with an average age of 41 years and the disease duration of 9.6 years. There were a total of 108 events of NP-SLE in 83 patients. The most common manifestations were seizures and cardiovascular disease. The total annual costs were US $ 13,307 per patient. Direct costs dominated total costs, and hospital care costs accounted for 52% of direct costs. Patients with NP-SLE incurred in direct and indirect costs significantly higher when they were compared to those without NP-SLE. The number of events NP-SLE was an independent variable associated with direct and indirect costs. So, the implementation of an intervention in the prevention of organ damage, especially in neuropsychiatric manifestations may reduce the costs of patients with SLE (21).

In another study, in 2009, Li et al estimated the direct medical costs to long-term of SLE patients and a subgroup of patients with SLE and LN. Active SLE patients of a large database and during this monitoring period, 2298 patients and a control group between 1999 and 2005 were included. The average annual medical costs for patients with SLE were higher than in the control group in the first year (US $ 16,089 vs. $ 6,831, respectively). Costs decreased slightly in the second year but increased 16% annually for five years to $ 23,860. LN patients (n = 489) were USD $ 13,228 - $ 34,907 higher than the control patients and the hospitalization rate in the subgroup with LN was 0.6 to one per capita, which was double compared with SLE patients without LN, and 3 to 4 times higher than the control group. This study concluded that SLE is an expensive condition, and medical expenses increased steadily over time, particularly for patients with LN SLE (22).

Zhu T et al in 2009 (23) assessed the direct and indirect costs of flare SLE patients and non-flare SLE patients from a social perspective in order to investigate the severity impact and the direct and indirect costs from flare clinical manifestations. The authors defined as activity 3 points or more in SELENA - SLEDAI, and 4 points or more in the BILAG, being this between 0 and 105 (maximum activity). Mild or moderate relapse was defined as one or more of the following:

1. Change in SELENA - SLEDAI of three points.
2. Worsening discoid lesions or new lesions, photosensitivity, cutaneous vasculitis, nasopharyngeal ulcers, pleuritis, pericarditis, arthritis or fever.
3. Increase of prednisolone dose without exceeding 0.5 mg / kg / day.
4. Necessity of adding or increasing NSAID or hydroxychloroquine.

While severe relapse was defined as:

1. Change in SELENA-SLEDAI twelve-points.
2. New or worsening vasculitis, nephritis, myositis, thrombocytopenia less than 60,000 or anemia with Hb less than 7, requiring increase prednisolone dose to 0.5 mg / kg / day
3. Use of new immunosuppressive agents.
4. Hospitalization for SLE.

A validated physical index consists of 41 items in 12 organs frequently used to measure the accumulated damage was used to measure damage (Systemic Damage Index -SDI). Damage was defined as any irreversible change occurred since the onset-disease of SLE which is observed for at least 6 months. The total SDI scores ranging from 0 to 49. They also defined each of the activities according to the organ involved.

This was a retrospective study of the disease costs; 306 Chinese patients between 18 and 65 with SLE were included and recruited between January 2006 and August 2007. Participants completed questionnaires on demographic data, employment status, and out-of-pocket expenses. The consumption of health resources was recorded in a questionnaire that patients self-reported. Total number of flares and the organs affected in the last 12 months were recorded. The authors found that patients with flare were younger with a shorter duration of illness and a higher disease activity at the evaluation time. The overall incidence of lupus flares was 0.24 episodes per patient-year. Patients with flares used more frequently health resources and increased significantly the direct and indirect annual costs.

The total average costs per patient-year were two times higher for patients with flare (USD 2006 $ 22,580 versus $ 10,870, p <0.0005). A multiple regression analysis showed that the number of relapse was an independent variable that leads to increase direct costs. Patients with renal / neuropsychiatric flare had higher direct costs compared with those with single-organ flare. The main conclusion of this study was that patients with flare incurred higher direct and indirect costs compared with those without crisis. The main organs affected by flares were renal and neuropsychiatric whose patients incurred higher costs for the disease than flares of other organs. The treatments that control effectively the disease activity and prevent relapses, especially the flare in vital organs, may reduce the high costs associated with relapse in SLE.

In Colombia, Quintana et al (24) conducted a study to determine the direct costs of health care for the first year of treatment for LN, based on the classification system of the

International Society of Nephrology / renal Pathology Society (ISN / RPS) (25); it is the first assessment that discriminates on type of renal histopathologic injury, finding a cost of $ 1,160 (USD, 2009) for LN type I and II; the type III and V share the same costs of $ 3,498 using the EUROLUPUS scheme in induction and maintenance with azathioprine (AZA). In case of use of mycophenolate (MMF), the costs increased to $ 13,646 for type III LN and $ 14,161 for the LN type V. In type IV the cost was $ 3,499 using the EUROLUPUS scheme and maintenance with AZA. The costs amount to $ 14,163 if is used MMF for induction and maintenance.

5. Complete pharmacoeconomic evaluations

Wilson et al in 2007 conducted a study that sought to determine whether the results of LN treatment with MMF, represented a positive impact on quality of life (QoL) and a better use of resources. The authors created a simulation model to estimate the costs of quality-adjusted life year (QALY) of a LN patient treated with intravenous Cyclophosphamide (CYC) or with MMF for an adjusted period of six months. The efficiency, quality of life, resource uses and cost data were obtained from literature and standard databases and where necessary, data were supplemented by expert opinion. The model predicts that the use of MMF improved the quality of life compared with intravenous CYC. In addition, MMF is less expensive than CYC, at a cost of £ 1.600 (€ 2,400, $ 3,100), a lower cost based on 2005 prices the National Health System. The additional price in the application of intravenous of CYC was the main determinant of this variation. The sensitivity analysis shows a 81% probability that the use of MMF is more cost effective compared with intravenous CYC, with a willingness to pay £ 30,000 (€ 44,700, $ 58,500) per QALY gained. The authors of this study concluded that the use of MMF represented an improvement in the quality of life, and is less expensive than intravenous CYC as induction therapy for LN (26).

6. Conclusions

SLE costs are primarily determined by factors related to disease state such as: duration, disease activity, damage, and also the state of physical and mental health of patients which are influenced by the disease progression and the accumulated damage. The compromise of major organs such as nephritis and neuropsychiatric lupus, and relapses are also known factors associated with increased direct and indirect costs, independent of demographic factors. It is well-known that interventions that lead to the control of disease activity, prevent relapses, and delay the progression of the disease, can potentially save large amounts of costs attributable to the damage and the compromise of target-organ.

In the studies reviewed in this chapter were found large discrepancies in both direct and indirect costs, a situation that cannot simply be explained by demographic and clinical differences, across different populations. These discrepancies can be attributed to the absence of defined guidelines for cost-effectiveness analysis. It should be noted that there are great differences in the context of the costs, methods of costing, the health system, and practice patterns through studies. It should also be considered, the studies reviewed are derived from several different types of studies from different countries over a period of at least 16 years. Changes in the state of knowledge about disease, medical technology and practice patterns can have substantial influence on the estimate of the costs. It is important

to set out more studies to highlight the magnitude of the problem of SLE to society and people in different countries, and these studies should have innovative designs that will be able to resolve methodological lack found in some studies.
Nowadays, there are new therapies specifically routed to the immune system (Belimumab); these therapies can control the activity of the disease and prevent exacerbations of target organ in SLE. Their costs are probably much higher than conventional therapies. Given the substantial costs associated with SLE, it is expected that the potential benefits of these therapies offset their costs and new economic evaluations will give more information about the properties.

7. Key point section

1. SLE costs are related to health statement which is influenced by the disease progression and the accumulated damage.
2. Direct and indirect costs are influenced mainly by major organs compromise such as nephritis and neuropsychiatric lupus and flares.
3. Save large amounts of costs can achieve through the control of disease activity, prevent relapses, and delay the progression of the disease.
4. There are discrepancies in the results of both direct and indirect cost studies which can be attributed to the absence of defined guidelines for cost-effectiveness analysis
5. New studies are necessaries to innovate designs in order to resolve methodological lack found in before studies, including the new therapies like Belimumab.

8. References

[1] Danchenko N, Satia JA, Anthony MS. Epidemiology of systemic lupus erythematosus: a comparison of worldwide disease burden. Lupus 2006;15:308–18.
[2] Rice DP. Estimating the cost of illness. Am J Public Health Nations Health. 1967 Mar;57(3):424-40
[3] Hodgson TA, Meiners MR. Cost-of-illness methodology: a guide to current practices and procedures. Milbank Mem Fund Q Health Soc 1982;60:429–62.
[4] Choi BCK, Pak AWP. A method for comparing and combining cost-of-illness studies: an example from cardiovascular disease. Chronic Dis Can 2002;23: 47–57
[5] Kascati KL. Measuring and estimating costs. In: Essentials of pharmacoeconomics. Philadelphia: Wolters Kluwer/ Lippincott Williams & Wilkins; 2009. p. 9–23.
[6] McInnes PM, Schuttinga J, Sanslone WR, Stark SP, Klippel JH. The economic impact of treatment of severe lupus nephritis with prednisone and intravenous cyclophosphamide. Arthritis Rheum. 1994 Jul;37(7):1000-6.
[7] Clarke AE, Petri MA, Manzi S, Isenberg DA, Gordon C, Senecal JL, et al. An international perspective on the well being and health care costs for patients with systemic lupus erythematosus. Tri-Nation Study Group. J Rheumatol. 1999 Jul; 26(7):1500-11.
[8] Zink A, Fischer-Betz R, Thiele K, Listing K, Huscher D, Gromnica-Ihle E, et al. Health care and burden of illness in systemic lupus erythematosus compared to rheumatoid arthritis: results from the national database of the German Collaborative Arthritis Centres. Lupus (2004) 13, 529–536.

[9] Clarke AE, Petri M, Manzi S, Isenberg DA, Gordon C, Senécal JL, et al. The systemic lupus erythematosus Tri-nation Study: absence of a link between health resource use and health outcome. Rheumatology (Oxford). 2004 Aug; 43(8):1016-24.
[10] Grootscholten C, Snoek FJ, Bijl M, van Houwelingen HC, Derksen RH, Berden JH; Dutch Working Party of SLE. Health-related quality of life and treatment burden in patients with proliferative lupus nephritis treated with cyclophosphamide or azathioprine/ methylprednisolone in a randomized controlled trial. J Rheumatol. 2007 Aug; 34(8):1699-707.
[11] Campbell R Jr, Cooper GS, Gilkeson GS. The impact of systemic lupus erythematosus on employment. J Rheumatol. 2009 Nov;36(11):2470-5.
[12] Clarke AE, Esdaile JM, Bloch DA, Lacaille D, Danoff DS, Fries JF. A Canadian study of the total medical costs for patients with systemic lupus erythematosus and the predictors of costs. Arthritis Rheum. 1993 Nov;36(11):1548-59.
[13] Clarke AE, Penrod J, St Pierre Y, Petri MA, Manzi S, Isenberg DA, et al. Underestimating the value of women: assessing the indirect costs of women with systemic lupus erythematosus. Tri-Nation Study Group. J Rheumatol. 2000 Nov;27(11):2597-604
[14] Sutcliffe N, Clarke AE, Taylor R, Frost C, Isenberg DA. Total costs and predictors of costs in patients with systemic lupus erythematosus. Rheumatology (Oxford). 2001 Jan;40(1):37-47
[15] Clarke A, Economic Impact of Lupus. The American Journal of managed care, 2001: S496:S501.
[16] Huscher D, Merkesdal S, Thiele K, Zeidler H, Schneider M, Zink A; German Collaborative Arthritis Centres. Cost of illness in rheumatoid arthritis, ankylosing spondylitis, psoriatic arthritis and systemic lupus erythematosus in Germany. Ann Rheum Dis. 2006 Sep;65(9):1175-83
[17] Panopalis P, Petri M, Manzi S, Isenberg DA, Gordon C, Senécal JL, et al. The systemic lupus erythematosus Tri-Nation study: cumulative indirect costs. Arthritis & Rheumatism (Arthritis Care & Research); 2007 Feb 15;57(1):64-70.
[18] Clarke AE, Panopalis P, Petri M, Manzi S, Isenberg DA, Gordon C, et al. SLE patients with renal damage incur higher health care costs. Rheumatology (Oxford). 2008 Mar;47(3):329-33.
[19] Panopalis P, Yazdany J, Gillis JZ, Julian L, Trupin L, Hersh AO, et al. Health care costs and costs associated with changes in work productivity among persons with systemic lupus erythematosus. Arthritis Rheum (Arthritis Care & Research). 2008 Dec 15;59(12):1788-95
[20] Carls G, Li T, Panopalis P, Wang S, Mell A, Gibson T, et al. Direct and Indirect Costs to Employers of Patients With Systemic Lupus Erythematosus With and Without Nephritis. J Occup Environ Med. *2009;51:66–79*
[21] Zhu T, Tam L, Lee V, Lee K, and Li E. Systemic lupus erythematosus with neuropsychiatric manifestation incurs high disease costs: a cost-of-illness study in Hong Kong. Rheumatology 2009;48:564–568
[22] Li T, Carls GS, Panopalis P, Wang S, Gibson TB, Goetzel RZ. Long-term medical costs and resource utilization in systemic lupus erythematosus and lupus nephritis: a five-year analysis of a large medicaid population. Arthritis & Rheumatism (Arthritis Care & Research); 2009 Jun 15;61(6):755-63

[23] Zhu T, Tam L, Lee V, Lee K and Li E. The Impact of Flare on Disease Costs of Patients With Systemic Lupus Erythematosus. Arthritis & Rheumatism (Arthritis Care & Research); 2009:1159–1167
[24] Quintana G, Coral-Alvarado P, Díaz J. Direct costs of health care of lupus nephritis in Colombia. Ann Rheum Dis 2011;70(Suppl3):694
[25] Weening JJ, D'Agati VD, Schwartz MM, Seshan SV, Alpers CE, Appel GB, et al. The classification of glomerulonephritis in systemic lupus erythematosus revisited. J Am Soc Nephrol. 2004 Feb;15(2):241-50.
[26] Wilson E, Jayne D, Dellow D and Fordham R. The cost-effectiveness of mycophenolate mofetil as first line therapy in active lupus nephritis. Rheumatology 2007;46;1096–1101

Part 2

Etiopathogenesis

3

Role of Bone Marrow in the Pathogenesis of Rheumatoid Arthritis

Shunsei Hirohata
Kitasato University School of Medicine
Japan

1. Introduction

Rheumatoid arthritis (RA) is a chronic inflammatory disease characterized by persistent synovial proliferation. Thus, joints in RA consist of massive proliferating synovium, forming an invading tissue termed pannus, which results in the destruction of cartilage and bone. One of the most important histologic characteristics of the synovium in RA includes cellular proliferation in the lining layer as well as in the sublining layer (Tak, 2004). In the lining layer, both type A and type B synoviocytes, alternatively called intimal macrophages and fibroblast-like synoviocytes, respectively, are found to proliferate (Tak, 2004). In the sublining layer, there is infiltration of a variety of cells, including dendritis cells (DC), lymphocytes, plasma cells, and polymorphnuclear leukocytes. Notably, lymphoid cluster in RA synovium sometimes forms pseudo-germinal center, consisting of CD20+ B cells in the center surrounded by CD4+ T cells (Tak, 2004; Hirohata, 2004). In the synovium of RA, neovascularization is usually accompanied by lining cell proliferation and inflammatory cell infiltration (Firestein, 1999). In fact, lining cells and inflammatory cells have been found to produce angiogenic growth factors (Koch, 1998). It should be noted, however, that the synovium of RA also showed neovascularization in the areas without either lining cell proliferation or inflammatory cell infiltration, suggesting that the neovascularization might be one of the primary abnormal features that are most proximal to the etiology of RA (Hirohata & Sakakibara, 1999).

A number of studies have suggested that abnormal activation of normal joint constituents, such as synovial lining cells, play a pivotal role in the synovial hyperplasia in RA (Shiozawa & Tokuhisa, 1992). However, increasing attention has emerged to the role of bone marrow in the pathogenesis of RA. The present article overviews an update on the role of bone marrow in the pathogenesis of RA.

2. Bone marrow and type A synoviocytes (intimal macrophages) in RA

2.1 Abnormalities in peripheral blood monocytes in RA

We previously showed that peripheral blood monocytes in patients with active RA are already activated to express higher densities of CD14 (Shinohara et al.,1992). It is also suggested that peripheral blood monocytes in patients with RA may have intrinsic abnormalities as evidenced by the enhanced expression of FcγR, which is repeatedly observed regardless of the disease activity of RA (Shinohara et al.,1992). It has been also demonstrated that CD14, FcγRI and FcγRII are involved in the regulation of various functions of monocytes, including the production of cytokines (Krutmann et al.,1990) and the expression of adhesion molecules (Lauener et al.,1990). Therefore, the observed abnormalities in our studies suggest that the recruitment of RA peripheral blood monocytes may result in further activation and adhesion of these cells in the synovial tissues, thus contributing to extending the rheumatoid disease process.

2.2 Accelerated generation of CD14+ monocyte-lineage cells from the bone marrow

Although previous studies have suggested a role of dysregulated proliferation of synoviocytes in synovial hyperplasia (Lafyatis et al.,1989), it was found that rheumatoid synovium had rarely evidence of mitosis, and that only 4% of rheumatoid synovial cells showed uptake of thymidine (Harris Jr.,1993). Thus, there has been no evidence for accelerated or dysregulated in situ proliferation of synoviocytes in rheumatoid synovium.

We have disclosed that the spontaneous generation of CD14+ cells from bone marrow CD14- progenitor cells was accelerated in RA patients compared with control patients (Hirohata et al.,1996). Moreover, the expression of HLA-DR on the bone marrow-derived CD14+ cells was also accelerated in RA patients compared with controls, confirming the accelerated maturation of macrophages in RA bone marrow. Consistently, CD14+ CD16+ blood monocytes with high expression of chemokine receptors and CD54 were found to be increased in active RA (Kawanaka et al., 2002). It should be also pointed out that the expression of a variety of chemokines and adhesion molecules is enhanced in vascular endothelium and fibroblast-like synoviocytes in the RA synovium (Oppenheimer-Marks & Lipsky,1998; Patel et al.,2001; Kanbe et al.,2002), possibly facilitating the entry of such CD14+ CD16+ blood monocytes into the synovium. These observations strongly support the hypothesis that the accelerated generation of CD14+ cells from bone marrow progenitor cells and the accelerated maturation of such CD14+ cells into tissue-infiltrative CD16+ monocytes before entry into the joint might play an important role in the pathogenesis of RA.

2.3 Evidence for recruitment of cells from systemic circulation in RA

It is noteworthy that accelerated angiogenesis has been demonstrated in RA synovium (Harris Jr.,1993), which might facilitate the recruitment of bone marrow-derived monocytes as well as lymphocytes into the synovium. In fact, the transendothelial migration of monocytes in RA synovium can be frequently observed under electron microscopy (Fig. 1).

Of interest, the formation of synovium-like tissue was also observed at the site of non-union formed after bone fracture as well as in the pericardial lesions in an RA patient (Fig. 2). Since such formation of the synovium-like tissue took place in the place without original synovial tissues, it is suggested that all the constituents of the newly formed tissue might be recruited from the systemic circulation. Finally, proliferative synovial tissues usually disappear at the site of bony ankylosis and total immobility. These observations strongly support the hypothesis that the accelerated generation and continuous recruitment of bone marrow-derived cells might play a critical role in the synovial hyperplasia in RA, thus accounting for the discrepancy between the marked synovial hyperplasia and the lack of evidence for accelerated proliferation of synoviocytes.

3. Origin of type B synoviocyte

3.1 Origin of type B synoviocytes

Type B synoviocytes, which are called fibroblast-like synoviocytes, have the morphologic appearance of fibroblasts as well as the capacity to produce and secrete a variety of factors,

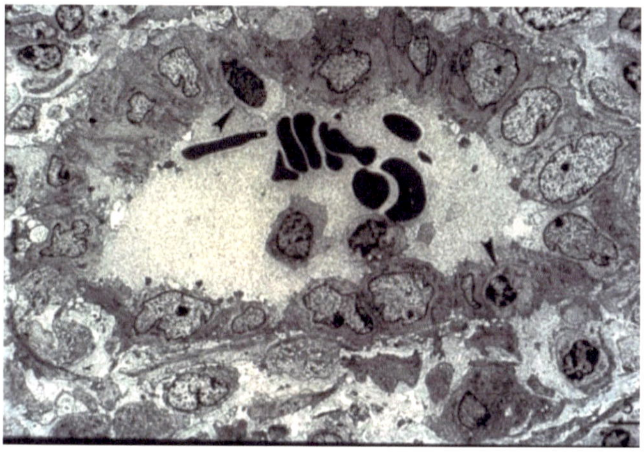

Monocyte-like cells are shown by arrow heads.
(Electron microscopy, the scale bar at the right-bottom corner indicates 5 μm)

Fig. 1. Transendothelial migration of monocyte into RA synovium.

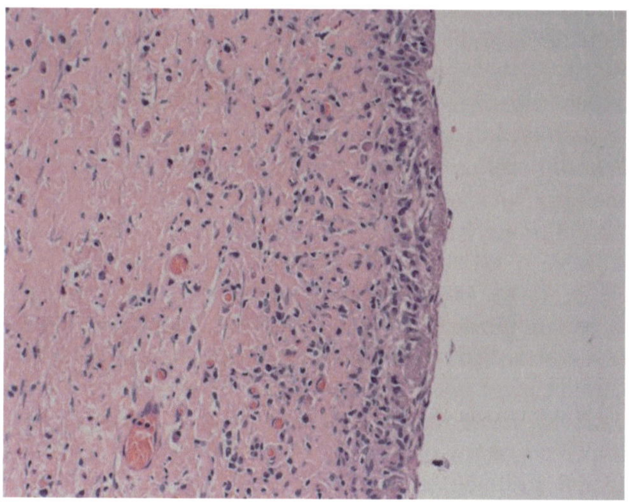

(Hematoxylin and eosin, original magnification x25)

Fig. 2. Synovium-like tissue at pericardium lesion in an RA patient

including proteoglycans, cytokines, arachidonic acid metabolites, and matrix metalloproteinases (MMPs), that lead to the destruction of joints (Firestein,1996). Unlike intimal macrophages, the precise origin of type B synoviocytes remains unclear, although they are thought to arise from the sublining tissue or other support structures of a joint (Firestein,1996). On the other hand, a number of studies have shown that peripheral blood dendritic cells (DC) accumulate in the synovium, where they undergo phenotypic and functional differentiation in situ (Zvaifler et al.,1985; Thomas et al.,1994). It has been also shown that synovial DC gradually lose their dinstinct morphologic appearance and become indistinguishable from fibroblasts in vitro (Hendler et al.,1985). Moreover, Kyogoku et al. identified the presence of DC-like cells that strongly express major histocompatibility complex (MHC) class II antigens and interact with T lymphocytes, in the sublining layers of the RA synovium (Kyogoku et al.,1992). They also showed that the sublining DC-like cells proliferate and differentiate into type A as well as type B synoviocytes to replace the lining layers (Kyogoku et al.,1992).

3.2 Generation of type B synoviocytes from bone marrow CD34+ cells in RA

Since it was shown that DC are derived from bone marrow CD34+ cells (Reid et al.,1992; Szabolcs et al.,1995; Chen et al.,2004), it was also likely that type B synoviocytes might be induced from bone marrow progenitors. In this regard, we previously demonstrated that bone marrow CD34+ cells from RA patients have abnormal capacities to respond to tumor necrosis factor-α (TNF-α) and to differentiate into fibroblast-like cells (FLC) producing MMP-1, suggesting that bone marrow CD34+ cells might generate type B synoviocytes and thus could play an important role in the pathogenesis of RA (Hirohata et al.,2001). Thus, CD34+ cells from the bone marrow of RA patients differentiated into cells with fibroblast-like morphology, which expressed prolyl 4-hydroxylase, in the presence of stem cell factor (SCF), GM-CSF, and TNF-α, much more effectively than CD34+ cells from the bone marrow of control subjects (Hirohata et al.,2001).

3.3 Capacity of bone marrow DC to differentiate into type B synoviocytes

We have recently demonstrated that bone marrow plasmacytoid DC (pDC) as well as myeloid DC (mDC), irrespective of their origin from RA bone marrow or osteoarthritis (OA) bone marrow, have prominent capacity to differentiate into FLC producing MMP-1 especially under influences of TNF-α (Hirohata et al.,2011). Of note, depletion of pDC from RA bone marrow CD34+ cells significantly diminished their capacities to differentiate into FLC, which were restored by addition of pDC in a dose-response manner (Hirohata et al.,2011).
It should be pointed out that generation of FLC from RA bone marrow CD34+ cells or pDC was correlated with MMP-1 levels in culture supernatants (Hirohata et al.,2001; Hirohata et al.,2011). On the other hand, it has been demonstrated that cadherin-11 is abundantly expressed in type B synoviocytes (Chang et al.,2010) compared with lung or dermal fibroblasts (Vandooren et al.,2008). Accordingly, the FLC induced from RA and OA bone marrow pDC expressed comparable amounts of cadherin-11 mRNA to RA and OA synovial FLC (Hirohata et al.,2011). These results indicate that DC are one of the progenitors of type B synoviocytes irrespective of RA or OA and suggest that bone marrow CD34+ cells might differentiate into type B synoviocyte-like cells via DC, since DC have been demonstrated to originate from CD34+ cells (Reid et al.,1992; Szabolcs et al.,1995; Chen et al.,2004). It is also likely that expansion of immature DC from bone marrow CD34+ cells might be upregulated in RA compared with in OA, accounting for the enhanced capacity of RA bone marrow CD34+ cells to differentiate into FLC upon stimulation with TNF-α, although further studies are required to confirm this point.

3.4 Recruitment of type B synoviocytes and their precursors into RA joints: Role of DC

It is thus suggested that the presence of abnormal precursors within the bone marrow progenitor cells might play an important role in the pathogenesis of RA by providing a repopulating reservoir of type B synoviocytes, as has been also suggested in other recent studies (Sen et al.,2000). Notably, the numbers of mDC and pDC have been found to be significantly decreased in RA peripheral blood, whereas both mDC and pDC are present in synovial fluid from RA (Jongbloed et al.,2006). In fact, previous study showed that pDC are recruited to RA synovial tissues and contribute into the local inflammatory environment (Lande et al,2004; Cavanagh et al.,2005). Recent studies have disclosed that the characteristic clinical phenomenon of destructive arthritis spreading between joints is mediated, at least in part, by the transmigration of activated RA synovial fibroblasts (Lefèvre et al.,2009). Thus, RA synovial fibroblasts showed an active movement from human RA synovial tissue or human cartilage-sponge complex containing RA synovial fibroblasts implanted into the SCID mouse to the naive cartilage implanted at the contralateral flank via the vasculature, leading to a marked destruction of the target cartilage (Lefèvre et al.,2009). The movement of DC-like cells from the sublining layer to the lining layer in RA synovium (Kyogoku et al.,1992) and the presence of DC in synovial fluid (Jongbloed et al.,2006; Lande et al,2004) strongly suggest that DC might be also released from the joint to the systemic circulation via draining veins. Since bone marrow pDC as well as mDC have capacities to differentiate into type B synoviocyte-like cells, it is possible that DC, as precursors for synovial fibroblasts, also contribute to the spread of destructive arthritis between joints in RA.

4. RA as a disease of antigen-presenting cells

A number of studies have demonstrated that RA is strongly associated with HLA-DR4 or DR1 (Nepom,2001), which are involved in the presentation of antigens to T cells. These results suggest that the antigen presentation involving HLA-DR4 or the shared epitope might play a critical role in the development of synovitis in human RA. In fact, the interactions between DC and T cells, possibly through MHC class II antigens, have been disclosed in the sublining layers of the RA synovium (Kyogoku et al.,1992). If the antigens presented by APC to T cells are perpetuating antigens, such as autoantigens or antigens of persistently infected virus, that are presented through MHC class II molecules, continuing activation of APC might take place. Further studies to explore such antigens that involve persistent interactions between APC and T cells would be still important for the complete understanding of the pathogenesis of RA.

As highlighted above, bone marrow derived monocytes and DC have been shown to be the precursors of type A synoviocytes and type B synoviocytes, respectively. It is therefore suggested that RA might be a disease of dysregulated activation of antigen-presenting cells (APC), leading to synovial proliferation. Lymphocytes activation in the synovium can also be triggered by the activation of APC, accounting for activation of T cells and B cells in the synovium. Triggering with arthritogenic antigens, followed by dysregulated generation of APC from the bone marrow might result in persistent recruitment of APC into the synovium.

5. Bone marrow abnormalities and angiogenesis in RA

A number of studies indicated that neovascularization is crucial to the synovial hyperplasia in RA (Koch,1998; Hirohata & Sakakibara,1999). Postnatal neovascularization has been attributed to so-called angiogenesis, a process characterized by the sprouting of new capillaries from preexisting blood vessels (Folkman & Shing,1992). However, recent studies have demonstrated that endothelial progenitor cells of bone marrow origin play a significant role in the de novo formation of capillaries without preexisting blood vessels, so-called vasculogenesis (Asahara et al.,1997; Gehling et al.,2000; Bhattacharya et al.,2000; Lin et al.,2000).

We also showed that RA bone marrow CD34+ cells have enhanced capacities to differentiate into endothelial cells in relation to synovial vascularization (Hirohata & Yanagida et al.,2004). Therefore, bone marrow CD34+ cells might contribute to synovial neovascularization by supplying endothelial precursor cells and, thus, play an important role in the pathogenesis of RA.

Neovascularization of the synovium is not unique to RA. It has also been observed in OA synovium and has been shown to play an important role in the development of new cartilage and mineralization (Brown et al.,1980; Giatromanolaki et al.,2003; Haywood et al.,2003). Of note, recent studies have revealed that levels of expression of the angiogenic factors VEGF and platelet-derived endothelial cell growth factor are increased in RA as well as in OA, relative to normal subjects, whereas the presence of an activated synovial vasculature was high only in RA (Giatromanolaki et al.,2003). Moreover, the vascular activation by VEGF/KDR was significantly lower in OA than in RA patients, although the activation of the hypoxia inducing factor α (HIFα) pathway was comparable in OA and RA patients (Giatromanolaki et al.,2003). These observations suggest the presence of intrinsic abnormalities in synovial endothelial cells in RA patients. Of note, we have disclosed that the expression of VEGFR-2/KDR mRNA in RA bone marrow CD34+ cells was significantly higher than that in OA bone marrow CD34+ cells (Hirohata & Yanagida et al.,2004). It is therefore likely that the differences in VEGF/KDR vascular activation in bone marrow CD34+ cells might result in differences in their capacity to generate endothelial progenitor cells between RA and OA patients (Koch et al.,1994; Giatromanolaki et al.,2001).

It has been shown that decreased numbers and impaired function of endothelial progenitor cells (EPCs) resulting in defective vasculogenesis are associated with RA, leading to premature atherosclerosis (Herbrig et al., 2006; Pakozdi et al., 2009). On the other hand, it has been recently disclosed that EPCs can be differentiated into 2 subpopulations, EPCs of monocytic versus hemangioblastic origin, which have been denoted as early-outgrowth and late-outgrowth EPCs, respectively (Jodon de Villeroché et al, 2010). More importantly, late-outgrowth EPCs have been found to be increased and have higher colony formation capacity in the active stage of RA. It is therefore likely that hemangioblastic EPC-dependent vasculogenesis might be associated with active inflammation and accelerated atherosclerosis in RA.

6. Abnormal gene expression in bone marrow CD34+ cells in RA

6.1 RA and hematopoietic stem cell transplantation

Although autologous hematopoietic stem cell transplantation (HSCT) has been used to treat severe RA in limited case reports (Joske,1997; Durez et al.,1998), a study with greater numbers of patients have disclosed that recurrence of RA is frequent after the autologous HSCT (Snowden et al.,2004; Bingham & Moore, 2004). Such frequent recurrence after autologous HSCT clearly indicates that abnormalities in bone marrow stem cells persist after the treatment. It has been proposed that bone marrow CD34+ progenitor cell reserve and function are defective in RA probably due, at least in part, to a TNF-α mediated effect, because significant restoration of the disturbed hematopoiesis was obtained following anti-TNF-α treatment (Papadaki et al.,2002; Porta et al.,2004). It should be noted, however, that blockade of TNF-α is not curative for RA in spite of its epoch-making impact on treatment of RA (Feldmann & Maini,2001). Thus, recurrence of RA is noted after discontinuation of blockade of TNF-α or even during anti-TNF-α therapy (Feldmann & Maini,2001). It is therefore likely that intrinsic abnormalities that were not secondary to the influences of TNF-α might be present in bone marrow progenitor cells, leading to recurrence of RA. In fact, although abnormal regulatory networks in the immune response and cell cycle categories were identified in bone marrow mononuclear cells from RA patients (Lee et al.,2011), it is possible that such changes might be secondary to systemic inflammation, presumably due to proinflammatory cytokines. In this regard, beyond its role in angiogenesis, the demonstration of the abnormal expression of VEGFR-2/KDR mRNA in RA bone marrow CD34+ cells (Hirohata & Yanagida et al.,2004) have brought an impact as the fist evidence for the intrinsic abnormality in RA bone marrow.

Mesenchymal stem cells (MSCs) have been shown to have potent anti-inflammatory and immunomodulatory properties through suppression of Th1/Th17 response and induction of Treg response (Macdonald et al., 2011). However, it remains unclear whether MSC therapy is beneficial for treatment of RA.

6.2 Nuclear factor kappa B1 (NFkB1)

As mentioned above, bone marrow CD34+ cells from RA patients have abnormal capacities to respond to TNF-α and to differentiate into FLC producing MMP-1, suggesting that abnormalities in bone marrow CD34+ cells might play a role in the pathogenesis in RA (Hirohata et al.,2001). TNF-α is one of the first triggers to be found effective for the activation of NFκ B (Müller-Ladner et al.,2002). Of note, we have recently demonstrated that RA bone marrow CD34+ cells showed enhanced expression of NFκ B1 (p50), silencing of which resulted in prevention of their differentiation into FLC (Hirohata et al.,2006).

6.3 FK506-binding protein5 (FKBP5)

Nakamura et al. recently disclosed that the expression of several genes including amphiregulin (AREG), chemokine receptor 4 (CXCR4), and FK506-binding protein 5 (FKBP5), was augmented in bone marrow mononuclear cells from RA patients compared with those from OA patients (Nakamura et al.,2006). Interestingly, FKBP5 was found to be involved in nuclear translocation and activation of NFκB by degradation of inhibitor of NFκB alpha (IκBα) in a human megakaryoblastic leukemia cell line (Bouwmeester et al.,2004; Komura et al.,2005). It is therefore suggested that the up-regulated expression of both NFκB1 and FKBP5 mRNAs in bone marrow CD34+ cells from RA patients might be involved cooperatively in their abnormal responses to TNF-α to differentiate into type B synoviocyte-like cells.

Although the expression of mRNAs for AREG, CXCR4 and FKBP5 has been shown to be augmented in RA bone marrow mononuclear cells (Nakamura et al.,2006), only FKBP5 mRNA expression was significantly upregulated in bone marrow CD34+ cells from RA (Matsushita et al.,2010). Therefore, it is suggested that the up-regulation of the expression of mRNAs for AREG and CXCR4 in RA bone marrow mononuclear cells might be sequelae of systemic inflammation of RA. By contrast, the up-regulation of FKBP5 mRNA expression in RA bone marrow CD34+ cells might not be secondary to systemic inflammation, but a primary abnormality in bone marrow CD34+ cells (Matsushita et al.,2010). It has been previously shown that TNF-α enhanced NFκB1 mRNA expression in bone marrow CD34+ cells from healthy individuals (Hirohata et al.,2006). However, TNF-α did not enhance FKBP5 mRNA expression in bone marrow CD34+ cells from healthy individuals (Matsushita et al.,2010). It is therefore confirmed that apart from NFkB1, the enhanced

FKBP5 mRNA expression in RA bone marrow CD34+ cells is not secondary to systemic inflammation of RA.

6.4 Krüppel like factor 5 (KLF-5)

Krüppel like factor 5 (KLF-5), a zinc finger-containing transcription factor, activates many genes, including platelet-derived growth factor (PDGF) A/B, plasminogen activator inhibitor-1, inducible nitric oxide synthase and VEGF receptors (Shindo et al.,2002; Nagai et al.,2005). KLF-5 has been shown to cooperate with NFkB1 to activate PDGF-A gene expression (Nagai et al.,2005; Aizawa et al.,2004), which might be involved in synovial fibroblast-like cell proliferation (Ohba et al.,1996). KLF-5 mRNA expression in bone marrow CD34+ cells was significantly higher in RA patients than in OA patients (Hirohata et al.,2009). It is thus likely that the upregulation of VEGFR-2/KDR mRNA expression might be secondary to the enhanced KLF-5 mRNA expression in RA bone marrow CD34+ cells. Of note, TNF-α enhanced NFkB1 mRNA expression, but not KLF-5 mRNA expression, in bone marrow CD34+ cells from normal individuals (Fig.3) (Hirohata et al.,2009).

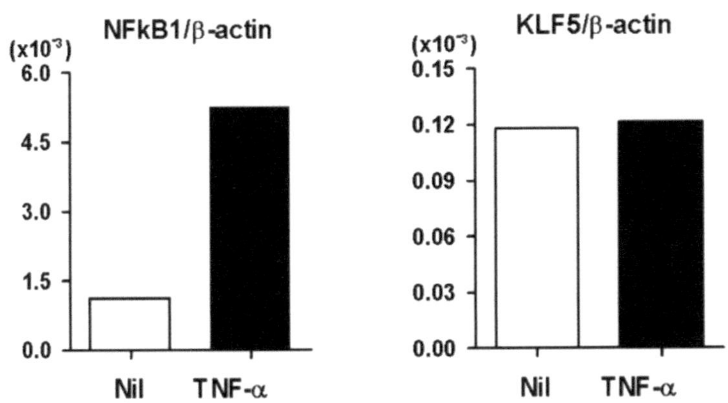

Fig. 3. Effect of TNF-α on the expression of mRNAs for NFkB1 and KLF-5 in bone marrow CD34+ cells from a healthy donor

Previous studies also demonstrated that the suppression of KLF-5 by silencing RNA resulted in a reduction of NFkB1 mRNA in IEC6 cells stimulated with lipopolysaccharide, indicating that KLF-5 is an upstream regulator for NFkB1 mRNA expression in IEC6 cells (Chanchevalap et al.,2006). Taken together, it is most likely that the upregulation of KLF-5 mRNA expression might lead to the enhanced expression of NFkB1 mRNA in bone marrow CD34+ cells, but not vice versa, in RA. In addition, the upregulation of KLF-5 mRNA as well as NFkB1 mRNA in RA bone marrow CD34+ cells might result in their abnormal capacities to differentiate into FLC. Although it is strongly suggested that KLF-5 might be an upstream regulator of NFkB1 mRNA in bone marrow CD34+ cells, further studies to explore the mechanism of abnormal expression of KLF-5 mRNA in BM CD34+ cells and its relation with FKBP5 would be important.

7. Conclusion

As summarized in Fig.4, accumulating evidence has been provided for the involvement of bone marrow in the pathogenesis of RA. Thus, all the constituents in the proliferating synovial tissues might be supplied from bone marrow CD34+ cells. Apparently, RA bone marrow CD34+ cells have abnormal mRNA expression for several genes, possibly resulting in abnormal differentiation of monocytes and DC. Moreover, it is strongly suggested that DC, as precursors for synovial fibroblasts, might also contribute to the spread of destructive arthritis between joints in RA (Hirohata et al.,2011; Lefèvre et al.,2009).

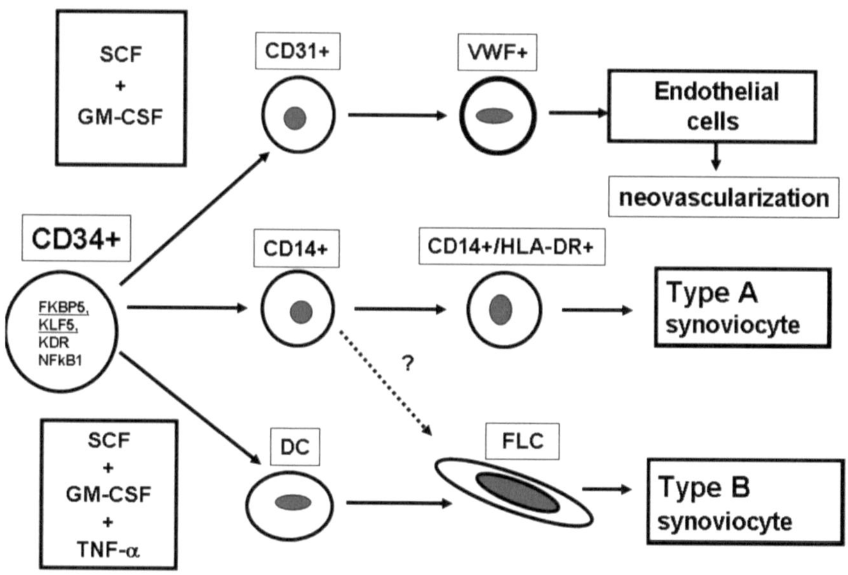

Fig. 4. Schema for the suggested role of bone marrow in the pathogenesis of RA

In the past decade, the importance of TNF-α in the pathogenesis of RA has come to be increasingly appreciated (Feldmann et al.,1996). We have revealed that CD34+ cells from bone marrow of RA patients have abnormal responsiveness to TNF-α (Hirohata et al.,2001). However, the precise sequelae of abnormal responses of CD34+ cells from bone marrow of RA patients to TNF-α remain unclear. KLF-5 might upregulate the expression of mRNAs for NFkB1 and VEGFR-2/KDR, whereas FKBP5 might enhance activation of NFkB, resulting in further upregulation of NFkB1 mRNA expression. Further studies that explore in detail the mechanism of abnormal expression of the genes, especially KLF-5 and FKBP5, in CD34+ cells from bone marrow of RA patients would be helpful in gaining a complete understanding of the etiology as well as the pathogenesis of RA. In this regard, we showed previously that GM-CSF-stimulated bone marrow CD34+ cells from 3 of 8 RA patients, but none from 7 OA patients, gave rise to spontaneous transformation of highly purified B cells of Epstein-Barr virus (EBV)-seronegative healthy donors, whereas neither GM-CSF-stimulated bone marrow CD34+ cells alone nor highly purified B cells alone gave rise to spontaneously transformed B cell lines (Hirohata et al.,2000). All the transformed B cell lines were positive for EBV-DNA. It is therefore possible that EBV might be involved in abnormalities in RA bone marrow CD34+ cells. Further studies to investigate the role of EBV in bone marrow abnormalities in RA would be interesting.

8. References

Aizawa K, Suzuki T, Kada N, et al. (2004). Regulation of platelet-derived growth factor-A chain by Krüppel -like factor 5: new pathway of cooperative activation with nuclear factor-kappa B. *J. Biol. Chem.* 279:70–6.

Asahara T, Murohara T, Sullivan A, et al. (1997). Isolation of putative progenitor endothelial cells for angiogenesis. *Science* 275: 964-7.

Bhattacharya V, McSweeney PA, Shi Q, et al. (2000). Enhanced endothelialization and microvessel formation in polyester grafts seeded with CD34(+) bone marrow cells. *Blood* 95: 581-5.

Bingham SJ, Moore JJ. (2004). Stem cell transplantation for autoimmune disorders. Rheumatoid arthritis. *Best Pract. Res. Clin. Haematol.* 17: 263-76.

Bouwmeester T, Bauch A, Ruffner H, et al. (2004). A physical and functional map of the human TNF-alpha/NF-kappa B signal transduction pathway. *Nat. Cell Biol.* 6: 97-105.

Brown RA, Weiss JB, Tomlinson IW, Phillips P, Kumar S. (1980). Angiogenic factor from synovial fluid resembling that from tumours. *Lancet* 1: 682-5.

Cavanagh LL, Boyce A, Smith L, et al. (2005). Rheumatoid arthritis synovium contains plasmacytoid dendritic cells. *Arthritis Res. Ther.* 7: R230-40.

Chanchevalap S, Nandan MO, McConnell BB, et al. (2006). Krüppel-like factor 5 is an important mediator for lipopolysaccharide-induced proinflammatory response in intestinal epithelial cells. *Nucl. Acids Res.* 34:1216–23.

Chang SK, Gu Z, Brenner MB. (2010). Fibroblast-like synoviocytes in inflammatory arthritis pathology: the emerging role of cadherin-11. *Immunol. Rev.* 233: 256-66.

Chen W, Antonenko S, Sederstrom JM, et al. (2004). Thrombopoietin cooperates with FLT3-ligand in the generation of plasmacytoid dendritic cell precursors from human hematopoietic progenitors. *Blood* 103: 2547-53.

Durez P, Toungouz M, Schandene L, Lambermont M, Goldman M. (1998). Remission and immune reconstitution after T-cell-depleted stem-cell transplantation for rheumatoid arthritis. *Lancet* 352: 881.

Feldmann M, Brennan FM, Maini RN. (1996). Role of cytokines in rheumatoid arthritis. *Annu. Rev. Immunol.* 14: 397-440.

Feldmann M, Maini RN. (2001). Anti-TNF alpha therapy of rheumatoid arthritis: what have we learned? *Annu. Rev. Immunol.* 19: 163-96.

Firestein GS. (1996). Invasive fibroblast-like synoviocytes in rheumatoid arthritis. Passive responders or transformed aggressors? *Arthritis Rheum.* 39: 1781-90.

Firestein GS. (1999). Starving the synovium: angiogenesis and inflammation in rheumatoid arthritis. *J. Clin. Invest.* 103: 3-4.

Folkman J, Shing Y. (1992). Angiogenesis. *J. Biol. Chem.* 267: 10931-4

Gehling UM, Ergun S, Schumacher U, et al. (2000). In vitro differentiation of endothelial cells from AC133-positive progenitor cells. *Blood* 95: 3106-12.

Giatromanolaki A, Sivridis E, Athanassou N, et al. (2001). The angiogenic pathway "vascular endothelial growth factor/flk-1(KDR)-receptor" in rheumatoid arthritis and osteoarthritis. *J. Pathol.* 194: 101-8.

Giatromanolaki A, Sivridis E, Maltezos E, et al. (2003). Upregulated hypoxia inducible factor-1alpha and -2alpha pathway in rheumatoid arthritis and osteoarthritis. *Arthritis Res .Ther.* 5: R193-201.

Harris ED Jr (1993). Etiology and pathogenesis of rheumatoid arthritis, in Kelley, W.N., Harris ED Jr., Ruddy S & Sledge CB. (eds.), *Textbook of Rheumatology 4th ed*, WB Saunders, Philadelphia.

Haywood L, McWilliams DF, Pearson CI, et al. (2003). Inflammation and angiogenesis in osteoarthritis. Arthritis Rheum. 48: 2173-7.

Hendler PL, Lavoie PE, Werb Z, Chan J, Seaman WE. (1985). Human synovial dendritic cells. Direct observation of transition to fibroblasts. *J. Rheumatol.* 12: 660-4.

Herbrig K, Haensel S, Oelschlaegel U, Pistrosch F, Foerster S, Passauer J. (2006). Endothelial dysfunction in patients with rheumatoid arthritis is associatedwith a reduced number and impaired function of endothelial progenitor cells. *Ann Rheum Dis.* 65:157-63.

Hirohata S, Yanagida T, Itoh K, et al. (1996). Accelerated generation of CD14+ monocyte-lineage cells from the bone marrow of rheumatoid arthritis patients. *Arthritis Rheum.* 39: 836-43.

Hirohata S, Sakakibara J. (1999). Angioneogenesis as a possible elusive triggering factor in rheumatoid arthritis. *Lancet* 353: 1331.

Hirohata S, Yanagida T, Nakamura H, Yoshino S, Tomita T, Ochi T. (2000). Bone marrow CD34+ progenitor cells from rheumatoid arthritis patients support spontaneous transformation of peripheral blood B cells from healthy individuals. *Rheumatol. Int.* 19:153-9.

Hirohata S, Yanagida T, Nagai T, et al. (2001). Induction of fibroblast-like cells from CD34(+) progenitor cells of the bone marrow in rheumatoid arthritis. *J. Leukoc. Biol.* 70: 413-21.

Hirohata S, Yanagida T, Nampei A, et al. (2004). Enhanced generation of endothelial cells from CD34+ cells of the bone marrow in rheumatoid arthritis: possible role in synovial neovascularization. *Arthritis Rheum.* 50: 3888-96.

Hirohata S. (2004). Involvement of B cells in the pathogenesis of rheumatoid arthritis (in Japanese). *Igakunoayumi* 209: 796-800.

Hirohata S, Miura Y, Tomita T, Yoshikawa H, Ochi T, Chiorazzi N. (2006). Enhanced expression of mRNA for nuclear factor kappaB1 (p50) in CD34+ cells of the bone marrow in rheumatoid arthritis. *Arthritis Res. Ther.* 8: R54.

Hirohata S, Miura Y, Tomita T, Yoshikawa H. (2009). Enhanced expression of mRNA for Krüppel -like factor 5 in CD34+ cells of the bone marrow in rheumatoid arthritis. *Ann. Rheum. Dis.* 68:763-4.

Hirohata S, Nagai T, Asako K, Tomita T, Yoshikawa H. (2011). Induction of type B synoviocyte-like cells from plasmacytoid dendritic cells of the bone marrow in rheumatoid arthritis and osteoarthritis. *Clin. Immunol.* 140: 276-83.

Jodon de Villeroché V, Avouac J, Ponceau A, et al. (2010). Enhanced late-outgrowth circulating endothelial progenitor cell levels in rheumatoid arthritis and correlation with disease activity. *Arthritis Res. Ther.* 12:R27.

Jongbloed SL, Lebre MC, Fraser AR, et al. (2006). Enumeration and phenotypical analysis of distinct dendritic cell subsets in psoriatic arthritis and rheumatoid arthritis. *Arthritis Res. Ther.* 8: R15.

Joske DJ. (1997). Autologous bone-marrow transplantation for rheumatoid arthritis. *Lancet* 350: 337-8.

Kanbe K, Takagishi K, Chen Q. (2002). Stimulation of matrix metalloprotease 3 release from human chondrocytes by the interaction of stromal cell-derived factor 1 and CXC chemokine receptor 4. *Arthritis Rheum.* 46: 130-7.

Kawanaka N, Yamamura M, Aita T, et al. (2002). CD14+,CD16+ blood monocytes and joint inflammation in rheumatoid arthritis. *Arthritis Rheum.* 46: 2578-86.

Koch AE, Harlow LA, Haines GK, et al. (1994). Vascular endothelial growth factor. A cytokine modulating endothelial function in rheumatoid arthritis. *J. Immunol.* 152: 4149-56.

Koch AE. (1998). Angiogenesis: implications for rheumatoid arthritis. *Arthritis Rheum.* 41: 951-62.

Komura E, Tonetti C, Penard-Lacronique V, et al. (2005). Role for the nuclear factor kappaB pathway in transforming growth factor-beta1 production in idiopathic myelofibrosis: possible relationship with FK506 binding protein 51 overexpression. *Cancer Res.* 65: 3281-9.

Krutmann J, Kirnbauer R, Kock A, et al. (1990). Cross-linking Fc receptors on monocytes triggers IL-6 production. Role in anti-CD3-induced T cell activation. *J. Immunol.* 145: 1337-42.

Kyogoku M, Sawai T, Murakami K, Ito J. (1992). Histopathological characteristics of rheumatoid arthritis —as a clue to elucidate its pathogenesis— (in Japanese). *Nippon Rinsho* 50: 483-89.

Lafyatis R, Remmers EF, Roberts AB, Yocum DE, Sporn MB, Wilder RL. (1989). Anchorage-independent growth of synoviocytes from arthritic and normal joints. Stimulation by exogenous platelet-derived growth factor and inhibition by transforming growth factor-beta and retinoids. *J. Clin. Invest.* 83: 1267-76.

Lande R, Giacomini E, Serafini B, et al. (2004). Characterization and recruitment of plasmacytoid dendritic cells in synovial fluid and tissue of patients with chronic inflammatory arthritis. *J. Immunol.* 173: 2815-24.

Lauener RP, Geha RS, Vercelli D. (1990). Engagement of the monocyte surface antigen CD14 induces lymphocyte function-associated antigen-1/intercellular adhesion molecule-1-dependent homotypic adhesion. *J. Immunol.* 145: 1390-4.

Lee H-M, Sugino H, Aoki C, Shimaoka Y, Suzuki R, Ochi K, Ochi T, Nishimoto N. (2011). Abnormal networks of immune response-related molecules in bone marrow cells from patients with rheumatoid arthritis as revealed by DNA microarray analysis. *Arthritis Res. Ther.* 13:R89.

Lefèvre S, Knedla A, Tennie C, et al. (2009). Synovial fibroblasts spread rheumatoid arthritis to unaffected joints. *Nat. Med.* 15:1414-20.

Lin Y, Weisdorf DJ, Solovey A, Hebbel RP. (2000). Origins of circulating endothelial cells and endothelial outgrowth from blood. *J. Clin. Invest.* 105: 71-7.

Macdonald GI, Augello A, De Bari C. (2011). Mesenchymal stem cells: Re-establishing immunological tolerance in autoimmune rheumatic diseases. *Arthritis Rheum.* [Epub ahead of print] PMID:21647863

Matsushita R, Hashimoto A, Tomita T, Yoshikawa H, Tanaka S, Endo H, Hirohata S. (2010). Enhanced expression of mRNA for FK506-binding protein 5 in bone marrow CD34 positive cells in patients with rheumatoid arthritis. *Clin. Exp. Rheumatol.* 28:87-90.

Müller-Ladner U, Gay RE, Gay S. (2002). Role of nuclear factor B in synovial inflammation. *Curr. Rheumatol. Rep.* 4: 201-7.

Nagai R, Suzuki T, Aizawa K, Shindo T, Manabe I. (2005). Significance of the transcription factor KLF5 in cardiovascular remodeling. *J. Thromb. Haemost.* 3:1569–76.

Nakamura N, ShimaokaY, Tougan T, et al. (2006). Isolation and expression profiling of genes upregulated in bone marrow-derived mononuclear cells of rheumatoid arthritis patients. *DNA Res.* 13: 169-83.

Nepom GT. (2001). The role of the DR4 shared epitope in selection and commitment of autoreactive T cells in rheumatoid arthritis. *Rheum. Dis. Clin. North. Am.* 27: 305-15.

Ohba T, Takase Y, Ohhara M, Kasukawa R. (1996). Thrombin in the synovial fluid of patients with rheumatoid arthritis mediates proliferation of synovial fibroblast-like cells by induction of platelet derived growth factor. *J. Rheumatol.* 23:1505-11.

Oppenheimer-Marks N, Lipsky PE. (1998). Adhesion molecules in rheumatoid arthritis. *Springer Semin. Immunopathol.* 20: 95-114.

Pakozdi A, Besenyei T, Paragh G, Koch AE, Szekanecz Z. (2009). Endothelial progenitor cells in arthritis-associated vasculogenesis and atherosclerosis. *Joint Bone Spine* 76:581-3.

Papadaki HA, Kritikos HD, Gemetzi C, et al. (2002). Bone marrow progenitor cell reserve and function and stromal cell function are defective in rheumatoid arthritis: evidence for a tumor necrosis factor alpha-mediated effect. *Blood* 99: 1610-19.

Patel DD, Zachariah JP, Whichard LP. (2001). CXCR3 and CCR5 ligands in rheumatoid arthritis synovium. *Clin. Immunol.* 98: 39-45.

Porta C, Caporali R, Epis O, et al. (2004). Impaired bone marrow hematopoietic progenitor cell function in rheumatoid arthritis patients candidated to autologous hematopoietic stem cell transplantation. *Bone Marrow Transplant.* 33: 721-8.

Reid CD, Stackpoole A, Meager A, Tikerpae J. (1992). Interactions of tumor necrosis factor with granulocyte-macrophage colony-stimulating factor and other cytokines in the regulation of dendritic cell growth in vitro from early bipotent CD34+ progenitors in human bone marrow. *J. Immunol.* 149: 2681-8.

Sen M, Lauterbach K, El-Gabalawy H, Firestein GS, Corr M, Carson DA. (2000). Expression and function of wingless and frizzled homologs in rheumatoid arthritis. *Proc. Natl. Acad. Sci. U S A* 97: 2791-6.

Shinohara S, Hirohata S, Inoue T, Ito K. (1992). Phenotypic analysis of peripheral blood monocytes isolated from patients with rheumatoid arthritis. *J. Rheumatol.* 19: 211-5.

Shindo T, Manabe I, Fukushima Y, et al. (2002). Krüppel-like zinc-finger transcription factor KLF5/BTEB2 is a target for angiotensin II signaling and an essential regulator of cardiovascular remodeling. *Nat. Med.* 8: 856–63.

Shiozawa S, Tokuhisa T. (1992). Contribution of synovial mesenchymal cells to the pathogenesis of rheumatoid arthritis. *Semin. Arthritis Rheum.* 21: 267-73.

Snowden JA, Passweg J, Moore JJ, et al. (2004). Autologous hemopoietic stem cell transplantation in severe rheumatoid arthritis: a report from the EBMT and ABMTR. *J. Rheumatol.* 31: 482-8.

Szabolcs P, Moore MA, Young JW. (1995). Expansion of immunostimulatory dendritic cells among the myeloid progeny of human CD34+ bone marrow precursors cultured with c-kit ligand, granulocyte-macrophage colony-stimulating factor, and TNF-alpha. *J. Immunol.* 154: 5851-61.

Tak PP. (2000). Examination of the synovium and synovial fluid, *in* Firestein GS, Panayi GS & Wollheim RA. (eds.), *Rheumatoid arthritis: Frontiers on pathogenesis and treatment*, Oxford University Press, New York, pp.55-68.

Thomas R, Davis LS, Lipsky PE. (1994). Rheumatoid synovium is enriched in mature antigen-presenting dendritic cells. *J. Immunol.* 152: 2613-23.

Vandooren B, Cantaert T, ter Borg M, et al. (2008). Tumor necrosis factor α drives cadherin 11 expression in rheumatoid inflammation. *Arthritis Rheum.* 58: 3051-62.

Zvaifler NJ, Steinman RM, Kaplan G, Lau LL, Rivelis M. (1985). Identification of immunostimulatory dendritic cells in the synovial effusions of patients with rheumatoid arthritis. *J. Clin. Invest.* 76: 789-800.

4

Estrogens Involvement in the Physiopathology of Articular Cartilage

Safa Moslemi, Magali Demoor, Karim Boumediene, Philippe Galera and Laure Maneix
Laboratory of Extracellular Matrix and Pathology, University of Caen/Lower-Normandy, Faculty of Medicine, Caen France

1. Introduction

Life expectancy increases in developed countries and results in a high prevalence of age-related diseases namely in women. Elderly subjects generate a huge demand on the social and health services linked to their disability and dependence. Besides the own effects of aging, the estrogenic deficiency, especially during menopause, is the major cause of degenerative diseases such as osteoporosis, skin aging, Alzheimer's disease and osteoarthritis (OA) (Antonicelli et al., 2008; Candore et al., 2006; Elders, 2000; Felson & Nevitt, 1998; Pietschmann et al., 2008; Stovall & Pinkerton, 2008). OA is a worldwide public health problem which may affect different sites of the skeleton. In the Western world, at least 10% of the population has OA symptoms and 80% of the population will be potentially affected after the age of 70 years. Knee OA represents one of the major causes of morbidity and disability in relation to the worsening of quality of life (Elders, 2000). Pathogenesis of knee OA involves multiple factors including gender, weight, and genetics. Although age-dependent degenerative pathologies, especially OA, involve complex mechanisms in which the imbalance of the cytokines/growth factors plays a crucial role, it is more and more obvious that estrogens participate, with their receptors and modulators, to all of these diseases affecting connective tissues (Calleja-Agius & Brincat, 2009). Estrogens are steroidal hormones irreversibly synthesized from androgens *via* a crucial enzyme of steroidogenesis called aromatase, a member of cytochrome P450 superfamily, encoded by the *CYP19* gene and being expressed in both sexes of many species (Simpson, 2003).

Although non genomic action of estrogens is now recognized but these sexual hormones act often as signaling molecules that exert their effects by binding to estrogen receptors (ER) within the cells.

The estrogen-receptor complex interacts then with DNA to change the expression of estrogen-responsive genes. The two known estrogen receptors, ERα and ERβ, are present in numerous tissues other than those associated with reproduction, including bone, liver, heart, brain and cartilage and being selectively expressed in some targets; for instance ERβ is selectively expressed in lung and intestine. The presence of ERα and ERβ was detected in articular chondrocytes of different species, especially in human, rat, pig, cow and rabbit

(Classen et al., 2001; Dayani et al., 1988; Oshima et al., 2007; Ushiyama et al., 1999). The action of 17β-estradiol (17β-E2) on the cartilage appears to be intimately linked to the sex of individuals since it was shown that the binding capacity of 17β-E2 to its receptor was significantly higher in chondrocytes derived from male rather than female individuals (Nasatzky et al., 1994). In addition, 17β-E2 can stimulate the nuclear expression of its own receptors in chondrocytes and create therefore a loop that reinforces the activation effects of the hormone in this cell type (Richmond et al., 2000). Moreover, a strong correlation was found between the polymorphism of *ESR1* gene encoding ERα and increased risk of OA in several populations (Bergink et al. 2003; Valdes et al., 2006). All these observations tend to prove that the cartilage is an estrogen-sensitive tissue, in which 17β-E2 would be likely to play a preponderant role in regulating chondrocyte homeostasis in joint diseases such as OA.

Even thought hormone replacement therapy (HRT) is the most efficient treatment against, at least, some of the degenerative pathologies mentioned above but studies confirm that risks linked to HRT can exceed the discounted benefits. As a consequence, it becomes important to address the question of the age-associated disorders and to find new targets to treat them. Selective Estrogen Receptor Modulators (SERM) like tamoxifen, raloxifen, fulvestrant and genistein have shown to be useful and attracted the attention of researchers (Cotter & Cashman, 2003; Khalil, 2010; Riggs & Hartmann 2003). A characteristic that distinguishes these substances from pure receptor agonists and antagonists is that their action is different in various tissues, thereby giving the possibility to selectively inhibit or stimulate estrogen-like action in various tissues. For instance tamoxifen (a first generation SERM) and raloxifen have been clinically used as antagonists of ER against breast cancer while they could be potentially agonists in bone and growth plate (Chagin et al, 2007; Nilsson et al, 2003). It has been proposed that these SERM could be used to replace natural estrogens to induce growth plate fusion reducing thereby the final height in girls expected to achieve extreme tall stature. Moreover, phytoestrogens (flavones, isoflavones, lignans) have aroused much interest as natural SERM and potential substitutes in the hormonal treatment of post-menopausal women, but they require much further investigation regarding their mechanism(s) of action and their safety (Dodin et al, 2003).

2. Estrogen synthesis and action

2.1 Estrogen synthesis *via* aromatase

Estrogens are steroidal hormones composed from 18 atoms of carbon and produced essentially in gonads, ovary and testis, but also in non reproductive tissues such as bone and adipose tissue. These lipophilic compounds irreversibly synthesized from androgens *via* a crucial enzyme of steroidogenesis called aromatase, a member of cytochrome P450 superfamily, encoded by the *CYP19* gene and being expressed in both sexes of many species. In pre-menopoausal women, estrogens such as 17β-E2 (the more estrogenic) and estrone are synthesized in ovary during follicular phase whereas estriol being produced essentially by placenta during pregnancy. After menopause, when ovary activity disappears, production of 17β-E2 from testosterone *via* aromatase is assumed by peripheral tissues like liver, adipose tissue, bone, vascular endothelium, chondrocyte and synovial cells (Simpson, 2003; Takeuchi et al., 2007; Tanko et al., 2008). Consequently, circulating 17β-E2 concentrations decrease drastically to 0.04-0.21 nM to reach those found in man (Chambliss & Shaul, 2002). Thus, estrogen action being localized and switch from endocrine to auto-, intra- and/or paracrine actions. Due to their lipophilic feature, estrogen can diffuse into the cell through plasma membrane and induce estrogen-dependent intracellular signaling pathways and/or bind the intracellular receptors especially ER stimulating an estrogen-dependent response in target cells.

2.2 ER structure

In mammals, estrogens produced locally in different tissues, may exert various biological effects but are also responsible of the development of some pathological process such as hormone-dependent cancers. Estrogens exert their physiological and pathological effects through specific receptors considered as nuclear factors by binding target genes at a specific *cis* sequence called Estrogen Responsive Element (ERE).

The first study on estrogen receptor, published by Toft & Groski in 1966, demonstrated that a specific protein of rat uterus was able to bind specifically estrogens. Later, the gene of this protein has been cloned (Walter et al., 1985) and sequenced (Green et al., 1986) from mammal cancer epithelium (MCF-7) of a patient suffering from breast cancer. This protein is now recognized as ERα. A second gene (ERβ) has been also cloned from a cDNA library of the rat prostatic cells (Kuiper et al., 1996), being expressed selectively in some tissues and presenting more affinity for phytoestrogens.

It is now established that the majority of the normal and pathological action of estrogens is generally mediated through these two estrogen receptors ERα and ERβ which are members of nuclear receptor super family including progesterone, glucocorticoids, androgens and vitamin D receptors (Nuclear Receptor Nomenclature Committee, 1999; Germain et al., 2006; Mangelsdorf et al., 1995). In human, ERα is encoded by *ESR1* gene located on chromosome 6 (6q25.1) whereas ERβ is encoded by *ESR2* gene located on chromosome 14 (14q23.2). Both *ESR1* and *ESR2* genes encoding the estrogen receptor may undergo alternative splicing of mRNA. Most of these transcripts differ only in their 5'UTR (Untranslated Region) and will be mainly translated into a long form of ERα, recognized as ERα66 (Flouriot et al., 1998). However, a second form of ERα protein, derived from alternative splicing of exon 1A mRNA or a site of alternative translation initiation (AUG codon 174) was discovered and named ERα46 (Barrailler et al. 1999; Flouriot et al., 2000). After translation, the 46 kDa isoform is truncated of the 173 first amino acids of the long form of 66 kDa. ERα46 protein is thus composed of 422 amino acids, whereas ERα66 has 595 amino acids. Both ER isoforms are capable of inducing a physiological response after ligand binding. The 46 kDa isoform can heterodimerize with ERα66 and competitively inhibit the functions of ligand-independent *trans* activation of the long form of the receptor (Flouriot et al., 2000).

ERα and ERβ (530 amino acids) are structurally organized in six distinct functional domains (A to F) (Fig. 1). There are structural and functional similarities more or less strong between ERα and ERβ whose homology percentages vary significantly depending on the area considered. DNA binding domain (DBD) is conserved at about 97%, which means that both receptors can bind the same *cis* nucleotide sequences and thus activate transcription of identical target genes. However, there is only 55% homology at the level of ligand binding domain (LBD), indicating that ERα and ERβ have different ligand binding specificity. Finally, ERβ has only a truncated form of ligand-independent *trans* activation domain (AF-1), thus limiting its *trans* activation ability (Hall & McDonnell, 1999; Pearce & Jordan, 2004).

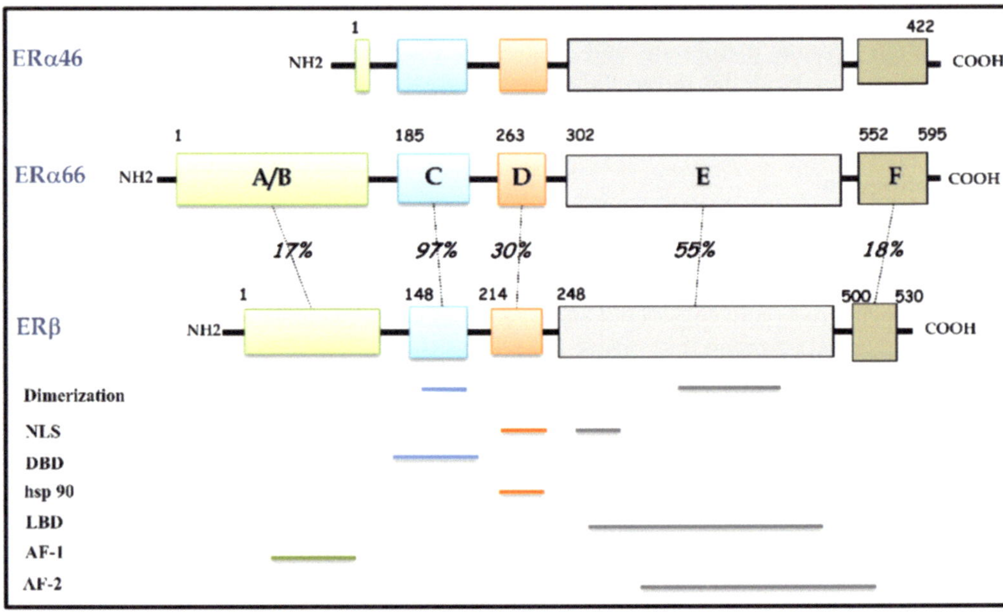

Fig. 1. Structures and functional domains of estrogen receptors (ER)

Structures, functional domains and sequence homology percentage (*italic*) of α and β isoforms. AF-1, ligand-independent *trans* activation domain; AF-2, ligand-dependent *trans* activation domain; DBD, DNA Binding Domain; hsp90, heat-shock protein 90; LBD, Ligand Binding Domain; NLS, Nuclear Localization Signal. These 3 isoforms, ERα46, ERα66 and ERβ are expressed in articular chondrocytes.

2.3 Genomic and non genomic action of estrogen

It is well established that estrogens act at target genes level to modulate their transcription *via* ER binding, so playing a transcriptional factor role recognized as ligand-dependent mechanism (Jensen & DeSombre, 1973). However, estrogen action becomes more complicated following the discovery of ERβ, or different ERα and ERβ isoforms but also with the identification of new plasma-associated membrane receptors. ERα and ERβ regulate thus estrogen-dependent genes expression through two distinct mechanisms: ERE-dependent genomic pathway and ERE-independent genomic pathway.

2.3.1 ERE-dependent genomic pathway

In this mechanism ERα and ERβ, following ligand fixation (estrogen, phytoestrogen, SERM), are subjected to homo- or hetero-dimerization, then ligand/ER complex move to the nucleus to bind directly ERE *cis* element (AGGTCAxxxTGACCT) (Hall et al., 2001) present in the promoter of target genes (Fig. 2). The determination of consensus sequences ERE and the fixation of ER will help to recruit transcriptional factors such as FOXA1 (Forkhead Box A1) or GATA4 (GATA binding protein 4), which will first ensure the chromatin remodeling necessary for ER binding. Ligand binding also allows the recruitment of transcription cofactors such as SRC-1 (Steroid Receptor Coactivator-1), GRIP-1 (Glucocorticoid Receptor Interacting Protein-1), CBP (CREB Binding Protein)/p300, or TRAP220 (Thyroid Hormone Receptor Activating Protein 220) (McKenna et al., 1999). The classic genomic pathway requires the activity of the two *trans* activation domains AF-1 and AF-2 that will allow the sequential and cyclic recruitment of different co-factors of transcription (Metivier et al., 2001).

2.3.2 ERE-independent genomic pathway

In this pathway, ERs will follow the classical mechanism described above except that they interact at the nuclear level with various transcriptional activator or repressor factors to regulate transcription of many estrogen-dependent genes that lack an ERE (Kushner et al., 2000; Paech et al., 1997; Sabbah et al., 1999; Safe, 2001).

Indeed, most estrogen-dependent genes have not necessarily in their regulatory regions a consensus ERE sequence. Therefore, estrogen will be involved in signaling pathways called ERE-independent which imply an interaction of ER with promoter of target gene through other transcription factors. In this case, the region of the receptor DBD does not bind to DNA, but participates in protein-protein interactions or recruitment of co-regulatory proteins to regulate expression of many genes. This mechanism of action is frequently used by nuclear receptors, which significantly complicates the decrypting of the effects induced by the ER (Gottlicher et al., 1998). Many of ER/protein interactions, which occur in cells to regulate transcription of many target genes, are composed for example of ER/AP-1 complex (c-Fos/c-Jun) (Ascenzi et al., 2006; Duan et al., 2008; Kushner et al. 2000; Matthews et al. 2006 ; Paech et al., 1997, Uht et al 1997; Webb et al., 1999,), ER/Sp complex (Ascenzi et al., 2006; He et al., 2005; Kim et al., 2003; Saville et al., 2000; Stoner et al., 2004), and ER/NF-κB complex (Galien & Garcia, 1997; Stein & Yang, 1995). This latter is the only known mechanism of transcriptional repression induced by ER (Fig. 2).

For instance, after being activated by 17β-E2 binding, ER interact with the transcription factor NF-κB to control the transcriptional repression of certain genes such as IL-6 gene, which is involved in cartilage catabolism. Furthermore, in articular chondrocytes, it has been shown that 17β-E2 can counteract the effects of IL-1β by inhibiting nuclear translocation of the p65 subunit of NF-κB and therefore, binding of p65 to inducible nitric oxide synthase (iNOS) gene promoter (Richette et al., 2007). In addition, it has been suggested that ER and NF-κB compete for binding to the same transcriptional co-activators (p300/CBP and PCAF), and that in the case of activation of transcription by 17β-E2 through ER, the pool of these co-activators is mobilized predominantly by ER at the expense of NF-κB (Ansari & Gandy, 2007).

Therefore, estrogen/ER complex allows developing multiple physiological responses following hormonal stimulation by different signaling pathways and inter-connections with different *trans* factors and *cis* elements at the DNA level of target cells.

2.3.3 Non genomic signaling pathway

The non-genomic effects are defined as any action that does not involve transcriptional activity resulting from direct or indirect interaction of a nuclear receptor with the regulatory sequences of hormone-regulated genes. These effects are very rapid (in the order of several seconds to several minutes), incompatible with gene activation or protein synthesis. The effects of non-genomic estrogen receptors are often linked to signaling pathways that involve G protein-coupled receptors, ion channels or receptors linked to enzymes. 17β-E2 could modulate intracellular calcium or cAMP production and activate MAPK/ERK, PLC, PKA, or that of PI3K signaling pathways (Marino et al., 2002) (Fig 2). All these effects are not modified by inhibitors of transcription (actinomycin D) or translation (cycloheximide) (Losel & Wehling, 2003), confirming that they do not depend on a genomic action. In 1998, Beyer and Raab, by coupling 17β-E2 to BSA (Bovine Serum Albumin), thereby preventing it from crossing the plasma membrane, observed that 17β-E2 modulates intracellular calcium. Thus,

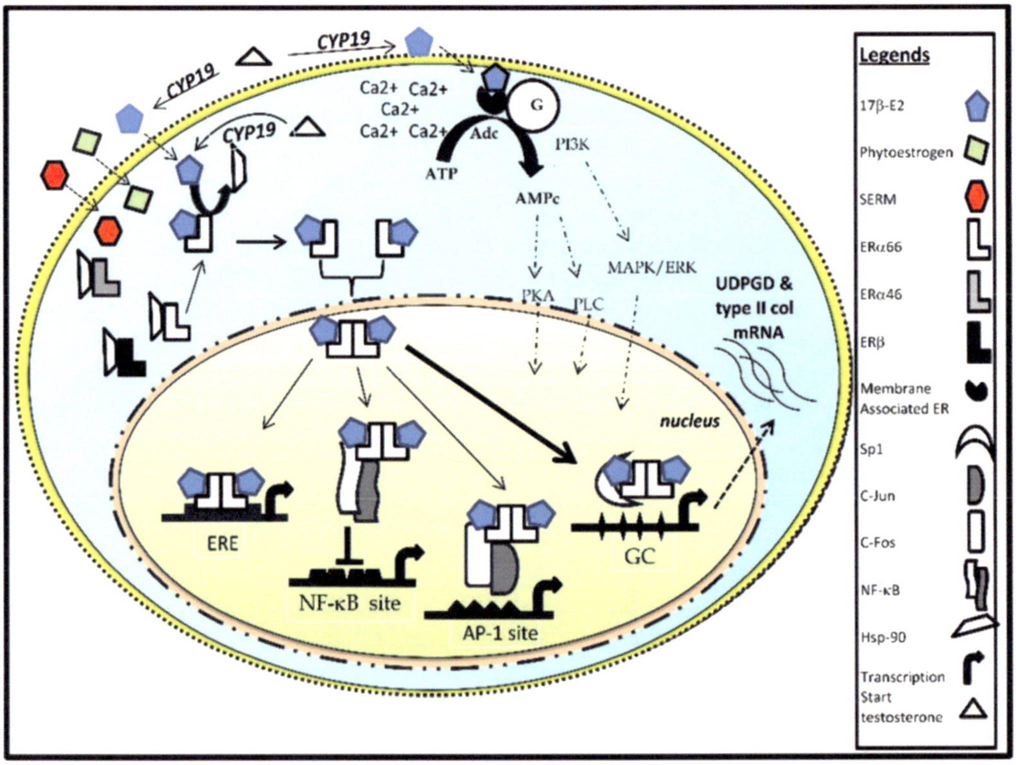

Fig. 2. Different pathways involved in estrogen receptors (ER) signaling.

These different pathways occur in estrogen sensitive cells including ERE-dependent genomic, ERE-independent genomic (*via* Sp1, AP-1 and NF-κB) and membrane associated ER/G protein mechanisms. NF-κB pathway is the only inhibitory mechanism. In articular chondrocytes ERα66 homodimer complex binds predominantly Sp1 proteins to activate GC-box mediated *trans* activation of target genes such as Uridine diphospho-glucose deshydrogenase (UDPGD) and type II collagen (type II Col). Other mechanisms mediated by ERα46 , ERβ, ERα and ERβ homo- and/or heterodimer and finally membrane associated ER / protein G need to be elucidated in articular chondrocytes. Note that 17β-E2 production from androgens like testosterone takes place *via* aromatase (*CYP19*) locally (intracrine effect) or in other cells (paracrine or endocrine effects). Adc, Adenylate cyclase; AP-1, Activating Protein-1; ERK, Extracellular signal Regulated Kinase; ERE, Estrogen Responsive Element; G, G protein; Hsp-90; Heat-shock protein 90; MAPK, Mitogen-Activated Protein Kinase; NF-κB, Nuclear Factor-κB; PI3K, Phosphatidyl Inositol 3-Kinase; PKA, Protein Kinase A; PLC, Phospholipase C; SERM, Selective Estrogen Receptor Modulator; Sp1, Specific Protein 1.

they confirm that this action is induced by a membrane ER. The existence of membrane estrogen receptor was discovered in the late 1970s in endometrial cells (Pietras & Szego, 1977). Various studies tempted to show that these membrane receptors are structurally similar to the classical cytoplasmic ER and that the α and β forms are represented (Chambliss & Shaul, 2002; Pappas et al., 1995; Razandi et al., 1999). More recently, a novel isoform of ERα was highlighted: ERα36. This 36 kDa protein lacks the *trans* activation domains AF-1 and AF-2 and has a DBD and a partial LBD, suggesting a membrane localization for this isoform (Wang et al., 2006). Also, estrogen binding sites localized at the membrane and the cytoplasm were detected in MCF-7 (Harrington et al., 2006). Since ER does not have a transmembrane domain, it appears that palmitoylation of the classical form of the receptor is necessary for its membrane addressing (Acconcia et al., 2005; Ellmann et al., 2009). In addition, it has been demonstrated that ERα could be anchored to the plasma membrane through interactions with many membrane proteins such as caveolin 1 and 2, striatine or with adapter proteins like Shc and p130 Cas (Crk -associated substrate) (Cheskis et al., 2007).

2.3.4 Ligand-independent signaling pathway

In absence of 17β-E2, ER can be activated by phosphorylation *via* protein kinases A or C by extracellular signals like growth factors or cytokines, neurotransmitters, or by cell cycle regulators (Le Goff et al., 1994). Epidermal growth factor (EGF) mimics the effects of 17β-E2 in the mouse uterus. Similarly, insulin, insulin-like growth factor-I (IGF-I), dopamine or transforming growth factor-α (TGF-α) may activate ER. The main targets of these growth factors are the many serine residues present in the AF-1 domain of ER particularly Ser118 and Ser167 (Nilsson et al., 2001).

In summary, estrogens are involved in many signaling pathways, allowing fine control of cell and tissue functions.

3. Estrogen involvement in osteoarthritis

3.1 Epidemiological observations and clinical data

OA is a worldwide public health problem which may affect different sites of the skeleton. In the Western world, at least 10% of the population present OA symptoms and 80% of the population will be potentially affected after the age of 70 years. Knee OA represents one of the major causes of morbidity and disability in relation to the worsening of quality of life. Pathogenesis of knee OA involves multiple factors including gender, weight, and genetics. Association between OA and estrogen deficiency during menopause has been firstly evoked by Cecil & Archer in 1925 following clinical observation.

The hypothesis that estrogen deficiency may promote the development of OA has then been relied on the results of observational epidemiological studies. It is known that the frequency of knee OA is higher in women than in men; it is worsened after menopause and is lower in women receiving hormone replacement therapy (HRT) (Oliveria et al., 1995; Wilson et al., 1990). Although contradictions exist, some studies have shown that hysterectomy may also be associated with OA suggesting the potential role of estrogens to prevent these age-related diseases (Inoue et al., 1995; Spector et al., 1988; Spector et al., 1991). In addition, women with metastatic breast cancer when treated with aromatase inhibitors develop joint pains and cessation of aromatase inhibitors therapy resolved this joint pain (Burstein & Winer, 2007; Crew et al., 2007); aromatase inhibitors are widely used as adjuvant therapy in postmenopausal women with ER positive breast cancer (for review see Moslemi & Seralini, 2005). Moreover, an association of estrogen receptor (ERα and ERβ) polymorphisms has been found in patients with OA compared to unaffected subjects. All these data suggest a protective role of estrogen and HRT on OA through functional isoforms of ER. Such a protective effect of estrogen on the development of OA may suggest two potential mechanisms: a direct effect on cartilage and an indirect effect through modifications of sub-chondral bone remodelling. Nevertheless, some clinical studies based on symptomatic parameters failed to report any effect of HRT on cartilage metabolism, that's why further studies are required to clearly demonstrate beneficial effects of estrogens on molecular regulations of articular cartilage homeostasis.

3.2 Biological *in vivo* and *in vitro* studies

In vivo animal studies indicate that estrogens may have a protective effect against OA, reversing or reducing the cartilage degradation in ovariectomized mice, rats, sheeps and monkeys (Cuzzocrea et al., 2003; Ham et al., 2002; Høegh-Andersen et al., 2004; Oestergaard et al., 2006). However, the way by which estrogens act to prevent the pathogenesis of OA in these models remains unclear. It is supposed that estrogens prevent cartilage degradation by increasing production of growth factors such as insulin growth factor-I (IGF-I) and suppressing pro-inflammatory cytokines expression such as interleukin-6 (IL-6). A few data exist about the role of estrogen in regulating the synthesis of matrix compounds. *In vivo*, 17β-E2 prevents the degradation of collagen type II in the women treated with HRT (Mouritzen et al., 2003) but *in vitro*, it does not seem capable of modulating neosynthesis nor secretion of type II collagen in articular chondrocytes in primary culture (Ab-Rahim et al., 2008; Claassen et al., 2006). The measurement of serum C-terminal telopeptide of type II collagen (CTX-II) in bovine articular cartilage explants has determined that 17β-E2 significantly protected the cartilage degradation induced by tumor necrosis factor-α (TNF-α) and oncostatin M (Oestergaard et al., 2006). In similar *ex vivo* experiments, 17β-E2 can increase glycosaminoglycan (GAG) content of articular explants (Englert et al., 2006). Finally, the double invalidation of ERα and ERβ gene receptors (double knock-out ERα -/-, ERβ -/-) in mice aged of 6 months increases the number and size of osteophytes as well as a thinning of the sub-chondral plate, without changing the cartilage degradation (Sniekers et al., 2009). We demonstrated recently that 17β-E2 (the most potent among all estrogens) at physiologic doses, and ERα66 (wild type receptor) but not ERα46 (AF-1 deleted receptor) could up-regulate at both mRNA and protein levels UDP-glucose dehydrogenase (UDPGD) in primary cultured articular chondrocytes *via* specific protein 1 (Sp1) binding sites (Maneix et al., 2008). This enzyme is responsible of UDP-glucuronate synthesis which is the main component of GAG chains polymerization in cartilage: it plays an essential role in the elongation of GAG chains and their attachment to the axial protein of proteoglycans (PGs). Its decarboxylation provides UDP xylose, which serves to anchor chains of chondroitin sulfate (CS), dermatan sulfate (DS) and heparan sulphate (HS). Moreover, we also established that 17β-E2 increases the gene expression of type II collagen (*COL2A1*), the main collagen of hyaline cartilage, *via trans* activation domains AF-1 of ERα66 in coordination with the transcription factors Sp1, Sp3, p300 and Soxs (Maneix et al, 2010). It would thus be a genomic mechanism ERE-independent. Finally, our preliminary results also showed that phytoestrogens such as apigenin and genistein could up-regulate the expression of UDPGD (unpublished data).

Overall, these data indicate that estrogen/phytoestrogens and their receptors can be considered as potent regulators of chondrocyte homeostasis and are pro-anabolic for extracellular matrix synthesis. This may have potential applications in the tissue engineering of articular cartilage and offer new perspectives to prevent and/or to treat OA.

4. Mechanisms of estrogen action in OA

4.1 Effects on growth factors and cytokines

17β-E2 can firstly interact with pathways affecting the synthesis and secretion of the key growth factors involved in the regulation of cartilage metabolism. So, TGF-β expression in the iliac crest chondrocytes is influenced by 17β-E2 in a biphasic manner: low concentrations of

17β-E2 increase TGF-β expression whereas supra-physiologic doses decrease strongly its expression (Saggese et al., 1993). The concept of dose-dependence is confirmed by the majority of the studies on 17β-E2 in the articular cartilage where physiological doses of the hormone show to be protective when considering the structural integrity of tissue while supra-physiologic concentrations are often deleterious (Richette et al., 2003) (Fig. 3). Experiments on chondrocytes from ovariectomized monkeys treated with 17β-E2 showed that this hormone increases concomitantly the expression of the binding protein of IGF-I (IGFBP-2) and synthesis of PG (Richmond et al., 2000). In addition, the synovial fluid of these animals contains IGF-I twice more than untreated animals. Thereafter, it was shown that estrogen deficiency increases the sensitivity of cell response to certain pro-inflammatory cytokines through an increase in the number of receptors or cytokine cofactors amplifying consequently the effects of catabolic cytokines in these cells. Estrogen treatment in ovariectomized animals significantly reduced the production and secretion of pro-inflammatory cytokines in articular chondrocytes. This anti-inflammatory effect of 17β-E2 was highlighted by Le Bail et al. (2001) who showed that the localized production of 17β-E2 by synovial cells has inhibited the IL-6 secretion by articular chondrocytes. In addition, 17β-E2 can also reduce production of pro-inflammatory prostaglandins through a decrease in the mRNA steady-state levels of cyclooxygenase-2 (COX-2) in bovine articular chondrocytes (Morisset et al., 1998).

4.2 Metalloproteinases (MMPs) expression and activity

The majority of the beneficial effects of 17β-E2 in articular chondrocytes is focused on the inhibition of catabolic pathways. Thus, Lee et al. (2003) found that 17β-E2 decreases the secretion of the metalloproteinase MMP-1 in human osteoarthritic articular chondrocytes. In addition, 17β-E2 can antagonize the degradation of PGs and the expression and activity of MMP-1, MMP-3 and MMP-13 enzymes induced by IL-1β in rabbit articular chondrocytes (Richette et al., 2004). Especially, the effects of 17β-E2 on the expression of MMP-13 seem to be transmitted through the indirect binding of ERα66 at an AP-1 site in the promoter of MMP-13 gene (Lu et al., 2006). Like the mode of action of 17β-E2 on the expression levels of TGF-β, the effects of the hormone on the expression of MMPs and their inhibitors TIMPs (tissue inhibitors of MMPs) appear to be dose-dependent. Low doses of 17β-E2 decreased MMP-1/TIMP-1 and MMP-3/TIMP-1 ratios while higher concentrations have the opposite effect (Song et al., 2003).

4.3 Anti-oxidant effects

The generation of reactive oxygen species (ROS) contributes actively to the cartilage ECM degradation in OA, in particular by inducing a decrease in the synthesis of PGs. However, due to the structure of their phenol nuclei, 17β-E2 and its metabolites have anti-oxidant features (Liehr & Roy, 1998) that protect the cartilage degradation induced by ROS (Claassen et al., 2005). It is now established that 17β-E2 is a modulator of the redox status of chondrocytes.

During the arthritic process, overproduction of nitric oxide (NO) is a consequence of the action of proinflammatory cytokines such as IL-1β or TNF-α that promote the activation of inducible nitric oxide synthase (iNOS) in OA chondrocytes. The iNOS gene is under the control of an estrogen-dependent promoter. Indeed, estrogen deficiency activates transcription of this promoter while a replacement therapy by 17β-E2 inhibits it in ovariectomized mice (Cuzzocrea et al., 2003). 17β-E2 can counteract the deleterious effects induced by IL-1β in rabbit articular chondrocytes by reducing the binding capacity of NF-κB

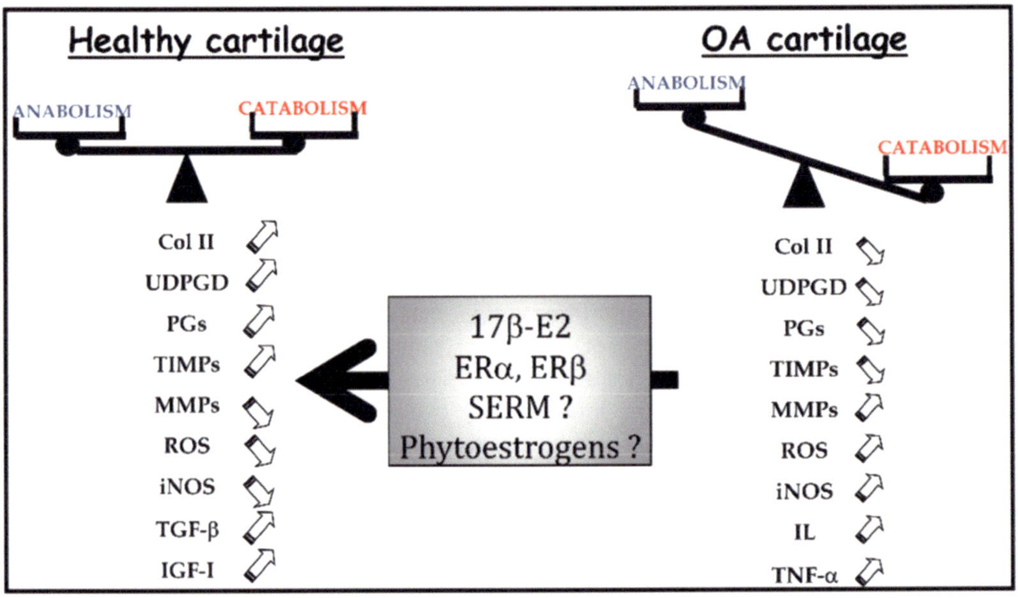

Fig. 3. Role of 17β-E2 and estrogen receptor ERα / ERβ on joint cartilage homeostasis.

Col II, type II collagen; IGF-I, Insulin-like Growth Factor-I; IL, Interleukin; iNOS, Inducible Nitrogen Oxide Synthase; MMPs, Metalloproteinases; PGs, Proteoglycans; ROS, Reactive Oxygen Species; SERM, Selective Estrogen Receptor Modulators; TIMPs, Tissue Inhibitors MMPs; TGF-β, Transforming Growth Factor-β; TNF-α, Tumor Necrosis Factor-α; UDPGD, Uridine Diphospho-Glucose Dehydrogenase. The roles of SERM and phytoestrogens need to be clarified.

in the promoter of iNOS gene resulting in inhibition of nuclear translocation of this factor (Richette et al., 2007). This results in an inhibition of iNOS gene transcription and a subsequent reduction in NO production by chondrocytes.

4.4 Matrix components turn-over

To better understand the physiopathology of articular cartilage in osteoarthritis, Høegh-Andersen et al. (2004) have validated an experimental model of ovariectomized rats with modification in cartilage structure representative of *in vivo* pathological changes observed in early human osteoarthritis. In animals aged from 5 to 7 months, estrogen deficiency increases the erosion of the articular surface and accelerates the renewal of matrix molecules. This animal model also showed that the effectiveness of HRT in the prevention of cartilage loss is increased when estrogen is administered to the animal from its operation and not after a period of 3 weeks (Oestergaard et al. 2006). These works need to be compared with the many epidemiological data which showed that the benefits of HRT are strengthened when patients are treated at the first signs of menopause and continued their treatment over a period exceeding 5 years. The importance of prevention in the treatment of damaged cartilage appears essential.

4.5 Sub-chondral bone regulation

Within the joint, cartilage is not the only target tissue for estrogens. 17β-E2 also controls the renewal of the sub-chondral bone by maintaining a balance between the two players in bone remodeling: osteoblasts that synthesize bone matrix and osteoclasts that are responsible for the resorption (bone loss) of existing bone. Estrogens inhibit osteoclasts activation and are therefore considered as inhibitors of bone resorption. The predominant mechanism that appears to be involved is the inhibition of IL-6 synthesis, the main cytokine involved in the activation of resorption. This inhibition of IL-6 synthesis by estrogens is mediated through the modification of NF-κB binding on IL-6 gene promoter; there is no direct binding of ER to DNA (Ray et al., 1994). Consequently, an increase of bone resorption, generally favoring the occurrence of osteoporosis, is frequently seen in women after menopause which is related to the decrease of circulating estrogen levels during this period (Reginster et al., 2003). In this context, HRT could effectively prevent postmenopausal osteoporosis.

Paradoxically, the frequency of OA and osteoporosis in postmenopausal women are most often inversely correlated, as reflected in the levels of osteocalcin, a marker of bone turnover, which are generally lower among women with OA than women without OA (for review: Dequeker et al., 2003). Patients suffering from OA of the knee are generally less subjected to bone loss. The increase in bone mass is a risk factor for incidence and development of knee and hip osteoarthritis. It was suggested that an increase in bone density in the area of the sub-chondral bone may induce bone stiffness and accelerate cartilage destruction. Thus, high bone density is associated with an increase of OA prevalence of the hip, hand and knee in postmenopausal women. However, high bone density increases risk of knee OA but protects against the progression of the disease once it is established. Therefore, bone loss in people with OA which is already established accelerates the progression of the disease. Indeed, Jacobsen et al. (2007) showed that the reduction of intra-articular space in the hip was correlated with the decrease in mineral density of sub-chondral bone in postmenopausal women. It was suggested that the alteration of bone structure can cause changes in the load distribution within the joint and promote the development of OA (Sniekers et al. 2008). In this case, the favorable effect of estrogen on cartilage may be due in part to the anti-resorption effect of 17β-E2 on bone.

5. Phytoestrogen and Selective Estrogen Receptor Modulators (SERM)

During the second half of the 20th century, HRT has been repeatedly promoted as the only pharmacological approach allowing a global prevention of all disorders related to or potentiated by estrogen deprivation. Recently, the risk/benefit profile of HRT has been severely challenged because of apparent increased risks of invasive breast cancer, coronary heart disease events, stroke and pulmonary embolism among treated women. These new findings imply a careful reassessment of the current evidence justifying the prescription of HRT for the prevention of the management of chronic disorders. The many contradictions recorded concerning benefit/risk effects of HRT are often related to differences in methodology and criteria used in measuring the effects of estrogen therapy in clinical studies. Indeed, analysis based strictly on symptomatic parameters showed that HRT had no effect or even adverse effects on the progression of OA (Von Muhlen et al., 2002). Conversely, more advanced techniques of magnetic resonance imaging showed that recipients of long term HRT (5 years or more) had a volume of articular cartilage largest in the knee than women having never taken any treatments (Wluka et al., 2001). As to the evolution of medical imaging techniques and advances in the diagnosis of OA, it appears that estrogens have a strong potential for preventing disease and preserving the structural integrity of the articulation among postmenopausal women. Thus, recent clinical trials of consortium "Women's Health Initiative" showed that women treated with equine estrogens over a period of 7 years had 17% lower risk to undergo a hip replacement compared to control group (Cirillo et al., 2006). Finally, an *in vivo* study performed on 180 ovariectomized monkeys for 3 years found that HRT reduced the severity of arthritic lesions, through attenuation of the PGs loss and reducing the number of osteophytes in these animals (Ham et al., 2002). Given its chondroprotective potential, it would seem that HRT is capable of modulating chondrocyte metabolism. Studies have also shown that SERM and phytoestrogens may have beneficial effect on cartilage metabolism and to alleviate OA symptoms (Arjmandi et al, 2004; Bassleer et al., 1996; Guiducci et al., 2005; Tsai et al., 1992). It has been shown that when administered at a clinically relevant dose in young male rats, tamoxifen causes persistent retardation of longitudinal and cortical radial bone growth through systemic suppression of IGF-I production and local effects on the growth plate cartilage; it increases in chondrocytes proliferation/apoptosis and decreases the number of hypertophic chondrocytes (Karimian et al., 2008). Similarly, raloxifen could act as estrogen agonist on the growth plate of ovariectomized immature rabbits, accelerating growth plate senescence and thus hastening epiphyseal fusion (Nilsson et al, 2003).

Besides estrogens, natural molecules such as phytoestrogens (estrogen-like compounds in plants) sharing structural and functional homologies with endogenous estrogens, could also act (even thought at micromolar concentrations) as agonists and/or antagonists in hormone-sensitive target cells. Scientists are now interested in the tissue-selective activities of phytoestrogens considering anti-estrogenic effects in reproductive tissue that could help to reduce the risk of hormone-associated cancers (breast, uterine, ovarian, and prostate), while estrogenic effects on bone and cardiovascular system for instance could favor the maintenance of bone density and protect against atherosclerosis respectively. Moreover, it has been suggested that the consumption of dietary phytoestrogens (soja isoflavones, lignans, etc.) may have beneficial effects on bone health at all stages of life. That's why phytoestrogens have aroused much interest as potential substitutes in HRT of postmenopausal women, but they require much further investigation regarding their mechanism of action and their safety. Like estrogens, phytoestrogens may act *via* genomic and non genomic pathways. The most relevant molecular actions of phytoestrogens are those mediated by ERs. They may act on protein tyrosine kinase, MAP kinase, topoisomerase II and at all stages of cell cycle and apoptosis. They can also change the response to growth factors and cytokines. Genistein up to 100 μM reduces the production of lipopolysaccharide (LPS)-stimulated pro-inflammatory molecules (COX-2, NO) but not that of COX-1 responsible of releasing prostaglandins in normal human chondrocytes (Hooshmand et al., 2007). When tested on human chondrocytes and chondrocytic cell line CHON-002, bavachin, a flavonid phytoestrogen isolated from *Psoralea corylifolia*, potentially protected cartilage from inflammation-mediated damage in joints of OA through decreasing IL-1beta-induced activation of IKK-IκB alpha-NF-κB signaling pathway (Cheng et al., 2010). Formononetin, a phytoestrogen isolated from *Astragalus membranaceus* showed to have biphasic positive effects on human normal osteoblasts and OA sub-chondral osteoblasts by modifying their biological synthetic capacities (Huh et al., 2010). Using female bovine articular chondrocytes, it has been demonstrated that the stimulating effect of insulin on GAGs sulfate incorporation was enhanced significantly after preincubation of cells with 10^{-11} -10^{-5} M daidzein or 10^{-9} -10^{-5} M genistein but not by 17β-E2 (Claassen et al., 2008). More recently, xanthohumol, a prenylflavonoid extracted from hop, showed to prevent hyaluronan overproduction as well as PG and collagen loss in bovine chondrocytes;

hyluronan overproduction is considered as an early reaction in OA followed by PG loss and collagen degradation (Stracke et al., 2001). However, additional research is critical to determine how phytoestrogens act on cartilage cells to obtain a more complete understanding of the effects.

6. Conclusion

From epidemiological, clinical, *in vivo* and *in vitro* studies, a huge amount of data consistent with the fact that estrogens and their receptors can now be considered among the main players involved in the chondrocyte homeostasis and participate in cartilage protection from degradation and erosion occurring during menopause. Indeed, once ligand/ER complex is formed, estrogens such as 17β-E2 could act with ER to induce or to inhibit *trans* activation of target genes of chondrocytes, the predominant cells of articular cartilage allowing expression of the specific chondrogenic markers such as UDPGD, PGs, type II collagen or inhibition of catabolic markers such as metalloproteinases and interleukins. There are different pathways by which estrogen and ER may interact with target genes in chondrocytes but it seems that Sp1 mediated *trans* activation being preferentially used in this cell type. In this mechanism ER needs AF-1 sequence (ligand-independent *trans* activation domain) to exert its action on GC boxes *via* Sp1 in target genes. In addition, some molecules sharing structural and functional features with estrogens like SERM and phytoestrogens can mimic estrogenic action and are therefore useful to repair cartilage erosion or might contribute at least to protect premenopausal joint cartilage and to maintain its homeostasis in a prevention strategy but these molecules need further investigation and deserves more attention from the scientific community to prove their safety and efficacy.

7. Key points

Osteoarthritis, cartilage, chondrocytes, estrogens, phytoestrogens, selective estrogen receptor modulators, hormone replacement therapy, menopause.

8. References

Ab-Rahim, S., Selvaratnam, L. & Kamarul, T. (2008). The effect of TGF-beta1 and beta-estradiol on glycosaminoglycan and type II collagen distribution in articular chondrocyte cultures. *Cell Biol. Int.,* Vol. 32, No. 7, (Jul 2008), pp. (841-847)

Acconcia, F., Ascenzi, P., Bocedi, A., Spisni, E., Tomasi, V., Trentalance, A., Visca, P. & Marino, M. (2005). Palmitoylation-dependent estrogen receptor alpha membrane localization: regulation by 17beta-estradiol. *Mol. Biol. Cell,* Vol. 16, No. 1, (Jan 2005), pp. (231-237)

Ansari, R.A. & Gandy, J. (2007). Determining the *trans*repression activity of xenoestrogen on nuclear factor-kappa B in Cos-1 cells by estrogen receptor-alpha. *Int. J. Toxicol.,* Vol. 26, No. 5, (Sep-Oct 2007), pp. (441-449)

Antonicelli R, Olivieri F, Morichi V, Urbani E, Mais V. (2008). Prevention of cardiovascular events in early menopause: a possible role for hormone replacement therapy. *Int J Cardiol.,* Vol. 130, No. 2, (Nov 2008), pp. (140-146), Review

Arjmandi, B.H., Khalil, D.A., Lucas, E.A., Smith, B.J., Sinichi, N., Hodges, S.B., Juma, S., Munson, M.E., Payton, M.E., Tivis, R.D. & Svanborg, A. (2004). Soy protein may alleviate osteoarthritis sympthoms. *Phytomedicine,* Vol. 11, No. 7-8, (Nov 2004), pp. (567-575)

Ascenzi, P., Bocedi, A. & Marino, M. (2006). Structure-function relationship of estrogen receptor alpha and beta: impact on human health. *Mol. Aspects Med.,* Vol. 27, No. 4, (Aug 2006), pp. (299-402), Review

Barrailler, P., Chinestra, P., Bayard, F. & Faye, J.C. (1999). Alternative initiation of translation accounts for a 67/45 kDa dimorphism of the human estrogen receptor ERalpha. *Biochem. Biophys. Res. Commun.,* Vol. 257, No. 1, (Apr 1999), pp. (84-88)

Bassleer, C.T., Franchimont, P.P., Henrotin, Y.E., Franshimount, N.M., Geenen, V.G. & Reginster, J.Y. (1996). Effects of ipriflavone and its matabolites on human articular chondrocytes cultivated in clusters. *Osteoarthritis Cartilage,* Vol. 4, No. 1, (Mar 1996), pp. (1-8)

Bergink, A.P., Van Meurs, J.B., Loughlin, J., Arp, P.P., Fang, Y., Hofman, A., Van Leeuwen, J.P., Van Duijn, C.M., Uitterlinden, A.G. & Pols, H.A. (2003). Estrogen receptor alpha gene haplotype is associated with radiographic osteoarthritis of the knee in elderly men and women. *Arthritis Rheum.,* Vol.48, No. 7, (Jul 2003), pp. (1913-1922)

Beyer, C. & Raab, H. (1998). Nongenomic effects of oestrogen: embryonic mouse midbrain neurones respond with a rapid release of calcium from intracellular stores. *Eur. J. Neurosci.,* Vol. 10, No. 1 (Jan 1998), pp. (255-262)

Calleja-Agius, J. & Brincat, M.P. (2009). Effects of hormone replacement therapy on connective tissue: why is this important? *Best Practice & Research Clinical Obstetrics and Gynaecology,* Vol. 23, No. 1, (Feb 2009), pp. (121–27)

Candore, G., Balistreri, CR., Grimaldi, M.P., Vasto, S., Listì, F., Chiappelli, M., Licastro, F., Lio, D. & Caruso, C. (2006). Age-related inflammatory diseases: role of genetics and gender in the pathophysiology of Alzheimer's disease. *Ann N Y Acad Sci,* Vol. 1089, (Nov 2006), pp. (472-486), Review

Cecil, R.L. & Archer, B.H. (1925). Arthritis of the menopause, *JAMA,* Vol. 84 pp. (75–79)

Chagin, A.S., Karimian, E., Zaman, F., Takigawa, M., Chrysis, D., Sävendahl, L. (2007). Tamoxifen induces permanent growth arrest through selective induction of apoptosis in growth plate chondrocytes in cultured rat metatarsal bone. *Bone,* Vol. 40, No. 5, (May 2007), pp. (1415-1424)

Cheng, C.C., Chen, Y.H., Chang, W.L., Yang, S.P., Chang, D.M., Lai, J.H. & Ho, L.J. (2010). Phytoestrogen bavachin mediates anti-inflammation targeting Ikappa B kinase-I kappaB alpha-NF-kappaB signaling pathway in chondrocytes in vitro. *Eur J Pharmacol.* Vol. 636, No. 1-3, (Jun 2010), pp. (181-188)

Chambliss, K.L. & Shaul, P.W. (2002). Estrogen modulation of endothelial nitric oxide synthase. *Endocr. Rev.,* Vol.23, No. 5, (Oct 2002), pp. (665-686), Review

Cheskis, B.J., Greger, J.G., Nagpal, S. & Freedman, L.P. (2007). Signaling by estrogens. *J. Cell Physiol.,* Vol. 213, No. 3, (Dec 2007), pp. (610-617), Review

Cirillo, D.J., Wallace; R.B., Wu; L. & Yood; R.A. (2006). Effect of hormone therapy on risk of hip and knee joint replacement in the Women's Health Initiative. *Arthritis Rheum.,* Vol. 54, No. 10, (Oct 2006), pp. (3194-3204)

Claassen, H., Briese, V., Manapov, F., Nebe, B., Schünke, M. & Kurz, B. (2008). The phytoestrogens daidzein and genistein enhance the insulin-stimulated sulfate uptake in articular chondrocytes. *Cell Tissue Res.*, Vol. 333, No. 1, (Jul 2008), pp. (71-79)

Claassen, H., Schunke, M. & Kurz, B. (2005). Estradiol protects cultured articular chondrocytes from oxygen-radical-induced damage. *Cell Tissue Res.*, Vol. 319, No. 3, (Mar 2005), pp. (439-445)

Claassen, H., Schluter, M., Schunke, M. & Kurz, B. (2006). Influence of 17beta-estradiol and insulin on type II collagen and protein synthesis of articular chondrocytes. *Bone*, Vol. 39, No. 2, (Aug 2006), pp. (310-317)

Cotter, A. & Cashman, K.D. (2003). Genistein appears to prevent postmenopausal bone loss as effectively as hormone replacement therapy. *Nutr Rev.*, Vol. 61, No. 10, (Oct 2003), pp. (346-351)

Cuzzocrea, S., Mazzon, E., Dugo, L., Genovese, T., Di Paola, R., Ruggeri, Z., Vegeto, E., Caputi, A.P., Van De Loo, F.A., Puzzolo, D. & Maggi, A. (2003). Inducible nitric oxide synthase mediates bone loss in ovariectomized mice. *Endocrinology*, Vol. 144, No. 3, (Mar 2003), pp. (1098-1107)

Dequeker, J., Aerssens, J. & Luyten, F.P. (2003). Osteoarthritis and osteoporosis: clinical and research evidence of inverse relationship. *Aging Clin. Exp. Res.*, Vol. 15, No. 5, (Oct 2003), pp. (426-439), Review

Dodin, S., Blanchet, C. & Marc, I. (2003). Phytoestrogens in menopausal women: a review of recent findings. *Med Sci (Paris)*, Vol. 19, No. 10, (Oct 2003), pp. (1030-1037), Review (French)

Duan, R., Ginsburg, E. & Vonderhaar, B.K. (2008). Estrogen stimulates transcription from the human prolactin distal promoter through AP1 and estrogen responsive elements in T47D human breast cancer cells. *Mol. Cell Endocrinol.*, Vol. 281, No. 1-2, (Jan 2008), pp. (9-18)

Elders, M.J. (2000). The increasing impact of arthritis on public health. *J Rheumatol Suppl*, Vol. 6, (Oct 2000), pp. (6-8)

Ellmann, S., Sticht, H., Thiel, F., Beckmann, M.W., Strick, R. & Strissel, P.L. (2009). Estrogen and progesterone receptors: from molecular structures to clinical targets. *Cell Mol. Life Sci.*, Vol. 66, No. 15, (Aug 2009), pp. (2405-2426)

Englert, C., Blunk, T., Fierlbeck, J., Kaiser, J., Stosiek W., Angele, P., Hammer, J. & Straub, R.H. (2006). Steroid hormones strongly support bovine articular cartilage integration in the absence of interleukin-1beta. *Arthritis Rheum.*, Vol. 54, No. 12, (Dec 2006), pp. (3890-3897)

Felson, D.T. & Nevitt, M.C. (1998). The effect of estrogen on osteoarthritis. *Curr Opin Rheumatol*, Vol. 10, No. 3, (May 1998), pp. (269-272)

Flouriot, G., Brand, H., Denger, S., Métivier, R., Kos, M., Reid, G., Sonntag-Buck, V. & Gannon, F. (2000). Identification of a new isoform of the human estrogen receptor-alpha (hER-alpha) that is encoded by distinct transcripts and that is able to repress hER-alpha activation function 1. *EMBO J.*, Vol. 19, No. 17, (Sep 2000), pp. (4688-4700)

Flouriot, G., Griffin, C., Kenealy, M., Sonntag-Buck, V. & Gannon, F. (1998). Differentially expressed messenger RNA isoforms of the human estrogen receptor-alpha gene are generated by alternative splicing and promoter usage. *Mol. Endocrinol.*, Vol. 12, No. 12, (Dec 1998), pp. (1939-1954)

Galien, R. & Garcia, T. (1997). Estrogen receptor impairs interleukin-6 expression by preventing protein binding on the NF-kappaB site. *Nucleic Acids Res,* Vol. 25, No. 12, (Jun 1997), pp. (2424-2429)

Germain, P., Staels, B., Dacquet, C., Spedding, M. & Laudet, V. (2006). Overview of nomenclature of nuclear receptors. *Pharmacol. Rev.,* Vol. 58, No. 4, (Dec 2006), pp. (685-704)

Gottlicher, M., Heck, S. & Herrlich, P. (1998). Transcriptional cross-talk, the second mode of steroid hormone receptor action. *J. Mol. Med.,* Vol. 76, No. 7, (Jun 1998), pp. (480-489)

Green, S., Walter, P., Kumar, V., Krust, A., Bornert, J.M., Argos, P. & Chambon, P. (1986). Human oestrogen receptor cDNA: sequence, expression and homology to v-erb-A. *Nature,* Vol. 320, No. 6058, (Mar 1986), pp. (134-139)

Guiducci, S., Del Rosso, A., Cinelli, M., Margheri, F., D'Alessio, S., Fibbi, G., Matucci Cerinic, M., Del Rosso, M. (2005). Rheumatoid synovial fibroblasts constitutively express the fibronolytic pattern of invasive tumor-like cells. *Clin Exp Rheumatol.,* Vol. 23, No. 3, (May 2005), pp. (364-372)

Hall, J.M., Couse, J.F. & Korach, K.S. (2001). The multifaceted mechanisms of estradiol and estrogen receptor signaling. *J. Biol. Chem.,* Vol. 276, No. 40, (Oct 2001), pp. (36869-36872)

Hall, J.M. & McDonnell, D.P. (1999). The estrogen receptor beta-isoform (ERbeta) of the human estrogen receptor modulates ERalpha transcriptional activity and is a key regulator of the cellular response to estrogens and antiestrogens. *Endocrinology,* Vol. 140, No. 12, (Dec 1999), pp. (5566-5578)

Ham, K.D., Loeser, R.F., Lindgren, B.R. & Carlson, C.S. (2002). Effects of long-term estrogen replacement therapy on osteoarthritis severity in cynomolgus monkeys. *Arthritis Rheum.,* Vol. 46, No. 7, (Jul 2002), pp. (1956-1964)

Harrington, W.R., Kim, S.H., Funk, C.C., Madak-Erdogan, Z., Schiff, R., Katzenellenbogen, J.A. & Katzenellenbogen, B.S. (2006). Estrogen dendrimer conjugates that preferentially activate extranuclear, nongenomic versus genomic pathways of estrogen action. *Mol. Endocrinol.,* Vol. 20, No. 3, (Mar 2006), pp. (491-502)

He, S., Sun, J.M., Li, L. & Davie, J.R. (2005). Differential intranuclear organization of transcription factors Sp1 and Sp3. *Mol. Biol. Cell,* Vol. 16, No. 9, (Sep 2005), pp. (4073-4083)

Høegh-Andersen, P., Tanko, L.B., Andersen, T.L., Lundberg, C.V., Mo, J.A., Heegaard, A.M., Delaisse, J.M. & Christgau, S. (2004). Ovariectomized rats as a model of postmenopausal osteoarthritis: validation and application. *Arthritis Res. Ther.,* Vol. 6, No. 2, (Feb 2004), pp. (R169-R180)

Hooshmand, S., Soung do, Y., Lucas, E.A., Madihally, SV., Levenson, C.W. & Arjmandi, B.H. (2007). Genistein reduces the production of proinflammatory molecules in human chondrocyes. *J Nut Biochem.,* Vol. 18, No. 9, (Sep 2007), pp. (609-614)

Huh, J.E., Seo, D.M., Baek, Y.H., Choi, D.Y., Park, D.S. & Lee, J.D. (2010). Biphasic positive effect of formononetin on metabolic activity of human normal and osteoarthritic subchondral osteoblasts. *Int Immunopharmacol.,* Vol. 10, No. 4, (Apr 2010), pp. (500-507)

Inoue, K., Ushiyama, T., Kim, Y., Shichikawa, K., Nishioka, J., Hukuda, S. (1995). Increased rate of hysterectomy in women undergoing surgery for osteoarthritis of the knee. *Osteoarthritis Cartilage,* Vol. 3, No. 3, (Sep 1995), pp. (205–209)

Jacobsen, S., Jensen, T.W., Bach-Mortensen, P., Hyldstrup, L. & Sonne-Holm, S. (2007). Low bone mineral density is associated with reduced hip joint space width in women: results from the Copenhagen Osteoarthritis Study. *Menopause,* Vol. 14, No. 6, (Nov-Dec 2007), pp. (1025-1030)

Jensen, E.V. & DeSombre, E.R. (1973). Estrogen-receptor interaction. *Science,* Vol. 182, No. 108, (Oct 1973), pp. (126-134), Review

Karimian, E, Chagin, AS., Gjerde, J., Heino, T., Lien, EA., Ohlsson, C. & Sävendahl, L. (2008). Tamoxifen impairs both longitudinal and cortical bone growth on young male rats. *J bone Miner Res.,* Vol. 23, No. 8, (Aug 2008), pp. (1267-1277)

Khalil, R.A. (2010). Potential approaches to enhance the effects of estrogen on senescent blood vessels and postmenopausal cardiovascular disease. *Cardiovasc Hematol Agents Med Chem.,* Vol. 8, No. 1, (Jan 2010), pp. (29-46)

Kim, K., Thu, N., Saville, B. & Safe, S. (2003). Domains of estrogen receptor alpha (ERalpha) required for ERalpha/Sp1-mediated activation of GC-rich promoters by estrogens and antiestrogens in breast cancer cells. *Mol. Endocrinol.,* Vol. 17, No. 5, (May 2003), pp. (804-817)

Kuiper, G.G., Enmark, E., Pelto-Huikko, M., Nilsson, S. & Gustafsson, J.A. (1996). Cloning of a novel receptor expressed in rat prostate and ovary. *Proc. Natl. Acad. Sci. U. S. A.,* Vol. 93, No. 12, (Jun 1996), pp. (5925-5930)

Kushner, P.J., Agard, D.A., Greene, G.L., Scanlan, T.S., Shiau, A.K., Uht, R.M. & Webb, P. (2000). Estrogen receptor pathways to AP-1. *J. Steroid Biochem. Mol. Biol.,* Vol. 74, No. 5, (Nov 2000), pp. (311-317)

Le Bail, J., Liagre, B., Vergne, P., Bertin, P., Beneytout, J. & Habrioux, G. (2001). Aromatase in synovial cells from postmenopausal women. *Steroids,* Vol. 66, No. 10, (Oct 2001), pp. (749-757)

Lee, Y.J., Lee, E.B., Kwon, Y.E., Lee, J.J., Cho, W.S., Kim, H.A. & Song, Y.W. (2003). Effect of estrogen on the expression of matrix metalloproteinase (MMP)-1, MMP-3, and MMP-13 and tissue inhibitor of metalloproteinase-1 in osteoarthritis chondrocytes. *Rheumatol. Int.,* Vol. 23, No. 6, (Nov 2003), pp. (282-288)

Le Goff, P., Montano, M.M., Schodin, D.J. & Katzenellenbogen, B.S. (1994). Phosphorylation of the human estrogen receptor. Identification of hormone-regulated sites and examination of their influence on transcriptional activity. *J. Biol. Chem.,* Vol. 269, No. 6, (Feb 1994), pp. (4458-4466)

Liehr, J.G. & Roy, D. (1998). Pro-oxidant and antioxidant effects of estrogens. *Methods Mol. Biol.,* Vol. 108, pp. (425-435)

Losel, R. & Wehling, M. (2003). Nongenomic actions of steroid hormones. *Nat. Rev. Mol. Cell Biol.,* Vol. 4, No. 1, (Jan 2003), pp. (46-56), Review

Lu, T., Achari, Y., Sciore, P. & Hart, D.A. (2006). Estrogen receptor alpha regulates matrix metalloproteinase-13 promoter activity primarily through the AP-1 transcriptional regulatory site. *Biochim. Biophys. Acta,* Vol. 1762, No. 8, (Aug 2006), pp. (719-731)

Maneix, L., Beauchef, G., Servent, A., Wegrowski, Y., Maquart, F.X., Boujrad, N., Flouriot, G., Pujol, J.P., Boumediene, K., Galéra, P. & Moslemi, S. (2008) 17β-Estradiol up-regulates the expression of a functional UDP-glucose dehydrogenase in articular chondrocytes: Comparison with effects of cytokines and growth factors. *Rheumatology (Oxford),* Vol. 47, No. 3, (Mar 2008), pp. (281-288)

Maneix, L., Boujrad, N., Flouriot, G., Demoor, M., Boumediene, K., Moslemi, S. & Galéra, P. (2010). 17β-estradiol-induced up-regulation of type II collagen expression is mediated by ERα/Sp/SOX9/p300 complex through COL2A1 promoter/first intron interactions in differentiated and dedifferentiated articular chondrocytes. *World Congress on osteoarthritis, OARSI,* Brussels, Belgium, September 2010

Mangelsdorf, D.J., Thummel, C., Beato, M., Herrlich, P., Schütz, G., Umesono, K., Blumberg, B., Kastner, P., Mark, M., Chambon, P. & Evans R.M. (1995). The nuclear receptor superfamily: the second decade. *Cell,* Vol. 83, No. 6, (Dec 1995), pp. (835-839), Review

Marino, M., Acconcia, F., Bresciani, F., Weisz, A. & Trentalance, A. (2002). Distinct nongenomic signal transduction pathways controlled by 17beta-estradiol regulate DNA synthesis and cyclin D1 gene transcription in HepG2 cells. *Mol. Biol. Cell,* Vol. 13, No. 10, (Oct 2002), pp. (3720-3729)

Matthews, J., Wihlen, B., Tujague, M., Wan, J., Strom, A. & Gustafsson, J.A. (2006). Estrogen receptor (ER) beta modulates ERalpha-mediated transcriptional activation by altering the recruitment of c-Fos and c-Jun to estrogen-responsive promoters. *Mol. Endocrinol.,* Vol. 20, No. 3, (Mar 2006), pp. (534-543)

McKenna, N.J., Lanz, R.B. & O'Malley, B.W. (1999). Nuclear receptor coregulators: cellular and molecular biology. *Endocr. Rev.,* Vol. 20, No. 3, (Jun 1999), pp. (321-344), Review

Metivier, R., Penot, G., Flouriot, G. & Pakdel, F. (2001). Synergism between ERalpha transactivation function 1 (AF-1) and AF-2 mediated by steroid receptor coactivator protein-1: requirement for the AF-1 alpha-helical core and for a direct interaction between the N- and C-terminal domains. *Mol. Endocrinol.,* Vol. 15, No. 11, (Nov 2001), pp. (1953-1970)

Morisset, S., Patry, C., Lora, M. & De Brum-Fernandes, A.J. (1998). Regulation of cyclooxygenase-2 expression in bovine chondrocytes in culture by interleukin 1alpha, tumor necrosis factor-alpha, glucocorticoids, and 17beta-estradiol. *J. Rheumatol.,* Vol. 25, No. 6, (Jun 1998), pp. (1146-1153)

Moslemi, S. & Seralini, S. (2005). Estrogens and breast cancer: Aromatase activity disruption. In: *Trends in Breast Cancer Research,* Editor: Andrew, P. Yao, pp. (101-127), ISBN, 1-59454-134-5, Nova Science Publishers, Inc., New York

Mouritzen, U., Christgau, S., Lehmann, H.J., Tanko, L.B. & Christiansen, C. (2003). Cartilage turnover assessed with a newly developed assay measuring collagen type II degradation products: influence of age, sex, menopause, hormone replacement therapy, and body mass index. *Ann. Rheum. Dis.,* Vol. 62, No. 4, (Apr 2003), pp. (332-336)

Nasatzky, E., Schwartz, Z., Soskolne, W.A., Brooks B.P., Dean D.D., Boyan B.D. & Ornoy A. (1994). Evidence for receptors specific for 17 beta-estradiol and testosterone in chondrocyte cultures. *Connect. Tissue Res.,* Vol. 30, No. 4, pp. (277-294)

Nilsson, O., Falk, J., Ritzén, E.M., Baron, J. & Sävendahl, L. (2003). Raloxifene acts as an estrogen agonist on the rabbit growth plate. *Endocrinology,* Vol. 144, No. 4, (Apr 2003), pp. (1481-1485)

Nilsson, S., Makela, S., Treuter, E., Tujague, M., Thomsen, J., Andersson, G., Enmark, E., Pettersson, K., Warner, M. & Gustafsson, J.A. (2001). Mechanisms of estrogen action. *Physiol Rev.,* Vol. 81, No. 4, (Oct 2001), pp. (1535-1565)

Nuclear Receptor Nomenclature Committee (1999). A unified nomenclature system for the nuclear receptor superfamily, *Cell,* Vol. 97, No. 2, (Apr 1999), pp. (161-163)

Oestergaard, S., Sondergaard, B.C., Hoegh-Andersen, P., Henriksen, K, Qvist, P., Christiansen, C., Tanko, L.B. & Karsdal, M.A. (2006). Effects of ovariectomy and estrogen therapy on type II collagen degradation and structural integrity of articular cartilage in rats: implications of the time of initiation. *Arthritis Rheum.,* Vol. 54, No. 8, (Aug 2006), pp. (2441-2451)

Oliveria, SA., Felson, D.T., Reed, J.I., Cirillo, P.A. & Walker, AM. (1995). Incidence of symptomatic hand, hip, and knee osteoarthritis among patients in a health maintenance organization. *Arthritis Rheum.,* Vol. 38, No. 8, (Aug 1995), pp. (1134-1141)

Paech, K., Webb, P., Kuiper, G.G., Nilsson, S., Gustafsson, J., Kushner, P.J. & Scanlan, T.S. (1997). Differential ligand activation of estrogen receptors ERalpha and ERbeta at AP1 sites. *Science,* Vol. 277, No. 5331, (Sep 1997), pp. (1508-1510)

Pappas, T.C., Gametchu, B. & Watson, C.S. (1995). Membrane estrogen receptors identified by multiple antibody labeling and impeded-ligand binding. *FASEB J.,* Vol. 9, No. 5, (Mar 1995), pp. (404-410)

Pearce, S.T. & Jordan, V.C. (2004). The biological role of estrogen receptors alpha and beta in cancer. *Crit. Rev. Oncol. Hematol.,* Vol. 50, No. 1, (Apr 2004), pp. (3-22), Review

Pietras, R.J. & Szego, C.M. (1977). Specific binding sites for oestrogen at the outer surfaces of isolated endometrial cells. *Nature,* Vol. 265, No. 5589, (Jan 1977), pp. (69-72)

Pietschmann, P., Rauner, M., Sipos, W. & Kerschan-Schindl K. (2008). Osteoporosis: an age-related and gender-specific disease - a mini-review. *Gerontology,* Vol. 55, No. 1, pp. (3-12)

Ray, A., Préfontaine, K.E. & Ray, P. (1994). Down-modulation of interleukin-6 gene expression by 17beta-estradiol in the absence of high affinity DNA binding by the estrogen receptor. *J. Biol. Chem.,* Vol. 269, No. 17, (Apr 1994), pp. (12940-12946)

Razandi, M., Pedram, A., Greene, G.L. & Levin, E.R. (1999). Cell membrane and nuclear estrogen receptors (ERs) originate from a single transcript: studies of ERalpha and ERbeta expressed in Chinese hamster ovary cells. *Mol. Endocrinol.,* Vol. 13, No. 2, (Feb 1999), pp. (307-319)

Reginster, J.Y., Kvasz, A., Bruyère, O. & Henrotin, Y. (2003). Is there any rationale for prescribing hormone replacement therapy (HRT) to prevent or to treat osteoarthritis? *Osteoarthritis Cartilage,* Vol.,11, No. 2, (Feb 2003), pp. (87-91)

Richette, P., Corvol, M. & Bardin, T. (2003). Estrogens, cartilage, and osteoarthritis. *Joint Bone Spine, Vol.* 70, No. 4, (Aug 2003), pp. (257-262)

Richette, P. Dumontier, M.F., Francois, M., Tsagris, L., Korwin-Zmijowska, C., Rannou, F. & Corvol, M.T. (2004). Dual effects of 17beta-oestradiol on interleukin 1beta-induced proteoglycan degradation in chondrocytes. *Ann. Rheum. Dis.,* Vol. 63, No. 2, (Feb 2004), pp. (191-199)

Richette, P., Dumontier, M.F., Tahiri, K., Widerak, M., Torre, A., Benallaoua, M., Rannou, F., Corvol, M.T. & Savouret, J.F. (2007). Oestrogens inhibit interleukin 1beta-mediated nitric oxide synthase expression in articular chondrocytes through nuclear factor-kappa B impairment. *Ann. Rheum. Dis.,* Vol. 66, No. 3, (Mar 2007), pp. (345-350)

Richmond, R.S., Carlson, C.S., Register, T.C., Shanker, G. & Loeser, R.F. (2000). Functional estrogen receptors in adult articular cartilage: estrogen replacement therapy increases chondrocyte synthesis of proteoglycans and insulin-like growth factor binding protein 2. *Arthritis Rheum.,* Vol. 43, No. 9, (Sep 2000), pp. (2081-2090)

Riggs, B.L. & Hartmann L.C. (2003). Selective estrogen-receptor modulators - mechanisms of action and application to clinical practice. *N Engl J Med,* Vol.,348, No.7, (Feb 2003), pp. (618–629)

Sabbah, M., Courilleau, D., Mester, J. & Redeuilh, G. (1999). Estrogen induction of the cyclin D1 promoter: involvement of a cAMP response-like element. *Proc. Natl. Acad. Sci. U. S. A.,* Vol. 96, No. 20, (Sep 1999), pp. (11217-11222)

Safe, S. (2001). Transcriptional activation of genes by 17 beta-estradiol through estrogen receptor-Sp1 interactions. *Vitam. Horm.,* Vol. 62, pp. (231-252)

Saggese, G., Federico, G. & Cinquanta, L. (1993). In vitro effects of growth hormone and other hormones on chondrocytes and osteoblast-like cells. *Acta Paediatr. Suppl,* Vol. 82, Suppl. 391, (Sep 1993), pp. (54-59)

Saville, B., Wormke, M., Wang, F., Nguyen, T., Enmark, E., Kuiper, G., Gustafsson, J.A. & Safe, S. (2000). Ligand-, cell-, and estrogen receptor subtype (alpha/beta)-dependent activation at GC-rich (Sp1) promoter elements. *J. Biol. Chem.,* Vol. 275, No. 8, (Feb 2000), pp. (5379-5387)

Simpson, E.R. (2003). Sources of estrogen and their importance. *J. Steroid Biochem., Mol. Biol., Vol.* 86, No. 3-5, (Sep 2003), pp. (225-230)

Sniekers, Y.H., Intema, F., Lafeber, F.P., Van Osch, G.J., Van Leeuwen, J.P., Weinans, H. & Mastbergen, S.C. (2008). A role for subchondral bone changes in the process of osteoarthritis; a micro-CT study of two canine models. *BMC Musculoskelet. Disord.,* (Feb 2008), pp. (9-20)

Sniekers, Y.H., Van Osch, G.J., Ederveen, A.G., Inzunza, J., Gustafsson, J.A., Van Leeuwen, J.P. & Weinans, H. (2009). Development of osteoarthritic features in estrogen receptor knockout mice. *Osteoarthritis Cartilage,* Vol. 17, No. 10, (Oct 2009), pp. (1356-1361)

Stein, B. & Yang, M.X. (1995). Repression of the interleukin-6 promoter by estrogen receptor is mediated by NF-kappa B and C/EBP beta. *Mol. Cell Biol.,* Vol. 15, No. 9, (Sep 1995), pp. (4971-4979)

Song, Y.J., Wu, Z.H., Lin, S.Q., Weng, X.S. & Qiu, G.X. (2003). The effect of estrogen and progestin on the expression of matrix metalloproteinases, tissue inhibitor of metalloproteinase and interleukin-1beta mRNA in synovia of OA rabbit model. *Zhonghua Yi. Xue. Za Zhi.,* Vol. 83, No. 6, (Mar 2003), pp. (498-503)

Spector, T.D., Brown, G.C. & Silman, A.J. (1988). Increased rates of previous hysterectomy and gynecological operations in women with osteoarthritis. BMJ, Vol. 297, No. 6653, (Oct 1988), pp. (899–900)

Spector, T.D., Hart, D.J., Brown, P., Almeyda, J., Dacre, J.E., Doyle, D.V. & Silman, A.J. (1991). Frequency of osteoarthritis in hysterectomized women. *J Rheumatol.,* Vol. 18, No. 12, (Dec 1991), pp. (1877–1883)

Stoner, M., Wormke, M., Saville, B., Samudio, I., Qin, C., Abdelrahim, M. & Safe, S. (2004). Estrogen regulation of vascular endothelial growth factor gene expression in ZR-75 breast cancer cells through interaction of estrogen receptor alpha and SP proteins. *Oncogene,* Vol. 23, No. 5, (Feb 2004), pp. (1052-1063)

Stovall, D.W. & Pinkerton, J.V. (2008). Estrogen agonists/antagonists in combination with estrogen for prevention and treatment of menopause-associated signs and symptoms. *Womens Health (Lond Engl),* Vol. 4, No. 3, (May 2008), pp. (257-268)

Stracke, D., Schulz, T. & Prehm, P. (2011). Inhibitors of hyaluronan export from hops prevent osteoarthritic reactions. *Mol Nutr Food Res.* Vol. 55, No. 3, (Mar 2011), pp. (485-494)

Takeuchi, S., Mukai, N., Tateishi, T. & Miyakawa, S. (2007). Production of sex steroid hormones from DHEA in articular chondrocyte of rats. *Am. J. Physiol. Endocrinol. Metab.,* Vol. 293, No. 1, (Jul 2007), pp. (E410-E415)

Tanko, L.B., Sondergaard, B.C., Oestergaard, S., Karsdal, M.A. & Christiansen, C. (2008). An update review of cellular mechanisms conferring the indirect and direct effects of estrogen on articular cartilage. *Climacteric,* Vol. 11, No. 1, (Feb 2008), pp. (4-16)

Toft, D. & Gorski, J. (1966). A receptor molecule for estrogens: isolation from the rat uterus and preliminary characterization. *Proc. Natl. Acad. Sci. U. S. A.,* Vol. 55, No. 6, (Jun 1966), pp. (1574-1581)

Tsai, C.L., Liu, T.K. & Chen, T.J. (1992). Estrogen and osteoarthritis: a study of synovial estradiol and estradiol receptor binding in human osteoarthritic knees. *Biochem Biophys Res Commun.*, Vol. 183, No. 3, (Mar 1992), pp. (1287-1291)

Uht, R.M., Anderson, C.M., Webb, P. & Kushner, P.J. (1997). Transcriptional activities of estrogen and glucocorticoid receptors are functionally integrated at the AP-1 response element. *Endocrinology,* Vol. 138, No. 7, (Jul 1997), pp. (2900-2908)

Valdes, A.M., Van Oene, M., Hart, D.J., Surdulescu, G.L., Loughlin, J., Doherty, M. & Spector, T.D. (2006). Reproducible genetic associations between candidate genes and clinical knee osteoarthritis in men and women. *Arthritis Rheum.,* Vol. 54, No. 2, (Feb 2006), pp. (533-539)

Von Muhlen, D., Morton, D., Von Muhlen, C.A. & Barrett-Connor, E. (2002). Postmenopausal estrogen and increased risk of clinical osteoarthritis at the hip, hand, and knee in older women. *J. Womens Health Gend. Based. Med.,* Vol. 11, No. 6, (Jul-Aug 2002), pp. (511-518)

Walter, P., Green, S., Greene, G., Krust, A., Bornert, J.M., Jeltsch, J.M., Staub, A., Jensen, E., Scrace, G., Waterfield, M. & Chambon P. (1985). Cloning of the human estrogen receptor cDNA. *Proc. Natl. Acad. Sci. U. S. A.,* Vol. 82, No. 23, (Dec 1985), pp. (7889-7893)

Wang, Z., Zhang, X., Shen, P., Loggie, B.W., Chang, Y. & Deuel, T.F. (2006). A variant of estrogen receptor-{alpha}, hER-{alpha}36: transduction of estrogen- and antiestrogen-dependent membrane-initiated mitogenic signaling. *Proc. Natl. Acad. Sci. U. S. A.,* Vol. 103, No. 24, (Jun 2006), pp. (9063-9068)

Webb, P., Nguyen, P., Valentine, C, Lopez, G.N., Kwok, G.R., McInerney, E., Katzenellenbogen, B.S., Enmark, E., Gustafsson, J.A., Nilsson, S. & Kushner, P.J. (1999). The estrogen receptor enhances AP-1 activity by two distinct mechanisms with different requirements for receptor *trans*activation functions. *Mol. Endocrinol.*, Vol. 13, No. 10, (Oct 1999), pp. (1672-1685)

Wilson, M.G., Michet, C.J. Jr., Ilstrup, D.M. & Melton, L.J. (1990). Idiopathic symptomatic osteoarthritis of the hip and knee: A population-based incidence study. *Mayo Clin Proc.*, Vol. 65, No. 9, (Sep 1990), pp. (1214-1221)

Wluka, A.E., Davis, S.R., Bailey, M., Stuckey, S.L. & Cicuttini, F.M. (2001). Users of oestrogen replacement therapy have more knee cartilage than non-users. *Ann. Rheum. Dis.*, Vol. 60, No. 4, (Apr 2001), pp. (332-336)

Part 3

Clinical Manifestations and Diagnosis of Rheumatic Diseases

5

Rheumatoid Arthritis Interstitial Lung Disease

Ophir Vinik, Theodore Marras, Shane Shapera and Shikha Mittoo
University of Toronto, Department of Medicine
Canada

1. Introduction

Rheumatoid arthritis (RA) is a systemic, autoimmune, inflammatory disorder affecting 0.5-1% of the North American population (Gabriel, 2001). It has a predilection for young women with an incidence rate of up to 130 per 100,000 compared with 70 per 100,000 in men [Minaur et al, 2004]. It is associated with a median survival decrease of up to 11 years compared to the general population (Minaur et al., 2004). The disease course may be complicated by extra-articular manifestations that confer an added burden of morbidity and mortality. RA-associated cardiovascular and infectious complications are commonly highlighted as major causes of morbidity and mortality in these patients (Maradit-Kremers et al., 2005). However, pulmonary involvement, the third leading extra-articular manifestation of RA, is now also recognized as a major cause of morbidity and mortality in RA patients. This was demonstrated in an autopsy study of 81 RA patients where the cause of death was determined to be infectious in 23.5%, cardiovascular in 17.3% and respiratory in 9.9% of patients (Suzuki et al., 1994). Pulmonary complications are the presenting manifestation of RA in up to 20% of patients (Brown, 2007). These complications include airway disease, pleural effusion, pulmonary nodules, and interstitial lung disease (ILD). This chapter will discuss the epidemiology, clinical features, management of RA-associated ILD (RA-ILD) and highlight the links between pulmonary involvement and autoimmunity.

2. RA-ILD

2.1 Scope and epidemiology

Reports of the prevalence of RA-ILD are widely variable and likely comprise significant underestimates owing to inconsistency of clinical criteria used to define the condition, methods used for disease detection, and heterogeneity of study populations. Identification of ILD is further confounded by the fact that many of the medications used for the treatment of RA have potential deleterious effects on the lungs. A recent population-based study from the Rochester Epidemiology Project suggested that as many as 1 in 10 patients with RA will be diagnosed with ILD over the course of the disease (Bongartz et al., 2010).

RA patients with extra-articular manifestations, in particular those with respiratory disease, are at increased mortality risk, with a standardized mortality ratio ranging from 2.5 to 5.0 (Brown, 2007). RA-ILD remains a major cause of death in RA; the median and 5-year survival is 3.5 years and between 37-39%, respectively (Hakala, 1988). The mortality risk was found to be most significant in the first 5 years after an initial hospitalization. In a more recent incident-based study from the Rochester cohort of 582 patients with RA, the risk of death was found to be three times higher in RA patients with ILD compared to patients without ILD; the median survival following ILD diagnosis was only 2.6 years (Bongartz et al., 2010). In general, treating connective tissue disease -associated ILD (CTD-ILD) early, with immunosuppressive medications, not only may halt ILD progression, but may improve quality of life. This may be true for RA-ILD as well, but these disease-specific data are scarce. The poor prognosis of RA patients with ILD highlights the need for clinicians to recognize the clinical features of this condition and be cognizant of its course and management.

2.2 Clinical features and course

Clinical detection of ILD in RA patients may be challenging. The challenge stems from the non-specific clinical features of this condition and, typically, symptoms that are often masked or manifest in an insidious manner. Patients most commonly present complaining of worsening shortness of breath on exertion and a dry cough. Since this patient population suffers from arthritis that often limits their physical activity, the presentation of exertional dyspnea may in fact already denote advanced lung disease. Moreover, since maximum ventilation at peak exercise is approximately 70% of maximum voluntary ventilation (MVV), in the absence of significant lung disease, there is significant pulmonary reserve and exercise should not be limited by dyspnea (Hansen et al., 1984). Therefore, a low clinical threshold of suspicion should be maintained with respect to complaints of dyspnea in these patients. Complaints of lower-extremity swelling, syncopal episodes, and exertional chest pain may represent an underlying pulmonary arterial hypertension with right-sided heart failure, a severe complication of ILD. Clinicians should also be mindful of the fact that RA patients, particularly elderly patients, may have other co-morbid conditions such as congestive heart failure or anemia that may present with similar symptoms. Therefore, clinicians must consider and actively search for ILD in the presence of these symptoms, rather than simply assigning them to other more common co-morbidities.

Physical exam in early ILD may be normal. A small proportion of patients may have digital clubbing (Rajasekaran et al., 2001). Most commonly, RA patients with ILD will have bilateral fine crackles heard best at the end of inspiration and tend to be more prominent at the lung bases. Expiratory wheezing, bronchial or upper airway sounds are uncommon and their presence can suggest either airway disease involvement or a concomitant respiratory condition such as chronic obstructive pulmonary disease (COPD) or asthma. The presence of hypoxemia may denote a more advanced disease process. Physical exam findings of an elevated jugular venous pressure with CV waves, an abnormal hepatojugular reflux, and lower-extremity pitting edema can represent an underlying right ventricular dysfunction relating to pulmonary arterial hypertension. A parasternal heave, a prominent second heart sound, and a tricuspid regurgitation murmur on precordial exam, as well as a pulsatile liver and ascites on abdominal exam, are all findings suggestive of underlying advanced pulmonary arterial hypertension. Although uncommon in RA-ILD without concomitant COPD, clinicians should be aware of these physical findings to facilitate early detection of this serious complication.

Evolving evidence points to the existence of another unique clinical entity of RA-associated ILD in which patients also present with signs and symptoms suggestive of COPD. The syndrome of combined pulmonary fibrosis and emphysema (CPFE) was first described by Cottin et al. in 2005. CPFE was characterized by the association of tobacco smoking, significant dyspnea, impaired diffusion capacity on pulmonary function test, exertional hypoxemia and radiological features of both emphysema and diffuse interstitial lung opacities. This clinical entity was also described in a retrospective study of 34 patients with a connective tissue disease (CTD), 18 of which had RA. This study demonstrated the presence of CPFE in patients with CTD, particularly RA, and identified several features that distinguish CPFE in patients with CTD compared to non-CTD CPFE (Cottin et al., 2011). These features include a female predilection, younger age, higher lung volumes but a lower diffusion capacity. Smoking was identified in the majority of CTD patients with CPFE, but not in all. The presence of these features led the authors to suggest that CPFE is a unique pulmonary manifestation in patients with CTD, particularly RA (Cottin et al., 2011). Therefore, when assessing RA patients with respiratory complaints, clinicians should inquire about tobacco smoking history and be cognizant of CPFE features as these patients would potentially need additional monitoring and screening for development of pulmonary hypertension.

RA-associated ILD is a chronic, progressive pulmonary manifestation that confers significant morbidity and mortality (see section 2.1). As will be described in the next section, RA-associated ILD is heterogeneous in its presentation, but can be further defined by its histologic features. The course, radiographic pattern, response to treatment, and prognosis of RA-ILD can be linked to the specific underlying histological pattern.

2.3 Histopathology

ILD is defined as varying levels of inflammation and fibrosis of the lung parenchyma (Cushley et al., 1999). The classification criteria for ILD has undergone revision over the past 10 years and is still evolving as there is increased awareness that different histopathologic subtypes correlate with specific clinical presentations and have differing prognostic and therapeutic consequences. Nevertheless, it is widely accepted that ILD associated with CTD constitutes a unique class within the spectrum of ILD. From histological perspective, virtually any of the known histological patterns of interstitial pneumonia (IP) can occur in association with CTD. However, certain histological patterns are known to be more commonly associated with certain subtypes of CTD. In the case of RA, the most common patterns identified are the usual interstitial pneumonia (UIP) followed by the non-specific interstitial pneumonia (NSIP) (Lee et al., 2005).

Infiltration of inflammatory cells (plasma cells, neutrophils, and different T cells subpopulations) as well as varying degrees of fibrosis of the alveolar wall can be found in both NSIP and UIP (Parra et al., 2007). The key differentiating histological feature between the two is the temporal uniformity of the lesions seen in NSIP versus the temporal heterogeneity found in UIP. Temporal heterogeneity refers to the presence of varying degrees of inflammation and fibrosis within the same diseased lung. Therefore, in UIP, areas of normal lung are adjacent to areas of active inflammation. There are expanding areas of fibrosis with fibroblastic foci at the leading edges. These fibroblastic foci are rich in dense collagen and proliferating fibroblasts and are considered the hallmark lesions of UIP (Katzenstein & Myers., 1998). Another parenchymal lesion associated with UIP is formation of interconnected cystic spaces, called honeycombing, which indicates end stage fibrosis without evidence of active inflammation. In contrast, lung tissue in NSIP typically shows a homogeneous pattern of lymphocytic infiltrates in the alveolar septae (Parra et al., 2007). These correspond with areas of ground glass attenuation on thoracic high-resolution computed tomography (HRCT) and are the most characteristic feature of NSIP (Katzenstein & Fiorelli., 1994, Travis et al., 2000).

RA- ILD can also infrequently present with acute interstitial pneumonia (AIP), a sub-acute to rapidly progressive respiratory failure, and diffuse alveolar damage (DAD). DAD is the histologic abnormality observed in the acute respiratory distress syndrome (ARDS), which may be triggered most commonly by lung infections, sepsis, drug-induced lung disease, and inhalational lung injury (Katzenstein et al., 1986). The term AIP is reserved for cases where the inciting factor is unknown. Histologically, DAD is characterized by diffuse distribution of a temporally homogeneous appearance with alveolar septal thickening and fibrosis including hyaline membrane formation (Katzenstein et al., 1986). Distinguishing AIP from DAD superimposed on a pre-existing ILD, such as UIP, can be technically challenging. Clinically, the histological findings of AIP confer a mortality risk exceeding 50%, typically within several months of diagnosis (Katzenstein et al., 1986; Parambil et al., 2006). Patients surviving the acute syndrome are commonly left with significant morbidity and are at risk of recurrences (Bouros et al., 2000; Vourlekis et al., 2000).

Finally, in addition to a vigilant search for possible infectious triggers, clinicians assessing RA patients with respiratory symptoms should also obtain detailed medication history as certain medications used for the treatment of RA, such as methotrexate, cyclophosphamide, sulfasalazine, and TNF-alpha inhibitors have potential pneumotoxic effects and can present with diffuse lung disease. These medications can lead to ILD, particularly the NSIP pattern, but also may lead to a histologic pattern known as hypersensitivity pneumonitis (HP); thus, the etiology of ILD in RA can present a challenge to clinicians. Careful history regarding the temporal relationship between initiation of drugs and onset of respiratory symptoms may be helpful in deciphering causality. Onset of pulmonary findings within a 2 month period of drug initiation and stability in lung function and/or radiologic damage upon discontinuation of the toxic culprit are findings that support a drug-related etiology of ILD (Dixon et al., 2010).

As an example, methotrexate, the most commonly used drug for the treatment of RA, can result in interstitial pneumonitis and pulmonary fibrosis at any time or dosage during the course of treatment (Hilliquin et al., 1996; St Clair et al., 1985; Swierkot & Szechiński 2006). And, while the clinical presentation may be identical to RA-ILD, methotrexate-related toxicity usually occurs within 6 months of initiation, often within 2-3 months, and does not involve progressive decline in pulmonary function test (PFT). Other clinical clues to methotrexate-induced ILD are fever and eosinophilia from serum or from bronchoalveolar lavage fluid. The histopathologic correlate of methotrexate-induced ILD may be one of HP, DAD or a cellular NSIP type pattern (Imokawa et al., 2000; Kremer et al., 1997; St Clair et al., 1985). In contrast, cyclophosphamide, another agent used for the treatment of RA, is usually associated with an insidious onset of pulmonary symptoms and typically occurs after prolonged use (Segura et al., 2001). Therefore, it is essential to be vigilant regarding pulmonary symptoms even among patients with stable treatment and those with established disease.

2.4 Evaluation and radiographic findings

The diagnostic gold standard for identification and classification of RA-ILD has traditionally been a surgical, open-lung biopsy. Yet, since chest imaging now has a good correlation with histopathology, such a biopsy is not always necessary for diagnosis (Yoshinouchi et al., 2005). In fact, chest imaging is now considered a critical diagnostic and prognostic modality when assessing patients with suspected RA-ILD. It is foreseeable that in the future, a composite of radiologic and histologic data may be used to predict outcomes as it relates to RA-ILD, as this composite measure is now used in idiopathic pulmonary fibrosis (Raghu et al., 2011).

The chest radiographic pattern may be a useful screening test in select cases (Gabbay et al., 1997). Chest radiograph findings consist of a bilateral, peripheral, reticular opacity pattern with basal predominance. It is not possible to reliably distinguish between UIP and NSIP on chest radiograph. It is critical to recognize that patients with clinically important RA- ILD may have a completely normal chest radiograph; thus, the sensitivity of this test is inadequate to rule out RA-ILD. Instead, the standard of care in assessing patients with suspected RA-ILD is a thoracic high-resolution CT (HRCT), a method which has a very high sensitivity and can detect even mild disease.

HRCT provides a non-invasive radiological characterization of lung abnormality that may correlate reasonably well to the underlying pathology (Lee et al., 2005; MacDonald et al., 2001; Yoshinouchi et al., 2005). The characteristic UIP pattern on HRCT demonstrates marked interlobular septal thickening and intra-lobular reticulation, traction bronchiectasis (tethering open of otherwise relatively normal airways by the increased elasticity of surrounding lung) and honeycomb cysts, in a peripheral and basilar distribution (Macdonald et al., 2001; Martinez 2006) (See Figure 1). 'Ground-glass' opacities may be seen, but are atypical and the extent of ground glass and other atypical findings (such as upper lobe or central involvement) reduce the confidence that the radiologic pattern represents UIP (Macdonald et al., 2001, Martinez 2006).

In contrast to UIP, NSIP usually features more prominent 'ground-glass' changes. The 'ground-glass' changes tend to be symmetric with a basal and sub-pleural predilection. About half of all patients with NSIP will also have significant reticulation and a minority will have honeycombing (Yoshinouchi et al., 2005). Reticulation and honeycombing, when present in NSIP, are usually associated with the fibrosing sub-type (fibrosing NSIP) rather than the cellular sub-type (cellular NSIP) (See figures 2 & 3). The distinction refers to the histologic appearance of the lung interstitium, where the former is associated with more collagen deposition and the latter with more mononuclear inflammatory cellular infiltration.

The distinction between UIP and NSIP on HRCT remains challenging in many cases, as demonstrated by a study of 50 patients with idiopathic ILD, where the HRCT pattern of NSIP was indistinguishable from UIP in 32% of patients (Hartman et al., 2000). The HRCT diagnosis of NSIP was found to have a sensitivity and specificity ranging from 60 to 70% (Hartman et al., 2000). The most distinguishing feature appeared to be the finding of more prominent 'ground-glass' changes in NSIP versus UIP (MacDonald et al., 2001). The radiographic appearance of AIP early in its course is quite distinct from UIP and NSIP, primarily by the presence of bilateral, frequently diffuse, airspace disease with air bronchograms. However, as AIP progresses, the airspace pattern becomes less prominent and instead it presents with 'ground glass' changes and reticular opacities, making the distinction between the various ILD patterns more difficult (Manjunatha et al., 2010). Overall, the diagnostic challenges using imaging modalities outlined so far highlight the underlying need of a more definitive tissue diagnosis by lung biopsy in select cases, which is further discussed in the next section.

2.5 Screening and diagnosis

The significant morbidity and mortality associated with ILD in RA patients calls for increased vigilance on the part of clinicians to respiratory complaints in these patients. Clinicians should inquire about the presence of any respiratory symptoms during both

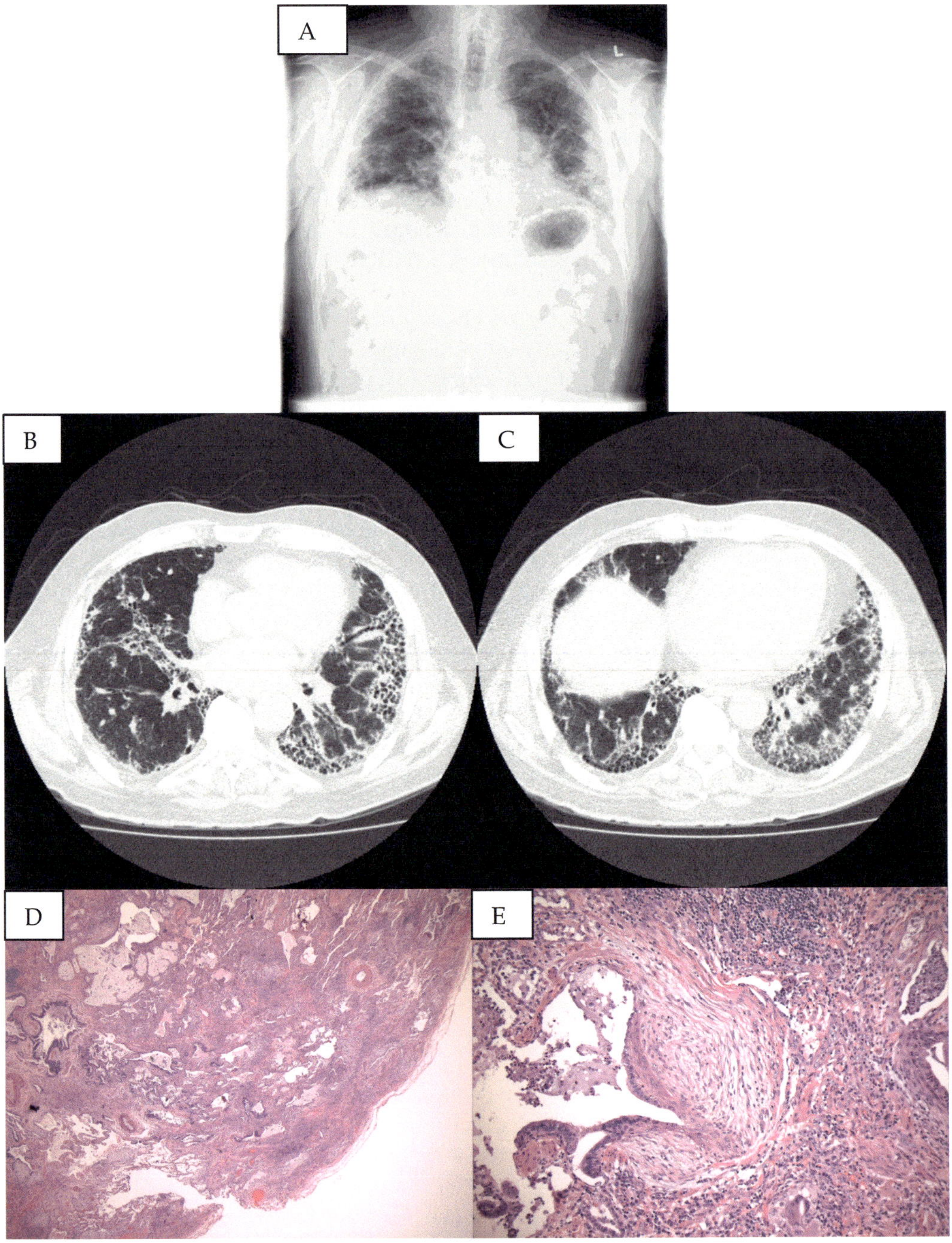

A. Chest radiograph (PA view) shows bilateral, peripheral reticulation and volume loss, B&C. HRCT shows bilateral, peripheral reticulation, traction bronchiectasis and honeycombing, D. Surgical lung biopsy; low magnification (16x H&E) view of UIP with sub-pleural areas of microscopic honeycomb change interspersed with areas of less affected lung parenchyma, E. Surgical lung biopsy; high magnification (100x H&E) view showing a fibroblast focus likely representing active fibrosis.

Fig. 1. RA-ILD UIP

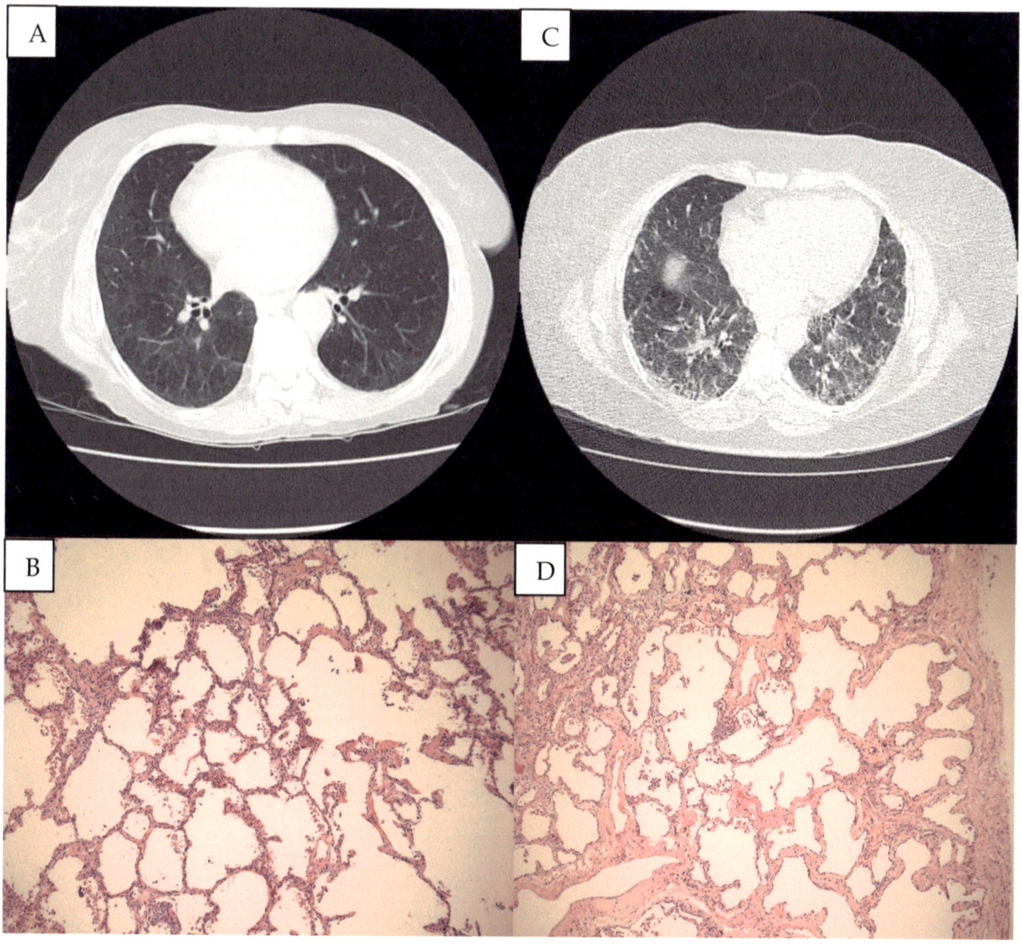

Fig. 2. A. HRCT of cellular NSIP in RA, showing predominantly peripheral and very subtle ground glass opacification, B. Surgical lung biopsy from patient in panel A; cellular NSIP with diffuse mild interstitial chronic inflammatory infiltrates (50x, H&E), C. HRCT of fibrotic NSIP in RA, showing predominantly reticulation, D. Surgical lung biopsy from patient in panel C; fibrotic NSIP with diffuse alveolar septal fibrosis without architectural distortion or remodeling (50x, H&E).

initial and follow-up visits, with particular emphasis on exertional dyspnea and persistent non-productive cough. Tobacco smoking history should be obtained from every RA patient and patients should be strongly encouraged to achieve smoking cessation and avoid passive (second-hand) smoking. A complete medication history should also be obtained to assess for any recent or current use of medications known to have potential pulmonary toxicity.

In the presence of respiratory symptoms, clinicians should also assess for any occupational or environmental exposures as well as for infectious stigmata. Examination of the respiratory system should be included in the routine follow-up of RA patients, with particular attention to the presence of bilateral inspiratory fine crackles as well as the less commonly encountered, inspiratory squeaks. In RA patients with known ILD, the physical examination should also include assessment for signs and symptoms of pulmonary hypertension.

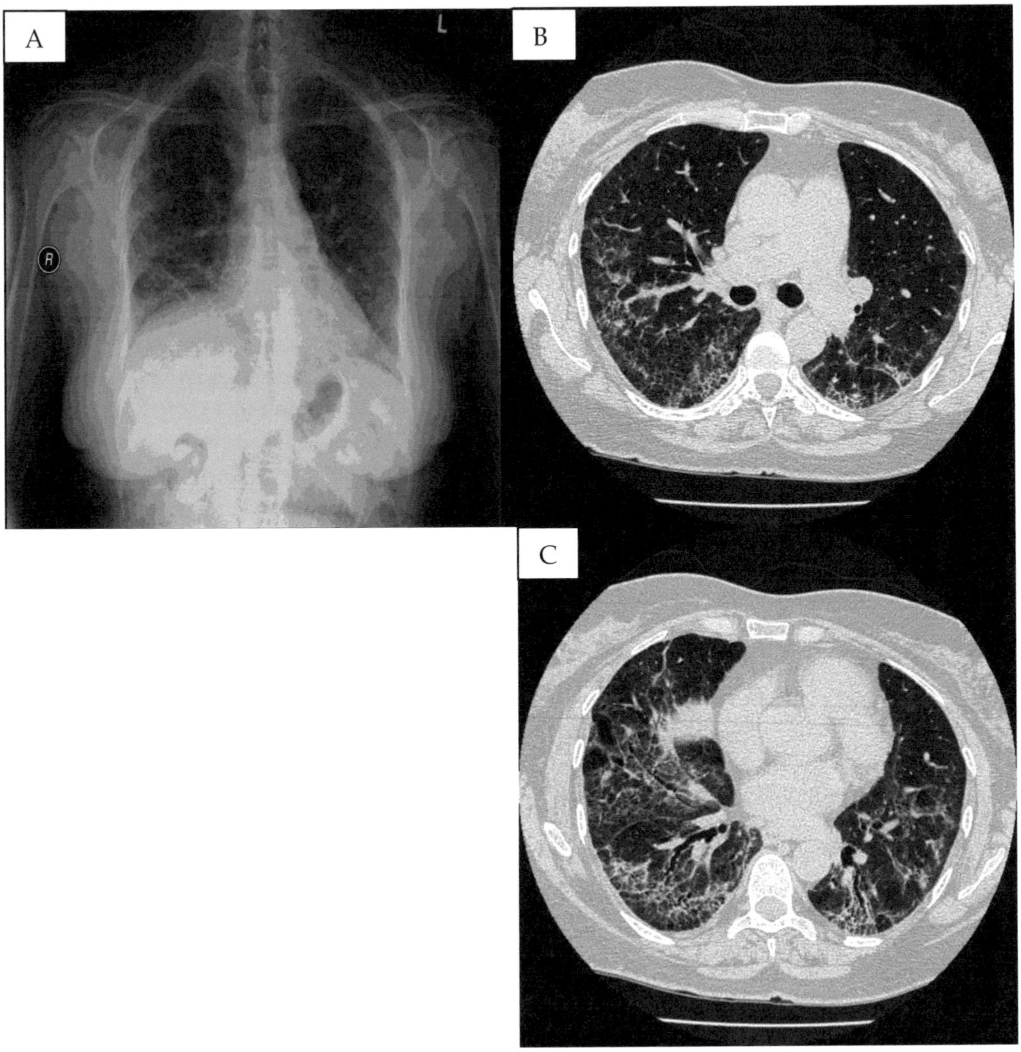

A. Chest radiograph (PA view) showing peripheral interstitial markings, B&C. HRCT showing peripheral and lower lobe predominant ground glass opacification and reticulation.

Fig. 3. RA-ILD mixed cellular and fibrotic

It is standard of care that newly diagnosed patients with RA should complete a baseline screening chest radiograph, especially before the initiation of methotrexate. In most cases, particularly in patients with pulmonary risk factors such as smoking, or those who are symptomatic with dyspnea and/or cough, a baseline pulmonary function test (PFT), including spirometry, lung volumes and diffusion capacity, should also be completed. Although evidence-based, formal guidelines are not available, it is considered standard of care to also perform a chest radiograph prior to initiation of a biologic therapeutic agent, in part to evaluate for stigmata of latent or active tuberculosis, but also to assess for the presence of ILD which may be adversely impacted by the therapy (Dixon et al., 2010). In the absence of any lung abnormality at time of RA diagnosis, further investigations should be guided by clinical context, particularly in preparation for treatment with potentially pneumotoxic medications. In the absence of specific evidence-based recommendations with regards to radiographic follow-up, clinical judgment should be exercised in making this decision.

Most commonly, ILD in RA is associated with PFT physiologic changes of restriction with a decreased diffusing capacity of carbon monoxide (Lee et al., 2005; Pappas et al., 2010). A decreased diffusing capacity is the most sensitive parameter for ILD on PFT. This may also be the sole PFT abnormality early in the course of ILD. A combination of obstructive and restrictive changes may co-exist in patients with other pulmonary co-morbidities such as asthma or COPD. As a result, some of these patients may present with combined obstructive and restrictive abnormalities or an isolated decreased diffusing capacity. For serial monitoring of PFTs, particular attention is paid to changes in absolute and percent predicted forced vital capacity (FVC) and diffusing capacity as markers of disease progression and response to treatment. A low diffusing capacity has been shown to be associated with disease progression and poor outcomes (Biederer et al., 2004, Hakala 1988). Less commonly, obstruction, as seen in obliterative bronchiolitis, is the hallmark of diffuse lung disease of RA. In this situation, forced expiratory volume in one second (FEV1) is reduced out of proportion to FVC, with an FEV1/FVC ratio < 0.8, and there may be hyperinflation and gas trapping. As a diagnostic tool, a PFT is insufficient and all RA patients with concern for ILD should undergo HRCT.

The superiority of HRCT over chest radiographs, PFTs, and bronchoalveolar lavage (BAL) in identifying ILD has been consistently demonstrated in research studies, although limited data exist regarding its exact sensitivity in detecting RA-associated ILD (e.g. Biederer et al., 2004) . Nevertheless, HRCT is the most sensitive non-invasive modality for the diagnosis of ILD in patients with RA.

The HRCT findings of UIP pattern, particularly in patients with a high pre-test probability based on clinical history, physical exam findings and an abnormal PFT, confirms the diagnosis of RA-ILD with great confidence (Martinez 2006). This is in part owing to the unique radiological features of UIP and it likely being the most common RA-associated ILD pattern (Lee et al., 2005). HRCT features of UIP in an RA patient are highly indicative of histologic findings of UIP on surgical lung biopsy, but could also be associated with fibrotic NSIP. Regardless, the presence of UIP findings unequivocally establishes the diagnosis of an ILD. The HRCT findings of NSIP pattern also has high diagnostic value albeit to a lesser extent, due to its less specific radiological features (MacDonald et al., 2001). Radiological uncertainty, inconsistency between diagnostic modalities or with clinical presentation, necessitates additional investigations including consideration of a surgical lung biopsy.

Surgical biopsy of lung parenchyma is now commonly performed by video-assisted thoracoscopic surgery (VATS). Although surgical risks should always be assessed for the individual patient, surgical lung biopsy, particularly VATS biopsy, is a relatively safe procedure that is well tolerated (Zhang & Liu, 2010). In light of its safety profile and high diagnostic yield, surgical lung biopsy should be strongly considered in the face of clinically important diagnostic uncertainty (See Figure 4 for summary of screening and diagnosis).

Bronchoalveolar lavage (BAL), a method to sample the lungs' terminal airways, transbronchial lung biopsy, and radiology-guided needle biopsy, usually provide samples that are generally insufficient to adequately characterize or classify ILD (Biederer et al., 2004). The main role of BAL in immunosuppressed patients with parenchymal

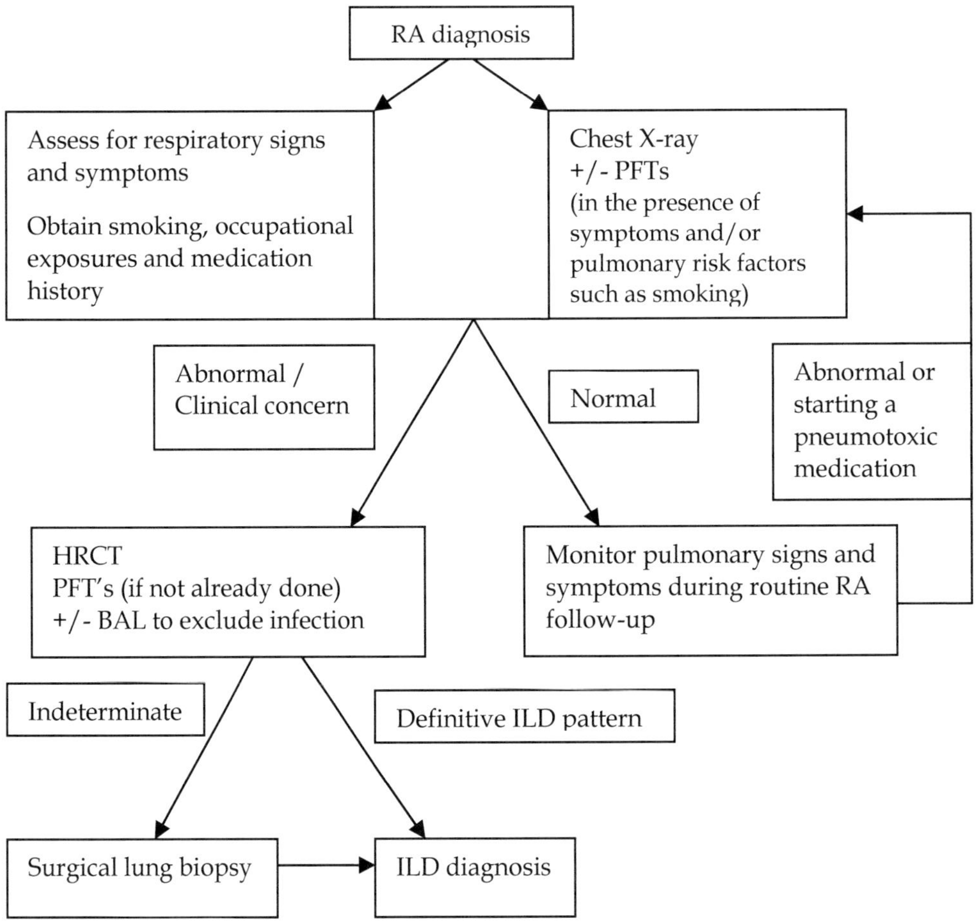

Fig. 4. Proposed screening protocol for RA-ILD and diagnosis flowchart

abnormalities on HRCT is to rule out infection and assess for malignancy. Therefore, unless infection is suspected, surgical lung biopsy is the preferred method of histologic detailed characterization of RA-associated ILD.

2.6 Management

A three-pronged approach should be considered for management of RA patients with ILD. The first phase of this approach is education and consideration of transplantation evaluation. RA patients diagnosed with ILD need to be counseled about the potentially progressive nature of this condition as well as its associated morbidity and mortality. In the setting of idiopathic pulmonary fibrosis (IPF), referral for lung transplantation evaluation should generally be considered relatively early in the disease course provided that there are no obvious contraindications for transplant. Predictors of poor prognosis and the need for more rapid assessment for lung transplant include a diffusing capacity less than 39%, documented deterioration in FVC by at least 10% or diffusing capacity by at least 15% over 6 months, new onset exertional oxygen desaturation below 88%, progression of symptoms, or advanced disease with evidence of significant honeycombing on HRCT at first presentation

(Orens et la., 2006). Although limited data is available for RA associated UIP, an analogous approach should be considered since UIP in RA patients seems to carry the same poor prognosis as IPF, worse than any other ILD (Park et al., 2007). RA patients with UIP are also more likely to experience acute exacerbations (Dawson et al., 2002, Park et al., 2007b), analogous to the recently defined acute exacerbations of IPF (Collard et al., 2007), and they seem to be less responsive to pharmacological treatments (Nannini et al., 2008). Patients with NSIP tend to have a better prognosis, and so transplant evaluation is usually reserved for patients with significant progression or more advanced disease that has not responded to therapy.

The second part of management is supportive care. Clinicians should ensure that patients receive annual influenza, as well as regular pneumococcal vaccinations. Smoking cessation and avoidance of passive smoke exposure are paramount as they exert a deleterious effect on disease progression. Assessment of the need for home oxygen should be done in the face of worsening respiratory status. For patients with impaired respiratory function, who plan to travel by air, clinicians should consider assessing their need for supplemental oxygen at altitude even in those who do not meet criteria for oxygen at sea level. Applications for disability, handicapped parking, and referrals to patient support groups should be implemented early in the management phase.

Finally, an immunosuppressive treatment regimen should be implemented. Currently, clinicians do not have the benefit of evidence-based guidelines to direct the pharmacological management of RA-associated ILD and current treatments rely to a great extent on clinical experience and evidence from management of ILD in other connective tissue diseases, such as scleroderma. In general, the use of glucocorticoids constitutes the basis of pharmacological management. However, their efficacy as monotherapy is limited and patients would typically require the addition of another immune modulating pharmacological agent. Oral prednisone is typically the first component of treatment with a starting dose ranging between 0.5 to 1 milligrams per kilogram of body weight daily. Patients should then be monitored closely for clinical changes as well as for possible adverse effects related to the use of high-dose glucocorticoids. It is prudent to obtain a baseline bone mineral density (BMD) and screen patients for the development of diabetes once treatment commences. Bone protection therapy with calcium and Vitamin D supplements should be given to all patients. Patients with an abnormal BMD at baseline should also be given a bisphosphonate. Prophylaxis against pneumocystis pneumonia (PCP) should be employed with long term prednisone use of at least 30 mg/day, in particular, if there is concomitant use of a cytotoxic agent (Yale & Limper, 1996).

Serial PFTs and chest HRCT scans are used to objectively assess clinical response to treatment. In the absence of clear guidelines as to the frequency of these tests, clinical judgment should be exercised. In general, a reasonable approach would be to have the initial follow-up at 8 to 12 weeks with repeat PFTs and subsequent follow-up every 3 to 6 months thereafter. Chest imaging might be initially repeated as early as 6 months after initiating immunosuppressive therapy, but typically follow-up imaging is performed annually with low-radiation dose CT scans. Repeat imaging should also be considered at any time when clinically important or unexplained changes occur in the patient's clinical course. Time to clinical response is variable and while some patients may experience improvement within a span of a few weeks, most will require several months, while still others may have very limited benefit.

A steroid-sparing immunosuppressive agent, should be considered relatively early in cases of RA-ILD. Clinical worsening on glucocorticoid monotherapy or significant burden of parenchymal involvement, as typically evidenced by >20% involvement on HRCT chest or <70% FVC, warrants the addition of a second immunosuppressive agent (Goh et al., 2008). Recommendations with respect to the second immunosuppressive agent are derived from studies of scleroderma-associated ILD (SSc-ILD). Oral cyclophosphamide, at doses between 1-2mg/kg body weigh daily, is used for extensive disease although its efficacy may be modest at best and its use associated with significant adverse effects. Monthly intravenous pulses of cyclophosphamide may be a reasonable alternative to oral cyclophosphamide as it has a similar efficacy profile, but lower toxicity when compared to oral therapy (Hoyles et al., 2006). Azathioprine can also be used, but may be reserved for patients with less severe disease or in those who are intolerant of cyclophosphamide, with an initial dose ranging between 2 - 3 milligrams per kilogram daily.

Various other immune-modulating therapies have been tried for the treatment of RA- ILD, none of which is sufficiently supported by empirical data to warrant routine use in practice. Application of these therapies to RA-ILD typically stems from clinical experience applying these treatments in other CTD-ILD.

One such example is mycophenolate, which has recently been described in case series to be associated with stabilization and potential improvement in lung function in patients with CTD-ILD (Saketkoo & Espinoza, 2008; Swigris et al., 2006) and SSc-ILD (Zamora et al., 2008). However, one limitation with the use of mycophenolate in the setting of RA is that while it might provide lung function benefit, it does not treat joint inflammation, and, therefore, often necessitates the use of higher corticosteroid use to manage RA disease activity. Thus, we recommend that mycophenolate should be used as a second-line agent in the management of RA-ILD. In contrast, methotrexate, a common agent used in many CTD, has been shown to not only provide no clinical benefit in RA-ILD, but may be potentially harmful by leading to ILD disease progression (Gochuico et al., 2008). Therefore, methotrexate should not be used in the setting of RA-ILD. The anti-CD20 antibody, Rituximab, has also been suggested based on its use in other CTD- and vasculitis- associated lung involvement (Brulhart et al., 2006, Stasi et al., 2006). However, caution is advised in light of concerns raised over the risk of pneumonitis with rituximab (Leon et al., 2004), including specifically in RA-ILD patients (Jadon et al., 2008). Anti-TNF alpha antibodies, tyrosine-kinase inhibitors (Distler et al., 2008) and anti-IL6 receptor antibody are also being considered for RA-associated ILD, but data is very limited and their safety in this setting has not been confidently established. The use of other agents, such as cyclosporine and hydroxychloroquine, has also been suggested yet with very limited empirical evidence (Chang et al., 2002).

Patients presenting with severe clinical symptoms, particularly with evidence of AIP, may receive an initial course of intravenous methylprednisolone pulses at 7 to 10 milligrams per kilogram of body weight. Intravenous cyclophosphamide at 10 to 15 milligrams per kilogram can be initiated concomitantly in this setting if no other contraindications exist (Kelly & Saravanan 2008). Once clinically stable, patients should then be switched to oral therapy.

Several adjuvant therapies have been suggested for RA- ILD, extrapolated from practices used to treat idiopathic or other CTD subtypes with ILD. One such treatment is N-acetylcysteine (NAC), which is commonly used in patients with idiopathic pulmonary fibrosis (IPF). It is believed to exert an anti-oxidant effect as well as have mucolytic properties. While limited evidence supports its efficacy in patients with IPF (Demedts et al., 2005), there is currently no evidence-based rationale for its use in RA- ILD. The use of anticoagulation in patients with RA- ILD has also been suggested in light of the increased risk of thrombosis associated with IPF (Hubbard et al., 2008). In the absence of empirical evidence, the decision to use anticoagulation should be made based on clinical risk assessment of each patient's individual risk factors and should not be initiated without direct guidance from a transplant centre in a patient being considered for lung transplantation.

3. Pulmonary inflammation and the pathogenesis of RA

RA has traditionally been conceptualized as an autoimmune disease of the synovium associated with an inappropriate excessive inflammatory response leading to systemic complications. Although the exact etiology of RA remains to be elucidated, it is now evident that RA's underlying pathophysiology is far more complex and extends beyond the traditional view that the disease begins in the synovium. Growing evidence suggest that the systemic inflammatory response and antibody formation precede synovial involvement and clinical symptoms of RA (van de Sande et al., 2011). In fact, antibodies associated with RA, including IgM rheumatoid factor and anti-citrullinated protein antibodies (ACPA) (a.k.a. anti-cyclic citrullinated protein, anti-CCP, antibodies) appear to be present in the serum of RA patients many years before the onset of clinical disease (Nielen et al., 2004, Rantapää-Dahlqvist et al., 2003).

The key to understanding the immunological processes believed to underlie the development of RA is the concept of citrullination. This refers to the post-translational modification of proteins whereby the amino acid arginine is de-aminated and converted to citrulline by the enzyme peptidylarginine deiminas (PAD) (Yamada et al., 2005). This conversion occurs intracellularly to affect the electrical charge of the protein, thereby altering its folding. In order to develop antibodies to citrullinated peptides, the immune system must be exposed to these altered proteins, which occurs following cell death, often incited by insult to the cell wall such as in the context of inflammation. The identity of citrullinated autoantigens is increasingly known, with the leading candidates for the development of RA being alpha-enolase, filaggren, and vimentin (Schellekens et al., 2000, van Venrooij WJ et al., 2008). Although it has been hypothesized that the primary tissue site of citrullination for development of RA is the joint (synovium), it is becoming increasingly recognized that other tissue sites may be involved in the pathogenesis of RA including the lung and oral mucosa (Bingham et al., 2010, Bongartz et al., 2007). In this section, we will highlight the mechanisms of how development of autoimmunity and RA is not restricted to processes in the joint and how pulmonary inflammation may incite the development of RA.

3.1 Genetic risk of pulmonary disease and of RA

Genetics is known to play an important role in the development of RA and its contribution is estimated to be around 30% and, in some studies, up to 60% (MacGregor et al., 2000). The strongest genetic association with RA has been mapped to a gene area on chromosome 6 known as the Human Leukocyte Antigen (HLA) locus (a.k.a. Major Histocompatibility Complex, MHC (Zanelli et al., 2000). These genes encode various proteins that play important immunological roles, including in the key distinction of self from foreign. Among the HLA loci, the HLA-DRB1 alleles have been shown to have strong association with RA

(Zanelli et al., 2000), although emerging data now also point to other loci, particularly HLA-DPB1, as independently conferring increased risk for ACPA-positive RA (Ding et al., 2009). Common to the multiple HLA-DRB1 alleles found to be associated with RA, is a shared amino-acid sequence, or motif, which was thus named the 'shared epitope' (SE) (Gregersen et al., 1987). The presence of SE alleles is known to be strongly associated with susceptibility to RA (du Montcel et al., 2005) and the presence of ACPA (Van der Helm-van Mil et al., 2006). The association between SE alleles and RA has been found to be significantly influenced by smoking, particularly, though not exclusively, in the presence of ACPA (Padyukov et al., 2004). Recent evidence suggests that the association between smoking and increased risk of ACPA-positive RA with SE alleles is dose-dependent, where individuals with over 20 pack-year smoking history have a 40 times increased risk of ACPA-positive RA if they carry the double SE alleles compared to non-smokers without the SE alleles (Källberg et al., 2011).

Finally, of note, existing evidence also suggest that certain other HLA-DR alleles, particularly HLA-DR4, are associated with the development of lung disease in RA patients, independent of smoking (Scott et al., 1987).

3.2 Importance of auto-antibodies to citrullinated peptides

In addition to being an apparent predictive marker for the development of RA, the presence of ACPA in patients also appear to be associated with a greater risk of developing extra-articular manifestations, including specifically lung serositis and pulmonary fibrosis (Alexiou et al., 2008, Turesson et al., 2007). Moreover, a recent study by Bongartz et al., (2007) included immunohistochemical examination of lung biopsies from 18 patients with RA-ILD and revealed the presence of citrullinated proteins in 8 (44%) of these patients (Bongartz et al., 2007). The exact identity of the citrullinated autoantigen was not identified; moreover, citrullination did not show any significant association with factors such as smoking, disease severity, histological subtype, degree of inflammation, or steroid use (Bongartz et al., 2007). The findings of citrullinated proteins in lung samples from non-RA patients with idiopathic ILD in the same study suggest that this process is not unique to RA and likely reflects a non-specific response to tissue injury and inflammation. The key difference, therefore, lies in the fact that, in RA patients, an aberrant immune response occurs by which ACPA are generated in response to these proteins, which in turn result in pathology. The challenge is then to identify the potential factors that might mediate this aberrant process.

3.3 Environmental triggers of pulmonary inflammation

Smoking has been firmly established as a causative agent in lung inflammation and injury. It has also been shown to be associated with both the development of RA, accounting for nearly 20% of the risk, and worse disease course of RA, even years after smoking cessation (Albano et al., 2001, Harrison, 2002). These two seemingly unrelated adverse effects of smoking on lung and RA are in fact intricately connected beyond the mere aggravated inflammatory response triggered by smoking. Smoking has been shown to be associated with an increase in pulmonary protein citrullination, which appears to be mediated by increase in PAD enzyme expression, particularly PAD2, in both parenchymal and bronchial tissue (Makrygiannakis et al., 2008). Moreover, as outlined previously (see section 3.1 Genetic risk of pulmonary disease and of RA) a strong, dose-dependent, association has been established between smoking and the presence of ACPA in RA patients (Källberg, et al., 2011). These findings point to a possible pathogenesis of pulmonary inflammation in RA patients in which ACPA react with the increased presence of citrullinated proteins in pulmonary tissue that were the result of pulmonary injury caused by environmental trigger such as smoking. Similar pathogenic processes were found with other environmental exposures such as silica (Stolt et al., 2010).

However, current evidence suggests that the interplay between synovium and lung is in fact far more complex. The findings of ACPA in ILD patients without clinical evidence of articular symptoms suggest that these antibodies can be generated independent of synovial involvement. This was further corroborated by a prospective study of ACPA-positive patients, who were found to have no radiological or histological evidence of synovial inflammation (van de Sande et al., 2011). In this study, 13 patients with positive RA serology (IgM rheumatoid factor and/or ACPA) but without clinical evidence of arthritis underwent knee MRI and arthroscopic synovial tissue biopsy with immuno-histochemistry testing. No significant differences were found when the results were compared to those obtained from a group of individuals with negative RA serology. After a median follow-up period of 3 months (range 1-6 months), 4 of these patients developed clinical evidence of arthritis. This demonstrated that the synovium in ACPA-positive patients is initially normal, even in patients who later develop clinical arthritis. In addition, existing evidence suggests that a proportion of patients with positive RA serology may already have HRCT parenchymal lung changes at time of RA diagnosis (Gabbay et al., 1997, Metafratzi et al., 2007, Reynsdottir et al., 2011). In fact, a retrospective study by Gizinski et al. (2009) showed that positive RA serology can be found in smokers with ILD without symptoms and signs of RA, but who may later develop RA. Therefore, clinicians assessing patients with positive RA serology but no articular symptoms should nevertheless inquire and be mindful of respiratory symptoms in these patients.

Taken together, these findings evoke a conceptual paradigm different from the long-held view of pulmonary inflammation being an extra-articular manifestation of synovial inflammation. In this paradigm, synovial inflammation is seen as a down-stream consequence of an aberrant immunological pulmonary process triggered by insults, such as smoking, that lead to the formation of ACPA. The ACPA, in turn, react to citrullinated proteins formed in the synovium due to a different, independent, insult such as mechanical or infectious joint injury (See figure 5). Further research is needed and is underway to elucidate this intricate interplay between the lung and the synovium as well as the possibility that such an interaction with the synovium may not only be limited to the lung.

3.4 Pre-RA and its clinical implications

The concept of 'early RA' has long been clinically utilized to denote patients in the early stages of the disease. However, the synovium of patients with 'early RA' already displays radiological (van der Heijde, 1995) and histological (Tak, 2001) evidence of chronic inflammation. Therefore, the concept of 'pre-RA' has been suggested to describe the time period before the onset of clinical signs and symptoms of synovial inflammation (van de Sande et al., 2011). During this time, patients may already have evidence of sub-clinical systemic inflammation, such as elevated non-specific inflammatory markers (e.g. C-reactive protein), and may be tested positive for the presence of ACPA. As previously described, the presence of ACPA can occur in the absence of synovial inflammation and may, in fact, precede clinical manifestation of arthritis by longer than a decade (Nielen et al., 2004). It is presumably during this time interval that the second, independent, injury occurs, which

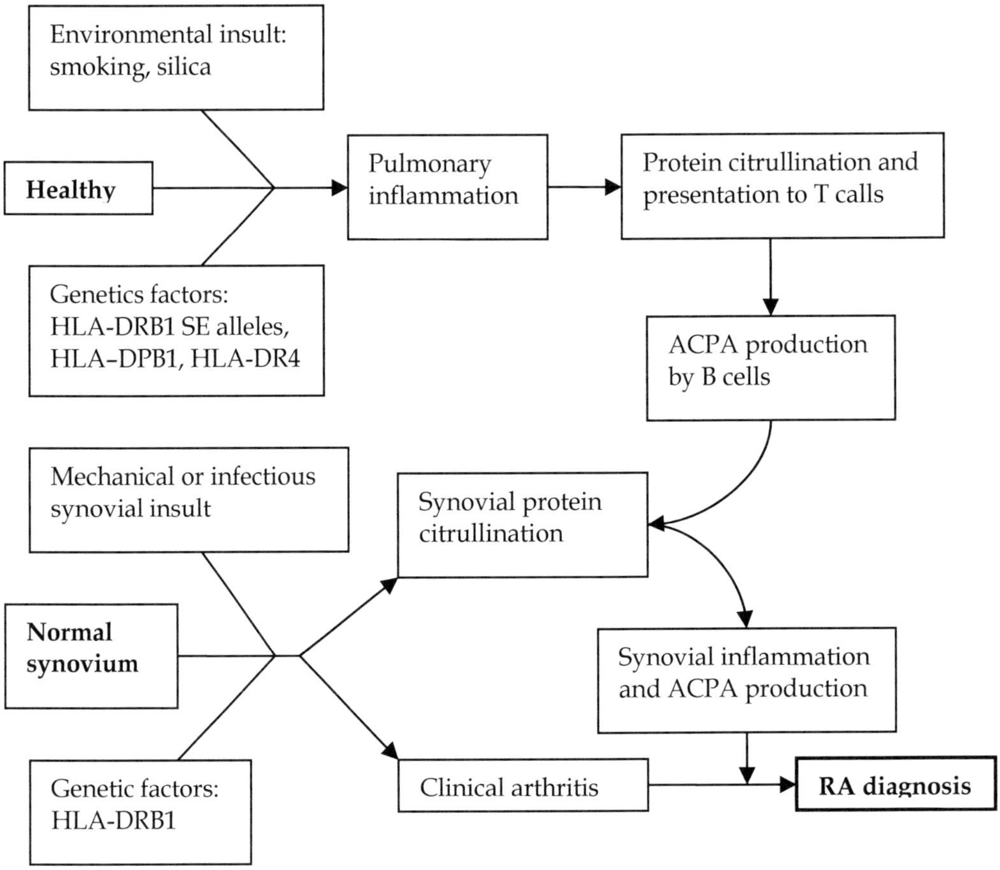

Fig. 5. The postulated interaction between genetics, environmental factors, pulmonary inflammation and protein citrullination in the pathogenesis of RA

leads to synovial protein citrullination and the resulting epitope spreading and development of synovial inflammation.

This multi-factorial model of RA development raises the potential for prevention, which may be aimed at averting, slowing, or potentially reversing the progression towards clinical RA. The first and foremost preventative measure based on the available evidence is avoidance of tobacco smoking. Since environmental exposures, such as smoking and silica inhalation, appear to play a key role in the initial formation of ACPA, avoidance of these triggers may potentially abort the development of RA in genetically susceptible individuals. Further research is necessary to better understand the initial development of ACPA and explore the potential for prevention, particularly in genetically susceptible individuals. The existence of a 'pre-RA' stage also provides an opportunity for potential pharmacological interventions that might prevent or delay the development of synovial inflammation. The identification of the second event that results in synovial protein citrullination should also be a focus of future research and preventative efforts.

The emerging evidence of the close interplay between the lungs and the synovium together with the growing recognition of the clinical significance of pulmonary complications in RA patients, including RA-ILD, suggest that RA patients may benefit from a multidisciplinary approach to their management. Although such collaboration appears to be most beneficial to RA patients with pulmonary complications, it may expand in the future to include patients with pulmonary inflammation at risk of RA by virtue of their genetics or ACPA presence, without yet having any articular manifestations.

4. Summary

Our understanding of RA and RA-ILD is quickly evolving in light of ongoing research. RA-ILD is increasingly recognized as a prevalent clinical entity with significant associated morbidity and mortality, which poses both diagnostic and therapeutic challenges to clinicians and calls for increased attention to pulmonary abnormalities in RA patients. In addition, as highlighted in this chapter, growing evidence also suggests that pulmonary inflammation plays an important role in the etiology of RA, particularly in autoantibody-positive patients, with evidence of lung injury preceding synovial inflammation. The complex interplay between the lung and the synovium remains to be further elucidated but it is clear that synovial inflammation can no longer be viewed as an isolated, independent process. The likely multi-factorial nature of this interplay not only raises the potential for new therapeutics targets in RA, but also raises the prospect for prevention. Furthermore, it also raises the question of whether similar complex interactions exist between the synovium and other organs. Future research is currently underway and would hopefully provide answers to these important questions, leading to a better understanding and management of RA.

5. Key points

1. RA is a common systemic inflammatory disorder affecting 1% of the general population
2. RA-ILD is a serious extra-articular manifestation that confers significant morbidity and mortality
3. Clinicians need to be vigilant to screen for respiratory signs and symptoms in RA patients as these may represent an underlying ILD
4. The diagnosis of RA-ILD can be made with HRCT but, in some cases, diagnostic uncertainty necessitates a surgical lung biopsy
5. UIP and NSIP are the most common histopathological patterns of RA-ILD
6. The treatment of RA-ILD is three-pronged, including education and transplant evaluation, supportive care and the use of immunosuppressive medications
7. Pulmonary inflammation, protein citrullination and the formation of auto-antibodies to citrullinated peptides may play a key role in the pathogenesis of RA
8. The interaction of genetics and environmental factors is fundamental to this process
9. Growing evidence point to a complex, multi-factorial interaction between the lung and the synovium, with lung injury preceding synovial inflammation
10. Further research is necessary to delineate this complex interplay and explore its clinical implications

6. Acknowledgment

Special thanks to Dr. David Hwang, department of pathology at the University of Toronto, for providing the histology images.

7. References

Albano SA, Santana-Sahagun E, & Weisman MH. (2001). Cigarette smoking and rheumatoid arthritis. *Semin Arthritis Rheum*, Vol.31, pp. 146–159.

Alexiou I, Germenis A, Koutroumpas A, Kontogianni A, Theodoridou K, & Sakkas L. (2008). Anti-cyclic citrullinated peptide-2 (CCP2) autoantibodies and extra-articular manifestations in Greek patients with rheumatoid arthritis. Clin Rheumatol, Vol. 27, pp. 511–513

Biederer J, A. Schnabel, C. Muhle, W. L. Gross, M. Heller, & M. Reuter. (2004). Correlation between HRCT findings, pulmonary function tests and bronchoalveolar lavage cytology in interstitial lung disease associated with rheumatoid arthritis. Eur Radiol, Vol. 14, pp.272–280

Bingham C, Reynolds M, Giles J, Felipe B, Fox-Talbot J, Halushka K, & Marc K. (2010). Citrullination and Peptidylarginine Deiminase (PAD) Expression Is Detected in the Oral Mucosa and Periodontium in the Absence of Rheumatoid Arthritis. Arthritis Rheum, Vol. 62 Suppl 10, pp. 1074

Bongartz T, Cantaert R, Atkins P, Harle J, Myers C, Turesson J, Ryu D, & and Matteson E. (2007). Citrullination in extra-articular manifestations of rheumatoid arthritis. *Rheumatology*, Vol. 46, pp. 70–75

Bongartz T, Nannini C, Medina-Velasquez Y, Achenbach S, Crowson C, Ryu J, Vassallo R, Gabriel S, & Matteson E. (2010). Incidence and Mortality of Interstitial Lung Disease in Rheumatoid Arthritis-A Population-Based Study. Arthritis & Rheumatism, Vol. 62, pp 1583–1591.

Bouros D, Nicholson A, Polychronopoulos V, du Bois R. Acute interstitial pneumonia (2000). *Eur Respir J* Vol. 15, pp. 412–418.

Brown K. (2007). Rheumatoid lung disease. Proc Am Thorac Soc, Vol. 4, pp.443–448.

Brulhart L, Waldburger JM, & Gabay C. (2006). Rituximab in the treatment of antisynthetase syndrome. *Ann Rheum Dis*, Vol. 65, pp. 974 -5

Chang HK, Park W, & Ryu DS. (2002). Successful treatment of progressive rheumatoid interstitial lung disease with cyclosporine: a case report. *J Korean Med Sci*, Vol.17, pp. 270-273

Collard H, Moore B, Flaherty K, Brown K, Kaner R, King T, Lasky J, Loyd J, Noth I, Olman M, Raghu G, Roman J, Ryu J, Zisman D, Hunninghake G, Colby T, Egan J, Hansell D, Johkoh T, Kaminski N, Kim D, Kondoh Y, Lynch D, Müller-Quernheim J, Myers J, Nicholson A, Selman M, Toews G, Wells A, & Martinez F. (2007). Acute Exacerbations of Idiopathic Pulmonary Fibrosis. Am. J. Respir. Crit. Care Med, Vol. 176, pp. 636-643

Cottin V, Nunes H, Mouthon L, Gamondes D, Lazor R, Hachulla E, Revel D, Valeyre D, & Cordier JF (2011). Combined Pulmonary Fibrosis and Emphysema Syndrome inConnective Tissue Disease. Arthritis & Rheumatism, Vol.63, pp. 295-304.

Cushley MJ, Davison AG, DuBois RM, Flower C, Greening A, Ibrahim N, Johnston I, Mitchell D, & Pickering A.(1999). The diagnosis, assessment and treatment of diffuse parenchymal lung disease in adults: British Thoracic Society recommendations. *Thorax*, Vol.54(suppl 1), pp.S1-14.

Dawson J, Fewins H, Desmond J, Lynch M, & Graham D. (2002). Predictors of progression of HRCT diagnosed fibrosing alveolitis in patients with rheumatoid arthritis. *Ann Rheum Dis*, Vol. 61, pp. 517–521

Demedts M, Behr J, Buhl R, Costabel U, Dekhuijzen R, Jansen H, MacNee W, Thomeer M, Wallaert B, Laurent F, Nicholson A, Verbeken E, Verschakelen J, Flower C, Capron F, Petruzzelli S, De Vuyst P, van den Bosch J, Rodriguez-Becerra E, Corvasce G, Lankhorst I, Sardina M, & Montanari M. (2005). High-dose acetylcysteine in idiopathic pulmonary fi brosis. *N Engl J Med*, Vol. 353, pp. 2229 -2242

Ding B, Padyukov L, Lundström E, Seielstad M, Plenge R, Oksenberg J, Gregersen P, Alfredsson L, & Klareskog L. (2009). Different Patterns of Associations With Anti-Citrullinated Protein Antibody-Positive and Anti-Citrullinated Protein Antibody-Negative Rheumatoid Arthritis in the Extended Major Histocompatibility Complex Region. *Arthritis Rheum*, Vol. 60, pp. 30–38.

Distler J, Manger B, Spriewald B, Schett G,& Distler O. (2008). Treatment of pulmonary fibrosis for 20 weeks with imatinib mesylate in a patient with mixed connective tissue disease. *Arthritis Rheum*, Vol. 58, pp. 2538-2542

Dixon W, Hyrich K, Watson K, Lunt M, BSRBR Control Centre Consortium, & Symmons D. (2010). Influence of anti-TNF therapy on mortality in patients with rheumatoid arthritis-associated interstitial lung disease: results from the British Society for Rheumatology Biologics Register. *Ann Rheum Dis*, Vol.69, pp. 1086–1091

du Montcel S, Michou L, Petit-Teixeira E, Osorio J, Lemaire I, Lasbleiz S, Pierlot C,Quillet P, Bardin T,Prum B, Cornelis F, & Clerget-Darpoux F. (2005). New Classification of HLA-DRB1 Alleles Supports the Shared Epitope Hypothesis of Rheumatoid Arthritis Susceptibility. Arthritis&Rheumatism, Vol. 52, pp. 1063–1068

Gabbay E, Tarala R, Will R, Carroll G, Adler B, Cameron D, & Lake F. (1997). Interstitial Lung Disease in Recent Onset Rheumatoid Arthritis. *Am J Respir Crit Care Med*, Vol. 156, pp. 528–535.

Gabriel SE. (2001). The epidemiology of rheumatoid arthritis. *Rheum Dis Clin North Am*, Vol. 27, pp. 269–281

Gizinski AM, Mascolo M, Loucks JL, Kervitsky A, Meehan RT, Brown KK, Holers V, & Deane KD. (2009). Rheumatoid arthritis (RA)-specific autoantibodies in patients with interstitial lung disease and absence of clinically apparent articular RA. *Clin Rheumatol*, Vol. 28, pp. 611-613.

Gochuico BR, Avila NA, Chow CK, Novero LJ, Wu HP, Ren P, MacDonald SD, Travis WD, Stylianou MP, & Rosas IO.(2008). Progressive preclinical interstitial lung disease in rheumatoid arthritis. Arch Intern Med, Vol. 168, pp. 159-166

Goh N, Desai S, Veeraraghavan S, Hansell D, Copley S, Maher T, Corte T, Sander C, Ratoff J, Devaraj A, Bozovic G, Denton C, Black C, du Bois R, & Well A. (2008). Interstitial Lung Disease in Systemic Sclerosis: a Simple Staging System. A*m J Respir Crit Care Med*, Vol. 177, pp. 1248 - 1254.

Gregersen PK, Silver J, & Winchester RJ. (1987). The shared epitope hypothesis: an approach to understanding the molecular genetics of susceptibility to rheumatoid arthritis [current comment]. Arthritis Rheum, Vol. 30, pp.1205–1213.

Hakala, M. (1988) Poor Prognosis in Patients with Rheumatoid Arthritis Hospitalized for Interstitial Lung Fibrosis. *Chest*, Vol. 93, pp. 114-118.

Hansen JE, Sue DY, & Wasserman K (1984). Predicted values for clinical exercise testing. *Am Rev Respir Dis*, Vol. 129(Suppl), pp. S49-S55.

Harrison BJ. (2002). Influence of cigarette smoking on disease outcome in rheumatoid arthritis. *Curr Opin* Rheumatol, Vol. 14, pp. 246–252.

Hartman T, Swensen S, Hansell D, Colby T, Myers J, Tazelaar H, Nicholson A, Wells A, Ryu J, Midthun D, du Bois R, & Mu¨ller N (2000). Nonspecific interstitial pneumonia: variable appearance at high-resolution chest CT. *Radiology* Vol. 217, pp. 701–705

Hilliquin P, Renoux M, Perrot S, Puéchal X, & Menkès CJ (1996). Occurrence of pulmonary complications during methotrexate therapy in rheumatoid arthritis. *Br J Rheumatol.* Vol. 35, pp. 441-445.

Hoyles RK, Ellis RW, Wellsbury J, Lees B, Newlands P, Goh NS, Roberts C, Desai S, Herrick AL, McHugh NJ, Foley NM, Pearson SB, Emery P, Veale DJ, Denton CP, Wells AU, Black CM, & du Bois RM. (2006). A multicenter, prospective, randomized, double-blind, placebo-controlled trial of corticosteroids and intravenous cyclophosphamide followed by oral azathioprine for the treatment of pulmonary fibrosis in scleroderma. *Arthritis Rheum*, Vol. 54, pp. 3962-3970.

Hubbard R, Smith C, Le-Jeune I, Gribbin J, & Fogarty A. (2008). The Association between Idiopathic Pulmonary Fibrosis and Vascular Disease A Population-based Study. Am J Respir Crit Care Med, Vol. 178, pp. 1257-1261

Imokawa S, Colby T, Leslie K, & Helmers R. (2000). Methotrexate pneumonitis: review of the literature and histopathological findings in nine patients. *Eur Respir J*, Vol. 15, pp. 373-381

Jadon D, Chan A, & McNally J.(2008). Life threatening leflunomide pneumonitis in a patient on rituximab. *Rheumatology*, Vol. 47(2), ii158 (no. 549)

Källberg H, Ding B, Padyukov L, Bengtsson C, Rönnelid J, Klareskog L,& Alfredsson L. (2011). Smoking is a major preventable risk factor for rheumatoid arthritis: estimations of risks after various exposures to cigarette smoke. *Ann Rheum Dis*, Vol. 70, pp. 508-511

Katzenstein AL, Myers JL, & Mazur MT. Acute interstitial pneumonia. A clinicopathologic, ultrastructural, and cell kinetic study. (1986) *Am J Surg Pathol* Vol. 10, pp. 256–267.

Katzenstein AL & Myers JL. (1998). Idiopathic pulmonary fibrosis: clinical relevance of pathologic classification. *Am J Respir Crit Care* Med, Vol. 157, pp. 1301–1315.

Kelly C & Saravanan V. (2008). Treatment strategies for a rheumatoid arthritis patient with interstitial lung disease. *Expert Opin. Pharmacothe*, Vol. 9, pp. 3221-3230.

Kremer JM, Alarcón GS, Weinblatt ME, Kaymakcian MV, Macaluso M, Cannon GW, Palmer WR, Sundy JS, St Clair EW, Alexander RW, Smith GJ, & Axiotis CA. (1997). Clinical, laboratory, radiographic, and histopathologic features of methotrexate-associated lung injury in patients with rheumatoid arthritis: a multicenter study with literature review. *Arthritis Rheum*. Vol. 40, pp. 1829-1837.

Lee HK, Kim DS, Yoo B, Seo J, Rho J, Colby T, & Kitaichi M. (2005). Histopathologic pattern and clinical features of rheumatoid arthritis-associated interstitial lung disease. *Chest*, Vol. 127, pp. 2019–2027

Leon RJ, Gonsalvo A, Salas R, & Hidalgo NC. (2004). Rituximab-induced acute pulmonary fibrosis. *Mayo Clin Proc*, Vol. 79, pp. 945 -56

MacDonald SLS, Rubens MB, Hansell DM, Copley SJ, Desai SR, du Bois RM, Nicholson AG, Colby TV, & Wells AU. (2001) Nonspecific interstitial pneumonia and usual interstitial pnuemonia: comparative appearances at and diagnostic accuracy of thin-section CT. Radiology Vol. 221, pp. 600–605.

MacGregor AJ, Snieder H, Rigby AS, Koskenvuo M, Kaprio J, Aho K, & Silman AJ. (2000). Characterizing the quantitative genetic contribution to rheumatoid arthritis using data from twins. *Arthritis Rheum*, Vol. 43, pp. 30-37.

Makrygiannakis D, Hermansson M, Ulfgren AK, Nicholas AP, Zendman AJ, Eklund A, Grunewald J, Skold CM, Klareskog L, & Catrina AI. (2008). Smoking increases peptidylarginine deiminase 2 enzyme expression in human lungs and increases citrullination in BAL cells. *Ann Rheum Dis*, Vol. 67, pp.1488-1492.

Manjunatha Y, Seith A, Kandpal H, & Das C. (2010). Rheumatoid Arthritis: Spectrum of Computed Tomographic Findings in Pulmonary Diseases. *Curr Probl Diagn Radiol*, Vol. 39, pp. 235-246.

Maradit-Kremers H, Nicola PJ, Crowson CS, Ballman KV, & Gabriel SE. (2005) Cardiovascular death in rheumatoid arthritis: a population-based study. *Arthritis Rheum*, Vol. 52, pp. 722–732.

Martinez F. (2006). Idiopathic Interstitial PneumoniasUsual Interstitial Pneumonia versus Nonspecific Interstitial Pneumonia. *Proc Am Thorac Soc*, Vol. 3, pp 81–95.

Metafratzi Z, Georgiadis A, Ioannidou C, Alamanos Y, Vassiliou M, Zikou A, Raptis G, Drosos A, & Efremidis S. (2007). Pulmonary involvement in patients with early rheumatoid arthritis. *Scandinavian Journal of Rheumatology*, Vol. 36, pp. 338-344

Minaur NJ, Jacoby RK, Cosh JA, Taylor G, & Rasker JJ. (2004) Outcome after 40 years with rheumatoid arthritis: a prospective study of function, disease activity, and mortality. *J Rheumatol Suppl*, Vol.69, pp.3–8.

Nannini C, Ryu JH, & Matteson EL. (2008). Lung disease in rheumatoid arthritis. *Curr Opin Rheumatol*, Vol. 20, pp. 340–346

Nielen M, van Schaardenburg D, Reesink H, van de Stadt R, van der Horst-Bruinsma I, de Koning M, Habibuw M, Vandenbroucke J, & Dijkmans B.*(2004)*. Specific autoantibodies precede the symptoms of rheumatoid arthritis: a study of serial measurements in blood donors. *Arthritis Rheum*, Vol. 50, pp. 380 -386.

Orens J, Estenne M, Arcasoy S, Conte J, Corris P, Egan J, Egan T, Keshavjee S, Knoop S, Kotloff R, Martinez F, Nathan S, Palmer S, Patterson A, Singer L, Snell G, Studer S, Vachiery J, & Glanville A. (2006). International Guidelines for the Selection of Lung Transplant Candidates: 2006 Update—A Consensus Report From the Pulmonary Scientific Council of the International Society for Heart and Lung Transplantation. J Heart Lung Transplant, Vol. 25, pp. 745–755

Padyukov L, Silva C, Stolt P, Alfredsson L, & Klareskog L. (2004). A Gene–Environment Interaction Between Smoking and Shared Epitope Genes in HLA–DR Provides a High Risk of Seropositive Rheumatoid Arthritis. *Arthritis&Rheumatism*, Vol. 50, pp. 3085–3092

Pappas D, Giles J, Connors G, Lechtzin N, Bathon J, & Danoff S. (2010). Respiratory symptoms and disease characteristics as predictors of pulmonary function abnormalities in patients with rheumatoid arthritis: an observational cohort study. *Arthritis Research & Therapy* , Vol. 12, pp. R104-114.

Parambi J, Myers J, & Ryu J. (2006) Diffuse Alveolar Damage: Uncommon Manifestation of Pulmonary Involvement in Patients With Connective Tissue Diseases. *Chest* Vol. 130, pp. 553-558

Park H, Kim S, Park N, Jang S, Kitaichi M, Nicholson A, & Colby T. (2007a). Prognosis of fibrotic interstitial pneumonia: idiopathic versus collagen vascular disease-related subtypes. Am J Respir Crit Care Med, Vol. 175, pp.705–711

Park IN, Kim D, Shim T, Lim C, Lee S, Koh Y, Kim WS, Kim WD, Jang S, & Colby T. (2007b). Acute exacerbation of interstitial pneumonia other than idiopathic pulmonary fibrosis. *Chest*, Vol.132, pp. 214–220

Parra E, Kairalla R, Ribeiro de Carvalho C, Eher E, & Capelozzi V. (2007) Inflammatory Cell Phenotyping of the Pulmonary Interstitium in Idiopathic Interstitial Pneumonia. Respiration Vol. 74 pp.159–169

Raghu G, Collard H, Egan J, Martinez F, Behr J, Brown K, Colby T, Cordier J, Flaherty K, Lasky J, Lynch D, Ryu J, Swigris J, Wells A, Ancochea J, Bouros D, Carvalho C, Costabel U, Ebina M, Hansell D, Johkoh T, Kim D, King T, Kondoh Y, Myers J, Mu¨ller N, Nicholson A, Richeldi L, Selman M, Dudden R, Griss B, Protzko S, & Schu¨nemann H. (2011). An Official ATS/ERS/JRS/ALAT Statement: Idiopathic Pulmonary Fibrosis: Evidence-based Guidelines for Diagnosis and Management. Am J Respir Crit Care Med, Vol. 183, pp. 788–824

Rajasekaran B, Shovlin D, Lord P, & Kelly C. (2001) Interstitial lung disease in patients with rheumatoid arthritis: a comparison with cryptogenic fibrosing alveolitis. *Rheumatology*, Vol.40, pp. 1022-1025.

Rantapaa-Dahlqvist S, de Jong B, Berglin E, Hallmans G, Wadell G, Stenlund H, Sundin U, & van Venrooij W. (2003). Antibodies against cyclic citrullinated peptide and IgA rheumatoid factor predict the development of rheumatoid arthritis. *Arthritis Rheum*, Vol. 48, pp. 2741 - 2749.

Reynsdottir G, Harju A, Engström M, Nyren S, Sköld M, Eklund A, Grunewald J, Klareskog L, & Catrina A. (2011). Lung changes are present in ACPA positive RA patients already at disease onset. *Ann Rheum Dis*, Vol. 70(Suppl 2), pp. A13

Saketkoo L & Espinoza L. (2008). Rheumatoid Arthritis Interstitial Lung Disease: Mycophenolate Mofetil as an Antifibrotic and Disease-Modifying Antirheumatic Drug. Arch Intern Med, Vol. 168, pp. 1718

Schellekens GA, Visser H, de Jong BA, van den Hoogen FH, Hazes JM, Breedveld FC, & van Venrooij WJ. (2000). The diagnostic properties of rheumatoid arthritis antibodies recognizing a cyclic citrullinated peptide. *Arthritis Rheum*, Vol.43, pp.155-163

Scott TE, Wise RA, Hochberg MC, & Wigley FM. (1987). HLA-DR4 and pulmonary dysfunction in rheumatoid arthritis. *Am J Med*, Vol. 82, pp. 765-771

Segura A, Yuste A, Cercos A, López-Tendero P, Gironés R, Pérez-Fidalgo JA, & Herranz C (2001). Pulmonary fibrosis induced by cyclophosphamide. *Ann Pharmacother*. Vol. 35, pp. 894-897

Stasi R, Stipa E, Del Poeta G, Amadori S, Newland A, & Provan D. (2006). Long-term observation of patients with anti-neutrophil cytoplasmic antibody-associated vasculitis treated with rituximab. *Rheumatology*, Vol. 45, pp.1432-1436

St Clair EW, Rice JR, & Snyderman R (1985). Pneumonitis complicating low-dose methotrexate therapy in rheumatoid arthritis. *Arch Intern Med*. Vol. 145, pp. 2035-2038.

Stolt P, Yahya A, Bengtsson C, Källberg H, Rönnelid J, Lundberg I, Klareskog L, & Alfredsson L. (2010). Silica exposure among male current smokers is associated with a high risk of developing ACPA-positive rheumatoid arthritis. *Ann Rheum Dis*, Vol. 69, pp. 1072-1076.

Suzuki A, Ohosone Y, Obana M, Mita S, Matsuoka Y, Irimajiri S, & Fukuda J. (1994) Cause of death in 81 autopsied patients with rheumatoid arthritis.*J Rheumatol, Vol.* 21, pp. 33–36.

Swierkot J, & Szechiński J. (2006). Methotrexate in rheumatoid arthritis. *Pharmacol Rep*, Vol. 58, pp. 473-492.

Swigris JJ, Olson AL, Fischer A, Lynch DA, Cosgrove GP, Frankel SK, Meehan RT, & Brown KK. (2006). Mycophenolate mofetil is safe, well tolerated, and preserves lung function in patients with connective tissue disease-related interstitial lung disease. *Chest*, Vol. 130, pp. 30-36.

Tak PP. (2001). Is early rheumatoid arthritis the same disease process as late rheumatoid arthritis? *Best Pract Res Clin Rheumatol*, Vol. 15, pp.17 - 26.

Travis WD, Matsui K, Moss JE, & Ferrans VJ. (2000). Idiopathic nonspecific interstitial pneumonia: prognostic significance of cellular and fibrosing patterns. Survival comparison with usual interstitial pneumonia and desquamative interstitial pneumonia. *Am J Surg* Pathol, Vol. 24, pp. 19–33.

Turesson C, Jacobsson L, Sturfelt G, Matteson E, Mathsson L, & Rönnelid J. (2007). Rheumatoid factor and antibodies to cyclic citrullinated peptides are associated with severe extra-articular manifestations in rheumatoid arthritis. Ann Rheum Dis, Vol. 66, pp.59–64

van der Heijde DM. (1995). Joint erosions and patients with early rheumatoid arthritis. *Br J* Rheumatol, Vol. 34 (Suppl 2): 74 - 78

Van der Helm-van Mil AH, Verpoort KN, Breedveld FC, Huizinga TW, Toes RE, & de Vries RR. (2006). The HLA–DRB1 shared epitope alleles are primarily a risk factor for anti–cyclic citrullinated peptide antibodies and are not an independent risk factor for development of rheumatoid arthritis. Arthritis Rheum, Vol. 54, pp. 1117–1121.

van de Sande M, de Hair M, van der Leij C, Klarenbeek P, Bos W, Smith M, Maas M, de Vries N, van Schaardenburg D, Dijkmans B, Gerlag D, & Tak P. (2011). Different stages of rheumatoid arthritis: features of the synovium in the preclinical phase. *Ann Rheum Dis*, Vol. 70, pp. 772–777

van Venrooij W, van Beers J, & Pruijn G. (2008). Anti-CCP Antibody, a Marker for the Early Detection of Rheumatoid Arthritis. *Ann N Y Acad Sci*, Vol.1143, pp.268-285

Vourlekis JS, Brown KK, Cool CD, Young DA, Cherniack RM, King TE Jr, & Schwarz MI. (2000). Acute Interstitial Pneumonitis. Case series and review of the literature. *Medicine (Baltimore)* Vol. 79, pp. 369–378.

Yale S, & Limper A. (1996). Pneumocystis carinii pneumonia in patients without human immunodeficiency syndrome: associated illness and prior corticosteroid therapy. *Mayo Clin Proc*, Vol.71, pp. 5-13

Yamada R, Suzuki A, Chang X, & Yamamoto K. (2005). Citrullinated proteins in rheumatoid arthritis. . *Front Biosci*, Vol. 10, pp. 54-64.

Yoshinouchi T, Ohtsuki Y,Fujita J, Yamadori I, Bandoh S, Ishida T, & Ueda R.

(2005). Nonspecific interstitial pneumonia pattern as pulmonary involvement of rheumatoid arthritis. *Rheumatol Int*, Vol. 26, pp. 121–125

Zamora AC, Wolters PJ, Collard HR, Connolly MK, Elicker BM, Webb WR, King TE Jr, Golden JA (2008). Use of mycophenolate mofetil to treat scleroderma-associated interstitial lung Disease. *Respir Med*, Vol. 102, pp.150-155.

Zanelli E, Breedveld FC, & de Vries RR. (2000). HLA class II association with rheumatoid arthritis: facts and interpretations. Hum Immunol, Vol. 61, pp. 1254–1261.

Zhang D & Liu Y. (2010). Surgical Lung Biopsies in 418 Patients with SuspectedInterstitial Lung Disease in China. *Inter Med*, Vol. 49, pp. 1097-1102

6

Juvenile Spondyloarthritis

Miroslav Harjaček[1], Lovro Lamot[1],
Lana Tambić Bukovac[1], Mandica Vidović[1] and Rik Joos[2]
[1]*Division of Rheumatology, Children's Hospital Srebnjak, Zagreb*
[2]*Division of Rheumatology, University Hospital Gent, Gent*
[1]*Croatia*
[2]*Belgium*

1. Introduction

Spondyloarthritis (SpA) is one of the most common chronic rheumatic diseases, with a prevalence of 0.3% in Western Europe (Braun, Bollow et al. 1998; Andersson Gare 1999; Saraux, Guedes et al. 1999; Fernandez-Sueiro, Alonso et al. 2004). Juvenile spondyloarthritis (jSpA) is a term that refers to a group of inflammatory disorders affecting children under the age of 16 years, with common clinical characteristics, all more or less HLA B27 associated, producing a continuum of clinical symptoms through adulthood. These diseases are characterized by enthesitis and arthritis affecting the joints of the lower extremities and seronegativity for IgM rheumatoid factor and antinuclear antibodies (Amor, Dougados et al. 1990; Dougados, van der Linden et al. 1991; Boyer, Templin et al. 1993; Fink 1995; Cury, Vilar et al. 1997; Petty, Southwood et al. 1998; Burgos-Vargas, Rudwaleit et al. 2002; Petty, Southwood et al. 2004; Heuft-Dorenbosch, Landewe et al. 2007; Colbert 2010). The SpA often begins as 'undifferentiated' disease, the presentation of which differs in children and adults; most notably, spinal involvement is uncommon, while hip arthritis is frequently seen in juvenile-onset disease. The SpA family of diseases includes ankylosing spondylitis (AS), reactive arthritis (ReA), psoriatic arthritis (PsA), arthritis associated with inflammatory bowel disease (IBD), undifferentiated SpA and a juvenile form of SpA. The latter are under ILAR (The International League of Associations for Rheumatology) classification of juvenile idiopathic arthritis (JIA) classified as enthesitis-related arthritis (ERA) or psoriatic arthritis (Petty, Southwood et al. 2004) Possible differences in the synovial immunopathologic features of jSpA, when compared to adult patients with SpA will be discussed. In addition, increasing evidence suggests that an anatomical zone referred to as the enthesis is a primary target of the pathological process. Genetic and environmental factors play important roles in the pathogenesis of the SpA, and will be discussed extensively. An update on treatment, as well pharmacological and physical therapies, will be made.

2. Epidemiology

The prevalence of spondyloarthritis among whites is estimated at 0.7 to 1.2%, and the female-to-male ratio is 1:2 (Rutkowska-Sak, Slowinska et al. 2010).

Estimates of the prevalence of juvenile SpA, and ERA specifically, are based on figures for juvenile arthritis, which vary considerably depending on geographic location and case definition (Colbert 2010). The worldwide prevalence of juvenile arthritis is reported between 7 and 400 per 100,000 children (0.007% to 0.4%), although the latter figure seems to be an outlier overestimating the number of cases (Manners and Bower 2002). ERA and PsA each comprise 2- 11% of those cases, which would give an estimated combined total of 0.28–88 cases per 100,000 children. Whether these figures include juvenile AS is not clear. The frequency of childhood-onset among AS patients, is estimated between one and nine percent, (Gomez, Raza et al. 1997; Hofer and Southwood 2002). In Croatian children, frequency of jSpA among other rheumatic diseases was 8.2% (Prutki, Tambic Bukovac et al. 2008). These data are similar to the results of American, Canadian and British studies where approximately 7.9 - 9.8 of all children referred to the pediatric rheumatology clinics were children with jSpA (Bowyer and Roettcher 1996; Malleson, Fung et al. 1996; Symmons, Jones et al. 1996). SpA is seen in approximately 20% of first-degree relatives of patients with jSpA (Burgos-Vargas, 2002).

3. Immunopathogenesis

In this section the actual knowledge on immunopathogenesis in SpA is discussed and was possible with referral to juvenile disease.

SpA is a multifactorial disease in which a disturbed interplay occurs between the immune system and environmental factors on a predisposing genetic background. One of the predisposing environmental factors could be bacterial infection. There is a well established association with different enteric pathogens (Schiellerup, Krogfelt et al. 2008) but also with Chlamydia (Gerard, Whittum-Hudson et al. 2010) and Clostridium (Birnbaum, Bartlett et al. 2008). In juvenile patients we found a relationship with *Mycoplasma pneumoniae* infection (Harjacek, Ostojic et al. 2006),.

Whether a key role is reserved for the innate immunity or the adaptive immune system or both is still not clear.

3.1 What is the possible role of the adaptive immune system?

Cellular infiltrates in SpA patients are localized at the sacroiliac joints, the synovium and the entheseal structures. The inifltrates are characterized by the presence of both CD4+ and CD8+ T lymphocytes, as well as B cells and macrophages (Saxena, Aggarwal et al. 2005; Singh, Aggarwal et al. 2007; Melis and Elewaut 2009). These infiltrated T cells are activated and require the active participation of costimulation pathways to play their role.

Dendritic cells (DCs) play a key role in discriminating between commensal microorganisms and potentially harmful pathogens as well as in maintaining the balance between tolerance and active immunity (Evans, Suddason et al. 2007). DCs as antigen-presenting cells, induce primary T cell activation. Upon activation, expansion, and maturation effector T helper (Th) cells derive from progenitor, naive CD4+ T cells. Committed CD4+ T cells may differentiate into Th1, Th2, Th 17 phenotypes (the effector Th cell triad), with distinct cytokine products and biological functions. They can also evolve into the inducible regulatory T (Treg) lineage, with immunomodulatory functions.

Treg's are important in the maintenance of immune homeostasis. Defects in Treg function or reduced numbers have been documented in several human autoimmune diseases, including RA and JIA (Nistala and Wedderburn 2009).

In patients with undifferentiated spondyloarthritis (e.g. ERA) the number of peripheral blood Th1, Th2, Th17, and Treg cells were found unchanged, but Th1 and Th17 cells were increased, and Th2 cells were reduced in the synovial fluid (SF) compared to blood. It appears that elevated levels of pro-inflammatory cytokines IL-1 and IL-6 in the SF may be responsible for increased Th17 cells in those patients (Mahendra, Misra et al. 2009).

3.2 What is the possible role of the innate immune system?

Accumulating evidence suggests that the majority of the IL-17 released in SpA arthritis is produced by innate immune cells rather than T cells, suggesting that the innate immune pathway might be of greater relevance than the Th17 mediated adaptive immune response in those patients (see below) (Appel, Maier et al. 2011).

In juvenile arthritis some differences in cytokine profile were noted compared to adults:

- SF levels of IL-1ss and IL-12p40 are increased in both Poly-JIA and ERA as compared to RA;
- IL-6 levels were higher in ERA compared to RA;
- the increase in IFN-g in children with ERA with undetectable IL-4 suggests a Th1-dominant immune response in this disease subset;
- additive or even synergistic effects with IL-1 and TNF-alpha in inducing cytokine expression and joint damage have been shown in vitro and in vivo;
- ERA patients with an antigen-specific response to pathogenic enteric bacteria had a higher ratio of SF/blood integrin, (CD103+) Treg's compared to those with no antigen-specific response. In those patients antigen-specific as well as mitogen-stimulated cytokine production showed a clear Th1 bias (Saxena, Misra et al. 2006).

Microbes initiate immune responses through Toll-like receptors (TLRs). TLRs are membrane-bound and frontline guardians in the human innate immune system. They primarily function to recognize pathogen-associated molecular patterns (PAMPs) of invading microorganisms, and on activation mount rapid, nonspecific innate responses and trigger sequential delayed specific adaptive cellular responses, which are mediated by complex signal transduction pathways involving adaptor molecules, costimulatory ligands and receptors, kinases, transcription factors, and modulated gene expression (Drexler and Foxwell 2010). Toll-like receptor 4 (TLR4) is a member of the Toll-like receptor family, and activation of the TLR4 signalling pathway may induce the release of proinflammatory cytokines such as tumour necrosis factor (TNF)-alpha and interleukin (IL)-12, which was considered to play an important role in pathogenesis of SpA. Serum TLR4 protein and mRNA levels, as well as *TLR-4* gene expression were found to be significantly higher in AS patients than in healthy controls (Yang, Liang et al. 2007; Assassi, Reveille et al. 2011). A bacterial trigger possibly causes disease exacerbation in ERA patients. A recent study has shown that increased TLR-2 and TLR-4 expression on PBMCs and SFMCs may recognize microbial/endogenous ligands and up-regulate IL-6 and MMP-3 leading to disease exacerbation (Myles and Aggarwal 2011).

3.3 Cartilage and bone destruction and bone remodeling

In chronic synovitis, cartilage and bone destruction occur as a consequence of synovial inflammation. Bone remodeling is a lifelong continuous process conducted by osteoblasts, synthesizing bone matrix, and its resorption by osteoclasts. Important regulators of osteoclast recruitment and function are the three key molecules Osteoprotegerin (OPG),

Receptor Activator of Nuclear factor -κB (RANK) and its ligand (RANKL). RANKL stimulates osteoclast production and survival via the membrane-bound receptor RANK, while OPG inhibits osteoclast differentiation and activation due to its function as a non-signaling decoy receptor for RANKL (Simonet, Lacey et al. 1997). The physiological balance between RANKL and OPG is regulated by various calcitropic cytokines and hormones, and alterations in their ratio are critical in the pathogenesis of bone diseases (Hofbauer and Schoppet 2004). Osteoblasts and T cells are important producer cells of RANKL. An inflammatory environment with T-cell activation may tilt the balance between OPG and RANKL and increase osteoclast activation and bone resorption. In SF of children ERA patients elevated soluble RANKL (sRANKL), reduced OPG levels, and elevated sRANKL/OPG ratio was found, resulting in an environment associated with bone loss (Schett 2009). Furthermore, ERA patients had a lower matrix metalloproteinase (MMP) level as well as a lower MMP/TIMP (tissue metalloproteinase inhibitors) ratio compared to poly JIA, which may partly explain the lesser degree of joint damage seen in ERA, as compared to poly JIA (Agarwal, Misra et al. 2009). In AS, a chronic and most severe form of SpA inflammation is associated with trabecular bone loss leading to osteoporosis, but also with cortical new bone formation (e.g. formation of bone spurs, such as syndesmophytes and enthesiophytes) leading to progressive ankylosis of the spine and sacroiliac joints. Excessive bone formation in AS leads to ankylosis of joints and poor physical function (Figure 1). This results in an apparent paradox of bone formation and loss taking place at sites closely located to each other. Osteoporosis can be explained by the impact of inflammation on the bone remodeling cycle. In contrast, new bone formation has been linked to aberrant activation of bone morphogenic protein (BMP) and Wingless-type like (WNT) signaling. (Figure 1 and Figure 2) (Lories, Derese et al. 2005; Lories, Luyten et al. 2009; Carter and Lories 2011). By contrast, tumor necrosis factor (TNF) does not appear to be the direct trigger for osteophyte formation in AS (Schett and Rudwaleit 2010).

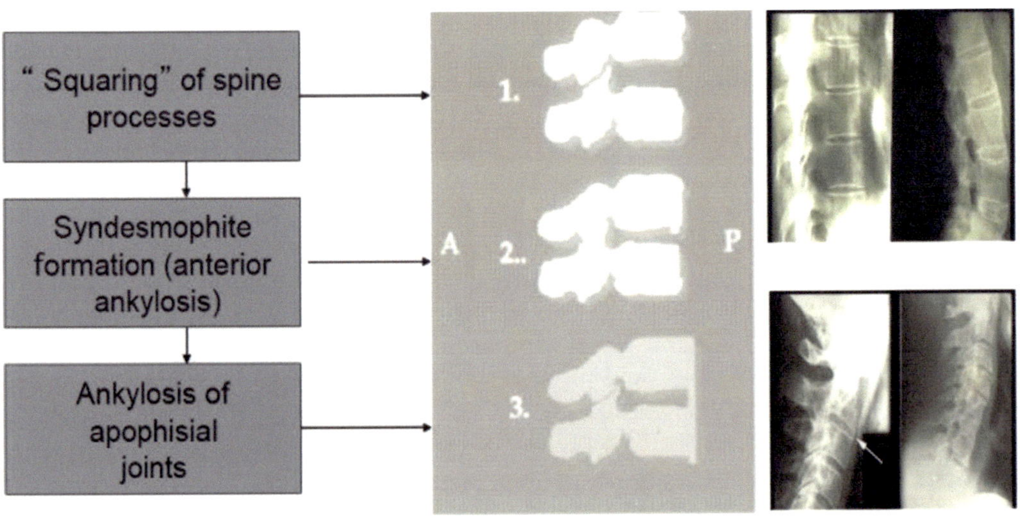

1. " Squaring" of spine processes; 2. Syndesmophyite formation (*anterior ankylosis*); 3. Ankylosis of apophyisial joints.

Fig. 1. The evolution of spine changes in jSpA patients with corresponding X-rays.

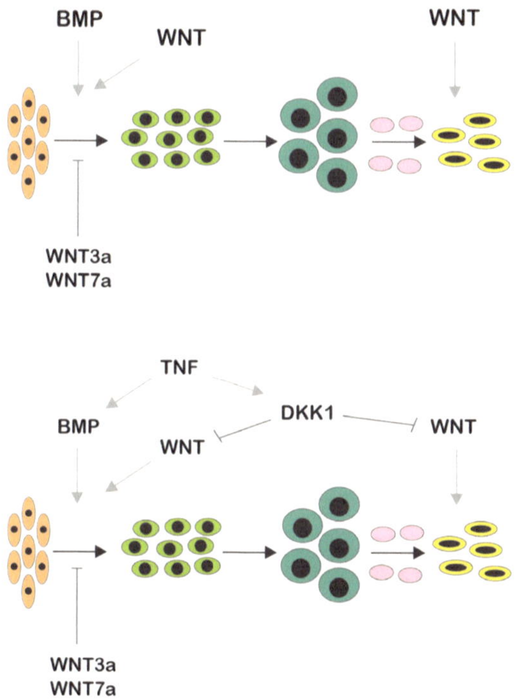

(a) Physiological endochondral bone formation is stimulated by bone morphogenetic proteins (BMPs). Wingless-type like (WNT) signaling plays a supportive role in relation to BMPs. However, some WNTs have a negative effect on early chondrocyte differentiation. **(b)** In the presence of inflammation, tumor necrosis factor (TNF) may stimulate BMP signaling but also the expression of DKK1, which acts a WNT antagonist. The balance between TNF, BMP and WNT signaling may determine the onset and progression of ankylosis. DKK, dickkopf. (Adapted from Arthritis Res Ther. 2009; 11(2): 221.Published online 2009 April 27. doi: 10.1186/ar2642.)

Fig. 2. Roles of BMPs and WNTs in ankylosis

3.4 Subclinical gut inflammation

Subclinical gut inflammation has been demonstrated in patients with all forms of SpA (Mielants, De Vos et al. 1996). In addition, several lines of evidence indicate that SpA may originate from the relocation to the joints of the immune process primarily induced in the gut (Fantini, Pallone et al. 2009). The transfer of the intestinal inflammatory process into the joints implicates that immune cells activated in the gut-draining lymph nodes can localize, at a certain point of the intestinal disease, either into the gut or into the joints. This is indicated by the overlapping expression of adhesion molecules observed on the surface of intestinal and synovial endothelial cells during inflammation. T cells activated in the Peyer's patches and mesenteric lymph nodes express the gut-addressing integrin α4/β7 and the chemokine receptor CCR9 (Campbell and Butcher 2002). Once activated, these cells reach the bloodstream through the efferent lymphatic's and the thoracic duct. In the gut mucosa, the interaction between α4/β7 integrin and its ligand, the mucosal addressin cell adhesion molecule 1 (MadCAM-1) expressed on the venular endothelial sheet (Berlin, Berg et al. 1993; Berlin, Bargatze et al. 1995) causes the initial rolling and subsequent arrest of activated T cells. MadCAM-1 is normally expressed on the intestinal mucosa and its expression is further enhanced during inflammation (Souza, Elia et al. 1999; Salmi and Jalkanen 2001). Once arrested on the surface of the intestinal venules, activated T cells transmigrate through the endothelial layer and move into the lamina propria following the gradient formed by the CCR-9-specific ligand CCL-25 (Johansson-Lindbom, Svensson et al. 2003; Stenstad, Ericsson et al. 2006). Therefore, the specific interaction between α4/β7 integrin with MadCAM-1, and CCR9 with CCL-25 is pivotal for T cell homing into the gut. However it is worth noting that other molecules mediate the cell-to-cell interaction in this process. For instance CD44, the very late antigen-4 (VLA-4, α4β1) and the lymphocytes function associated antigen-1 (LFA-1, αLβ2) expressed by activated T cells play a role in the recruitment of T cells into the gut (Salmi and Jalkanen 1998).(Figure 3).

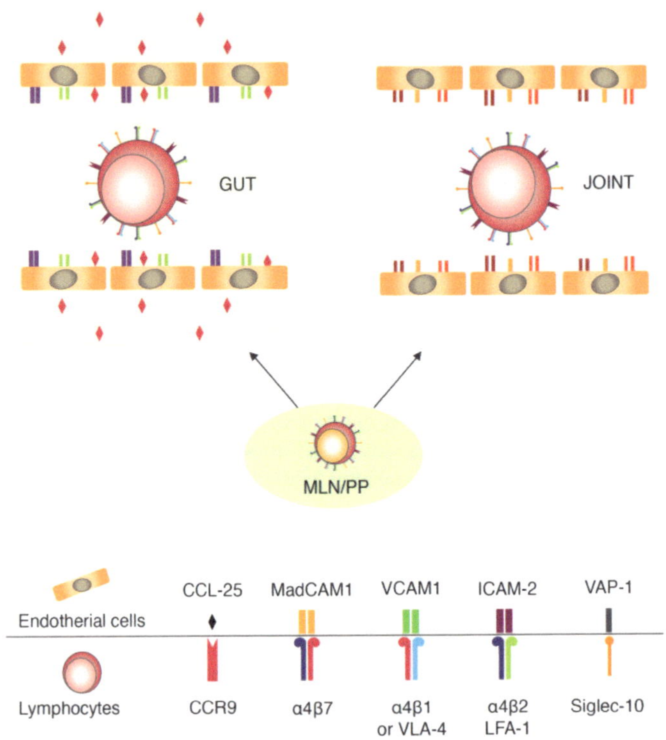

CCR9: Chemokine receptor-9; CCL-25: Chemokine ligand 25; MadCAM1: Mucosal addressin cell-adhesion molecule-1; VCAM1: Vascular cell adhesion molecule-1; ICAM: intracellular adhesion molecule; VLA-4: Very late antigen-4; LFA-1: Lymphocyte function associated antigen-1; VAP-1: Vascular adhesion protein-1 (adapted modified from Fantini, Pallone et al. 2009, Kivi, Elima et al. 2009; Aalto, Autio et al. 2011)

Fig. 3. The heterogeneous expression of adhesion molecules allows T cells activated in the gut to home into joints.

Conti *et al* (Conti, Borrelli et al. 2005) investigated a group of 129 children for suspected inflammatory bowel disease (IBD), 31 of whom had signs of axial and/or peripheral arthropathy, and after ileo-colonoscopy with biopsy, 7 children had classic IBD, 12 had indeterminate colitis, and 12 had lymphoid nodular hyperplasia of the distal ileum as the main feature. All children were HLA-B27 negative. These patients may be a population at risk of developing a full IBD phenotype. A recent study has shown that active Treg cell response, mainly dominated by IL-10 production, occurs in the gut of AS patients and is probably responsible for the absence of a clear Th17 polarization in the ileum of AS patients. Interestingly, a 5-fold increase in the proportion of Treg cells was observed in the gut of patients with AS, as compared to healthy subjects, with 70-80% of these cells also producing IL-10 (Ciccia, Accardo-Palumbo et al. 2010).

4. Histopathology

4.1 Enthesitis

Enthesitis is a distinctive pathological feature of spondyloarthritis and may involve synovial joints, cartilaginous joints, syndesmoses and extra-articular entheses (Benjamin and McGonagle 2007). This has traditionally been viewed as a focal abnormality, even though the inflammatory reaction intrinsic to enthesitis may be quite extensive. Entheses together with adjacent tissues may form mini organs, dubbed "enthesis organs or complex". According to this scenario the enthesis fibrocartilages that occupy a location adjacent to synovium (in joint or bursae or tendons) are dependent on the synovium for lubrication, oxygenation and removal of microdebris. The enthesis insertion being itself fibrocartilagenous is avascular, and does not have a resident population of macrophages. Therefore derangements in the enthesis would be expected to trigger an inflammatory response in the adjacent vascular synovium (Braun, Khan et al. 2000) (Figure 4).

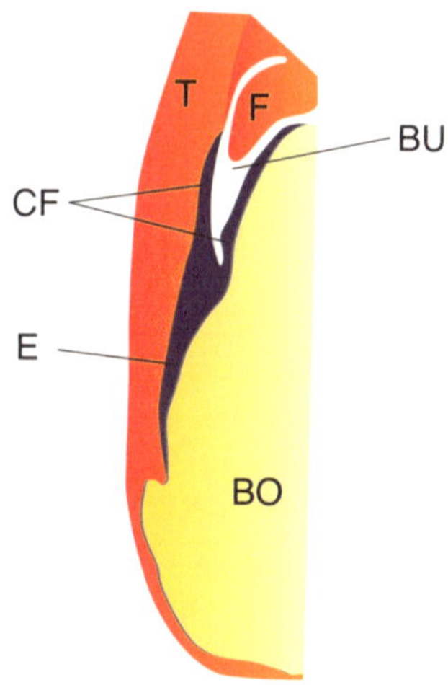

It consists of the enthesis itself (E), two complementary fibrocartilages (CF), an intervening bursa (BU) and a pad of synovium-covered protruding fat (F). The complementary fibrocartilages line the deep surface of the tendon (T) and cover the adjacent bone (BO) and protect these surfaces from compression when the foot is dorsiflexed. The bursa allows free movement of tendon relative to bone and the fat pad acts as a 'variable plunger' to prevent pressure changes from occurring in the bursa as the foot changes position. (adapted from (McGonagle and Benjamin 2009).

Fig. 4. A diagrammatic representation of an enthesis organ, modeled on that of the Achilles tendon.

This means that pathology related to the enthesis could trigger synovitis. Indeed, normal entheses are riddled with microdamage in aged subjects; this can be associated with microscopic synovitis, including villus formation and microscopic inflammatory cell infiltration in the immediately adjacent synovium, which is conceptualized in relationship to a synovio-entheseal complex (Braun, Khan et al. 2000). In man, there is an anatomical, biomechanical and temporal uncoupling between the inflammatory phase of disease and new bone formation and it appears that the bone formation follows on from the inflammation and may be a distinct phase.

4.2 Synovitis

Synovitis in juvenile SpA is characterized by marked lining layer hyperplasia, clear hypervascularity, and pronounced inflammatory cell infiltration with lymphocytes and macrophages, independent of disease duration or time of sampling. Despite some similarities with adult SpA, the findings with regard to lining layer hyperplasia and CD163+ macrophage (defined by the expression of the group B scavenger receptor CD163) infiltration are indicative of important differences in the synovial immunopathologic features of juvenile-onset SpA. The partial overlap with other JIA subtypes, with the exception of slightly lower vascularity in juvenile polyarthritis and higher inflammatory cell infiltration in juvenile oligoarthritis, emphasizes the need for further biologic characterization of JIA in order to define pathophysiologic, rather than phenotypic, subgroups (Kruithof, Van den Bossche et al. 2006). It is of interest that resident tissue macrophages, PMNs, and lining layer thickness, did correlate with global disease activity in adult SpA, and that changes in expression of synovial macrophage subsets, PMNs, and MMP-3 clearly reflected response to treatment (Kruithof, De Rycke et al. 2006).

5. Genetics

5.1 MHC genes

The central genetic factor recognized in SpA is the major histocompatibility complex (MHC) (Figure 5). While the risk for specific HLA allele in SpA may vary from one population group to another, the association of HLA-B27, and SpA has been well known for over 30 years. The HLA-B27 represents a family of 38 closely related cell surface proteins (encoded by the alleles HLA-B*2701-39) called subtypes of HLA-B27, most of which have evolved from the ubiquitous HLA-B*2705 (specifically the B*27052 allele) (Reveille and Maganti 2009). More recently, similar role for the HLA-B-7 has been proposed (Reynolds and Khan 1988; Cedoz, Wendling et al. 1995). Both antigens display significant levels of polymorphism, and the region of amino acid positions 63-71 in HLA-B27 appears to participate in the formation of at least three distinct epitopes shared by B27 and B7 identified as ME1, GSP5.3 and GS145.2, respectively (el-Zaatari, Sams et al. 1990; el-Zaatari and Taurog 1992). The proportion of B27-positive patients in the different SpA forms decreases from 95% in primary AS; to 70–80% in ReA; 50% in PsA and IBD with sacroiliitis/spondylitis, and to 0–10% in undifferentiated SpA. Findings of human family studies of twins and sibpairs support the notion that genetic factors other than B27 determine which B27-positive individuals develop arthritis. In Croatian patients with jSpA we have shown that the odds ratio (OR) for HLA-B*07 was 2.61, while the highest OR for a single HLA specificity was found for HLA-B*27 (OR=5.60). The HLA-B*07/B*27 combination found in 6/74 children showed higher risk (OR=14.82), but the combination of specificities: HLA-B*07/HLA-B*27, and D6S273-134 microsatellite locus, located in the HSP70-2 region, demonstrated the highest risk (OR=26.83) (Table 1.) (Harjacek, Margetic et

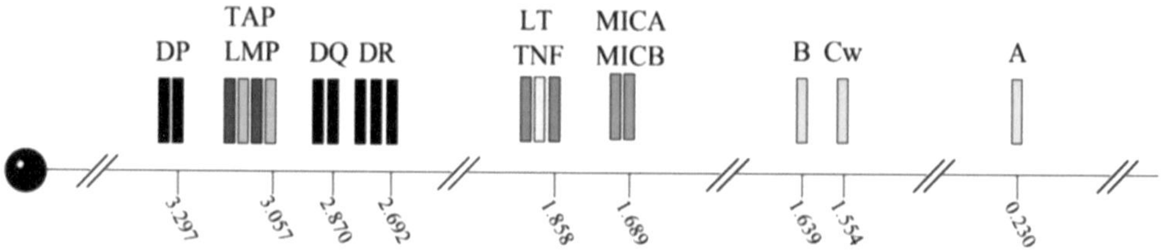

Fig. 5. HLA region on chromosome 6.

MARKER	OR	CI (95%)
B*07	2.61	1.40 - 4.87
B*27	5.69	2.93 - 11.06
D6S273-134	2.68	1.37 - 4.33
B*07; D6S273-134	2.72	1.34 - 5.53
B*27; D6S273-134	8.57	3.44 - 21.38
B*07/B*27	14.82	1.75 - 125.45
B*07/ B*27; D6S273-134	26.83	N/A*

OR – odds ratio: CI-confidence interval; * Not calculated due to the zero cell in table (Harjacek, Margetic et al. 2008).

Table 1. The odds ratio (OR) of 74 Croatian jSpA patients conferred by selected alleles alone or in combination.

al. 2008). During the genome-wide scan with polymorphic microsatellites, in addition to HLA-B27, D6S273 microsatellite locus was found to be highly relevant (LOD 3.8, $p < 0.00001$) in patients with AS (Brown, Pile et al. 1998).

Some recent progress has been made in understanding how B27 alleles confer such susceptibility, but the mechanism(s) continues to remain largely unknown, and may require new experimental approaches, and are beyond the scope of this review (Colbert, DeLay et al. 2010) (van der Heijde and Maksymowych 2010). B27-transgenic animals develop arthritis, and this directly involves B27 in the development of the disease (Khare, Bull et al. 1998). However, backcross studies in animal models of SpA suggest that multiple genes contribute to disease susceptibility (Laval, Timms et al. 2001; Brown, Brophy et al. 2003; Adarichev and Glant 2006). It is well known that the majority of SpA patients do not carry any of the known susceptibility HLA alleles. Furthermore, findings of human family studies in twins and sib pairs support the notion that genetic factors other than B27 determine which B27-positive individuals develop arthritis (Tsuchiya, Shiota et al. 1998; Brophy, Hickey et al. 2004).

5.2 Non MHC genes

There is little definitive knowledge about non- MHC in SpA. The ultimate goal in the mapping of diseases to particular genes is to isolate and clone the disease-causing gene itself. To clone such a gene successfully, it is necessary to map the disease gene to a very small region, which can be difficult in the case of complex diseases. In fact, it may require analyzing several hundreds or even several thousands of individuals (affected and unaffected) to detect the genes that are involved in SpA. Global gene expression profiling is a molecular technique that measures in parallel genome-wide expression of thousands of genes in a sample of cells. Genome scanning using SNP's (Single nucleotide polymorphisms) has been carried out to identify regions of the genome that show evidence of linkage to SpA outside the MHC (Sharma, Choi et al. 2009; Vegvari, Szabo et al. 2009; Reveille, Sims et al. 2010) (Table 2). In adult SpA, many other regions and genes have been implicated in candidate gene or linkage mapping studies, but will not be reviewed in depth here. In one large study SNP'S were used in JIA patients (n = 1,054); subtype specific association of the *eraP1* gene (endoplasmic reticulum aminopeptidase 1) with ERA JIA, and the *IL23R* gene with juvenile-onset psoriatic arthritis (jPsA), were found (Hinks, Martin et al. 2011). *eraP1* encodes a multifunctional aminopeptidase, but its role in the pathogenesis in any of the associated diseases has yet to be determined. It may play a role in trimming peptides, in the endoplasmic reticulum, for binding to HLA class I molecules where they are transported to the cell surface for presentation to T cells. Alternatively it may be important through its function in cleaving pro-inflammatory cytokine receptors, such as tumor necrosis factor receptor 1 (TNFR1) to generate soluble TNFR1. It is also thought to play a role in the cleavage of interleukin 1 receptor 2 (IL1R2) and interleukin 6 receptor alpha (IL6Rα), leading to increased soluble IL1R2 and IL6Rα (Haroon and Inman 2010).

GENE:	Name of gene:
IL-1β locus	Interleukin 1 beta
MMP	Matrix metalloproteinases
CASP1	Caspase 1
IL18	Interleukin 18
IL10R	Interleukin 10 receptor
TLR-4	Toll-like receptor 4
RGS1*	Regulator of G-protein signaling
eraP1	Endoplasmic reticulum aminopeptidase 1
IL23R	Interleukin 23 receptor
IL1R2	Interleukin 1 receptoc, type II
ANTXR2**	Anthrax toxin receptor 2

Adapted from: (Gu, Wei et al. 2009; Sharma, Choi et al. 2009; Vegvari, Szabo et al. 2009; Haroon and Inman 2010; Reveille, Sims et al. 2010; Hinks, Martin et al. 2011).

Table 2. The list of genes found by genome-wide expression profiling in SpA patients using SNP's (with exception of RGS1 that was found in undifferentiated SpA all other genes were identified in AS patients).

Studies of gene expression with the use of DNA microarray technologies offers a novel approach to determining pathogenesis of disease. In two pediatric studies, ability of microarray-based methods (Affymetrix platform) to identify genes with disease-specific expression patterns in peripheral blood mononuclear cells (PBMC) and synovial fluid mononuclear cells (SFMC) of JIA patients (including ERA patients), and healthy controls

was used. When compared to healthy controls, they found relevant gene expression in JAK/STAT cascade and chemokine pathway, lower levels of angiostatic CXCL10 chemokine, higher leevels of ELR^+ angiogenic chemokines and VEGF (vascular endothelial growth factor) in ERA PBMC, and decreased adult hemoglobin gene expression (Barnes, Aronow et al. 2004). They concluded that expression analysis identified differentially expressed genes in PBMC's obtained early in the disease from patients with different subtypes of JIA and in healthy controls, providing evidence of immunobiologic differences between these forms of childhood arthritis (Barnes, Grom et al. 2009). Our preliminary data have shown that jSpA patients exhibit complex patterns of gene expression for functions related to inflammatory and defense response, MAP kinase and cell cycle, chromatin modulation and transcription, cell death, apoptosis, and interestingly, gene closely linked to autoinflammatory diseases (NRLP3) (Harjacek M. 2010).
However, one should be cautious because microarray analysis produces vast amounts of data that can be analyzed and interpreted in many different ways.

6. Classification

Classifying juvenile spondyloarthritis is a "work in progress" and clearly problematic (Burgos-Vargas 2002; Colbert 2010). Since the recognition in 1982 by Rosenberg and Petty of the seronegative enthesopathy and arthropathy (SEA) syndrome (Rosenberg and Petty 1982) many attempts have been made to classify JSpA or SpA like diseases in children. The International League of Associations for Rheumatology (ILAR) Taskforce on Classification of Childhood Arthritis included the category of enthesitis-related arthritis (ERA) in the 1995 classification of juvenile idiopathic arthritis (JIA) (Fink 1995; Petty, Southwood et al. 1998) among the seven subgroups of juvenile arthritides. However when psoriasis, or dactylitis and nail pits along with arthritis are present, these children are excluded from ERA and may be classified as psoriatic arthritis or even undifferentiated arthritis (Burgos-Vargas, Rudwaleit et al. 2002; Colbert 2010). The classification criteria for ERA are excluding psoriatic arthritis (PsA), while reactive arthritis is not even mentioned. Moreover IBD is only maintained as a descriptor of the disease (Burgos-Vargas 2002). So, quite early in the discussion this led to several propositions for revision (Fantini 2001; Manners, Lesslie et al. 2003).
Another set of criteria for spondyloarthritis was developed by the European Spondyloarthropathy Study Group (ESSG) (Dougados, van der Linden et al. 1991). The ESSG criteria have been validated in children, but the emphasis on inflammatory spinal pain is problematic because such a symptom is uncommon in children in the first five years of disease (Prutki, Tambic Bukovac et al. 2008). Also, their sensitivity, positive predictive value and accuracy are lower than in adults (Prieur 1990). This classification includes PsA, ReA, IBD arthropathies as part of the SpA group and ranks the two most important characteristics of adult-onset SpA - inflammatory spinal pain and synovitis as major criteria. Since spinal pain is a less common feature at the onset of the disease in younger children, these criteria may be limited in children with jSpA.
Amor and coworkers (Amor, Dougados et al. 1990) also developed criteria for the classification of spondyloarthritis in adults that could be applicable in children, but like ESSG classification have lower sensitivity in childhood. According to Amor the features of spondyloarthropathy are associated with points, and if six or more points are present the diagnosis of SpA is confirmed.

A recent study showed that Garmisch-Partenkirchen criteria have the highest sensitivity and proposed them for identifying spondyloarthritis in juvenile patients (Hafner 1987; Joos, Dehoorne et al. 2009). According to these criteria probable spondyloarthritis is considered if two major criteria or major criterion one or two plus two minor criteria are present.

SpA usually begins in children as an undifferentiated form of the disease: a peripheral asymmetric oligoarthritis predominantly involving the lower limbs and/or with peripheral enthesitis and/or with dactylitis, and progress to differentiated forms over time (Colbert 2010). Most of these children could be classified as undifferentiated SpA (uSpA) according to the Amor (Amor, Dougados et al. 1990) and the ESSG criteria (Dougados, van der Linden et al. 1991).

Children with the SEA syndrome or with ERA are at risk of developing the other manifestations of the B27 associated disease process including axial involvement. In 1989, Burgos-Vargas and Clark reported that 75% of their Mexican patients with the SEA syndrome met the New York criteria for ankylosing spondylitis (AS) after 5 years of disease (Burgos-Vargas and Clark 1989).

Experts from the Assessment of Spondyloarthritis International Society (ASAS), recently developed definition criteria for inflammatory back pain (IBP), which is an important clinical symptom in adult patients with SpA (Sieper, van der Heijde et al. 2009). In addition, although revisions to the ILAR criteria have addressed some weaknesses Burgos-Vargas, R., M. Rudwaleit, et al. (2002; (Duffy, Colbert et al. 2005) several problems remain, some of which might have been exaggerated by the recent development of criteria that identify pre-radiographic 'axial SpA' in adults. (Rudwaleit, Landewe et al. 2009; Rudwaleit, van der Heijde et al. 2009). To best of our knowledge, these criteria are still not validated in children.

Different classification criteria for SpA are shown in Table 3.

ESSG criteria (Dougados, van der Linden et al. 1991)
Inflammatory low back pain
OR Synovitis asymmetrical or predominantly of the lower limbs
AND at least one of the following criteria: familial history of spondyloarthropathy, uveitis or inflammatory bowel disease; psoriasis, inflammatory bowel disease, enthesopathy, radiological sacroiliitis
AMOR criteria (Amor, Dougados et al. 1991)
A. Clinical signs or history of:
1. nocturnal pain lumbar or dorsal and/or morning stiffness (1 point);
2. asymmetrical oligoarthritis (2 point);
3. Indefinite buttock pain or alternating buttock pain (1 or 2 point);
4. Sausage finger or toe (2 point);
5. heel pain or any other enthesopathy (2 point)
6. iritis (2 point);
7. non gonoccocal urethritis or cervicitis within one month before the onset of the arthritis (1 point);
8. Diarrhea within one month before the onset of the arthritis (1 point);
9. Presence or history of psoriasis, and/or balanitis and/or chronic enterocolopathy (2 points).
B. Radiological signs:
10. Sacroiliitis (stage 2 ≥ if bilateral, or stage ≥ 3 if unilateral) (3 points)
C. Genetics:
11. Presence of HLA B27 and/or familial history of ankylosing spondylitis and/or Reiter's syndrome and/or psoriasis and/or uveitis and/or chronic enterocolopathy (2 points)
D. Reaction to treatment:
12. Improvement of pain within 48 hours by NSAIDs or relapse within 48 hours after stop of NSAIDs (2 points)

A spondyloarthropathy is declared in a patient having a score equal of greater than 6 as sum of the points on the 12 criteria.
SEA syndrome (Rosenberg and Petty 1982)
SERONEGATIVITY = absence of RF and ANA ENTHESOPATHY = tendonitis of the Achilles tendon, fascia plantaris or quadriceps tendon ARTHROPATHY = inflammatory arthritis of the axial skeleton or oligoarthropathy
ERA (Durban criteria) (Petty, Southwood et al. 1998)
Arthritis OR Enthesitis PLUS two or more of the following: A. Sacroiliac joint tenderness AND/OR inflammatory spinal pain; B. Presence of HLA-B27; C. Family history involving one or more first or second degree relatives with an HLA-B27 related disease, confirmed by a physician; D. Anterior uveitis (typically with pain, redness and/or photophobia); E. Onset of arthritis in a boy > 8 years of age AND none of the following: A. Presence of psoriasis in a first or second degree relative, confirmed by a dermatologist; B. Presence of a systemic arthritis.
Atypical spondyloarthritis in children (Hussein, Abdul-Khaliq et al. 1989)
MAJOR CRITERIA: 1. SA or oligoarthritis in family; 2. enthesopathy; 3. Arthritis of digital joints; 4. Sacroiliitis; 5. HLA B27 positive; 6. Recurrent arthritis or arthtalgia. MINOR CRITERIA: 1. Begin after age od 10 years 2. Male sex; 3. Only lower extremities affected; 4. Acute iridocyclitis or conjunctivitis; 5. Arthritis of hips; 6. Begin following unproven enteritis. Atypical spondyloarthritis was considered as probable when three major and two minor criteria were present.
Juvenile spondarthritis (Garmisch-Partenkirchen criteria) (Hafner 1987)
MAJOR CRITERIA: 1. Asymmetrical oligoarthritis with involvement of hip, knee or ankle joint; 2. Enthesopathy; 3. Pain of the lumbar spine or sacroiliac region; 4. acute idirocyclitis. MINOR CRITERIA: 1.Peripheral arthritis of 5 or more joints; 2. Male sex; 3, Disease inset after the age of 6 years; 4. HLA B27 positivity; 5. (Suspicion of) spondarthritis in family history Probable spondarthritis was considered if two major criteria or major criterion one or two plus two minor criteria were present.

ILAR = International League of Associations for Rheumatology; JIA = Juvenile Idiopathic Arthritis; ERA = Enthesitis related arthritis; ESSG = European Spondyloarthropathy Study Group;

Table 3. Classification criteria for spondyloarthritis.

None of the criteria evaluated above are perfect for the classification of JSpA. However, the Garmisch-Partenkirchen criteria are the major candidates for future research in identifying spondyloarthritis in juvenile patients (Kasapcopur, Demirli et al. 2005; Joos, Dehoorne et al. 2009).

7. Clinical manifestations

In this section we will try to give an overview of the different characteristics of the diseases. The authors consider several subforms of jSpA:

1. Reactive arthritis: resulting from an infection or inflammation on a distant location of the arthritis. It is merely an acute phenomenon, possibly relapsing and in a part of the patients evolving chronically.
2. Undifferentiated SpA: a chronic form of asymmetrical oligoarthritis, affecting the lower limbs, often accompanied by entheisitis and a number of extra-articular manifestations.
3. Juvenile ankylosing spondylitis: affecting preferentially the axial skeleton and can be considered as a clear precursor to the adult ankylosing spondylitis.
4. Juvenile psoriatic arthritis.
5. Inflammatory bowel disease-related arthritis
6. Juvenile ankylosing tarsitis
7. Clavicular cortical hyperostosis

These forms are discussed extensively below.

7.1 Reactive arthritis (ReA)

a. **Reactive arthritis** (ReA) comprises a number of diseases following infection or inflammation on a distant location in the body. The term is usually restricted to HLA-B27 associated disease triggered in about 80% of patient by arthritogenic bacteria such as *Salmonella, Yersinia, Shigella,* and *Campylobacter. Mycoplasma pneumonia* and *Chlamydia pneumonia* are less frequently responsible for the disease. Primary infection, regardless of the triggering agent, may be completely asymptomatic or with mild symptoms, and it usually precedes arthritis onset up to four weeks.
   Reactive arthritis commonly involves joints (knees, ankles) and entheses of the lower limbs. It can also affect temporomandibular joints and the cervical spine (Arabshahi, Baskin et al. 2007). It is marked with severe pain and swelling, sometimes with erythema over the affected joints, rarely with only mild symptoms. ReA following Salmonella or Yersinia infection sometimes presents with polyarthritis that affects small joints of the hands. Arthralgias may precede the onset of arthritis.
   Extra-articular manifestations of ReA include conjunctivitis, anterior uveitis, balanopostitis, urethritis, cervicitis (occurring more frequently in adolescent age with sexually acquired ReA caused by Chlamydia), aphthous stomatitis, diarrhea (as part of a generalized mucositis), erythema nodosum (particularly in Yersinia triggered ReA), and keratoderma blenorrhagicum (which clinically and histologically resembles psoriasis)
b. If arthritis, conjunctivitis and urethritis are present as a triad, reactive arthritis might be referred to as **Reiter's syndrome**.
c. A number of children, particularly those with HLA-B27, develop a **chronic course**, and may even develop AS (Leirisalo, Skylv et al. 1982; Hussein 1987; Artamonov, Akhmadi et al. 1991; Cuttica, Scheines et al. 1992; Yli-Kerttula, Tertti et al. 1995; Leirisalo-Repo,

Helenius et al. 1997; Leirisalo-Repo 1998). Children without HLA-B27 who have ReA, particularly when the disease is triggered by Yersinia or Campylobacter, usually have a rather short and benign course.
Diagnosis of ReA in children has usually been made in patients developing arthritis after a specific episode of infection, or those having positive serological tests against bacteria (Cassidy and Petty 2001). However, diagnostic tests (serology, PCR, etc.) may identify the etiologic agent in about 50% of the cases depending on the clinical picture and tests selected (Fendler, Laitko et al. 2001; Sieper, Rudwaleit et al. 2002). On the other hand, bacterial DNA has been identified in synovial fluid cells of patients with long-standing juvenile onset AS or undifferentiated SpA (Pacheco-Tena, Alvarado De La Barrera et al. 2001). In this sense, ReA constitutes a link rather than exclusion to ERA and SpA.

d. **Poststreptococcal reactive** arthritis (PSRA) has been proposed as a homogeneous clinical entity, distinct from acute rheumatic fever (ARF) and from other forms of reactive arthritis. However, available literature at present supports the idea that PSRA is in reality a heterogeneous group of clinical entities, some of which share clinical features with ARF and others with HLA B27-related spondyloarthritis. The assumed causal role of streptococcal infection is far from proven. Joint involvement is typically non-migratory and affects the large joints, particularly those of the lower limb. Mono, oligo and polyarthritis are equally represented (Moorthy, Gaur et al. 2009). The published data support the possibility, however, that there may be a subset of patients with PSRA who are HLA-B27-positive and are more likely to develop sacroiliitis (Mackie and Keat 2004). Elevated antistreptolysin titers may support but not definitely diagnose a poststreptococcal complication. The more specific and expensive antibody tests may be warranted, including antihyaluronidase, antideoxyribonuclease B, and antistreptokinase antibodies. American Heart Association, and the Red Book of the AAP suggest that antibiotic prophylaxis be given to all proven PSRA patients for 1 year, and if no carditis is observed, then prophylaxis should be discontinued. Moreover, physicians should be aware that antibiotic therapy might prevent the development of an antibody response (Barash, Mashiach et al. 2008).

7.2 Undiffentiated spondyloarthritis (ERA)

The onset of ERA is usually insidious and characterized by intermittent musculoskeletal pain and stiffness or inflammation of peripheral joints, mostly of the lower limbs, with enthesitis at one or more sites around the knee or foot. Axial skeleton symptoms are not common at the disease onset, but might become manifest in the later course (Burgos-Vargas 2002).

Arthritis and enthesitis are the hallmark of jSpA. Peripheral joint involvement at onset is present in over 80% of these patients, while inflammatory spinal pain in only 20-25%. This is one of the major differences between adult- and juvenile-onset spondyloarthritis. In most patients arthritis is either unilateral or asymmetrical oligoarthritis at onset. Distal joints of lower extremities (knee, ankle, tarsus) are affected more frequently than proximal joints. Polyarthritis is not common at disease onset and its distribution is generally asymmetrical (Burgos-Vargas 2002). At this stage of the disease it is difficult to differentiate jSpA from other forms of juvenile arthritides.

The sites of attachment of ligament, tendon, fascia or joint capsule to bone are characteristic sites of inflammation in the jSpA. In contrast to arthritis its specificity and diagnostic value are much more significant in jSpA. Enthesitis is frequently associated with tenosynovitis and bursitis, particularly of the foot, where arthritis also occurs. Foot enthesitis, including tarsal and calcaneal entheses (Achilles' tendon, plantar fascia), is the most common sign of jSpA and one of the most disabling conditions in these children. Its clinical manifestation is pain on standing and walking, and foot swelling, pressure tenderness at the insertion of tendons and ligaments to bone. Soft tissue swelling is the result of inflammation of tendon sheets and adjacent bursae. Enthesitis in the later course of the disease varies from rare episodes of active inflammation of one or few entheses to frequent recurrence of inflammation involving many sites, particularly the feet. Persistent enthesitis is associated with bone edema and overgrowth, cartilaginous proliferation, bone bridging and ankylosis. Subcortical bone cysts and erosions at tendon insertions are rare.

The severity, duration and consequences of arthritis and enthesitis may not parallel each other throughout the clinical course of the disease.

The most common extraarticular manifestation of ERA is uveitis, while mucositis, skin disease (excluding psoriasis), or cardiopulmonary and nervous system disease happens occasionally.

Uveitis in ERA is characterized by redness and pain in the eye with photophobia. It is usually unilateral, frequently recurrent and rarely leaves ocular residua. The occurrence of uveitis in children with ERA is less than 20% (lower incidence than in adults), but longer follow-ups reveal higher figures (Packham and Hall 2002; Petty, Smith et al. 2003).

Musculoskeletal examination should be focused on entheses, peripheral joints and axial skeleton including joints of the pelvis, spine and chest.

Marked localized tenderness on the patella at 2-, 6-, and 10-o'clock positions (Figure 6A), at the tibial tuberosity, at the attachment of the Achilles tendon (Figure 6B) or plantar fascia to the calcaneus (Figure 6C), at the attachment of the plantar fascia to the base of the fifth metatarsal (Figure 6C), and at the heads of the metatarsal bones (Figure 6C) suggests enthesitis. Tenderness as the sign of enthesitis is rarely demonstrable at the great trochanter of the femur, superior anterior iliac spine and iliac crest, pubic symphisis, ischial tuberosity, costochondral junctions, and entheses of the upper extremities. Walking on the toes and heels usually demonstrates altered weight bearing as the patient avoids pressure on inflamed entheses.

Peripheral joints in ERA are commonly affected asymmetrically and predominantly involve the lower limbs. Unilateral hip involvement is more likely to be a manifestation of ERA than the presenting feature of other forms of JIA. Knee involvement is often present both in ERA and oligoarticular JIA, but the child's age and sex, as well as the presence of HLA-B27, could be helpful in distinguishing the diagnosis. Small joint involvement of the foot and toes, especially intertarsal joints (tarsitis) may be characteristic of ERA, while polyarthritis with the involvement of small joints of the hands suggests another type of JIA (Berntson, Damgard et al. 2008).

Axial skeleton involvement is rarely present in the younger age and in the early stage of the disease. However, it is one of the major manifestations in the later course of ERA. Pain by direct pressure over one or both sacroiliac joints, compression of the pelvis, or distraction of the sacroiliac joints by Patrick test (Faber test) highly suggests sacroiliac inflammation. Lower back pain is usually present and associated with morning stiffness. Abnormalities in spine contour, such as reduction in the normal lumbar lordosis, exaggeration of the thoracic kyphosis, or increased occiput-to-wall distance can be revealed by simple inspection of the back. Restriction of hyperextension or inclination, loss of the normal curve in the lower part

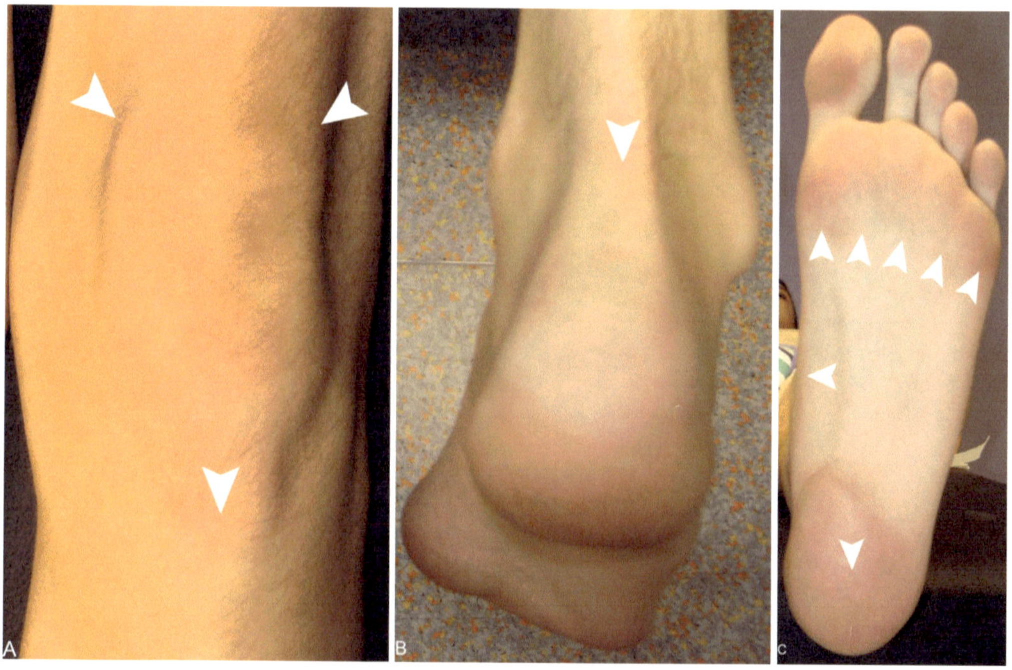

Fig. 6. A, Arrows indicate the most common sites of tenderness associated with enthesitis at the insertion of the quadriceps muscles into the patella and the attachments of the patellar ligament to the patella and tibial tuberosity. B, Arrow indicates the site of tenderness at the insertion of the Achilles tendon into the calcaneus. C, Arrows indicate the most common sites of tenderness associated with enthesitis at the insertion of the plantar fascia into calcaneus, base of the fifth metatarsal, and heads of the first through fifth metatarsals. Swelling in this area is best visualized by having the child lie prone on the examining table with the feet over the edge.

of thoracolumbar spine in the full forward flexion position is the usual sign of axial involvement. The rigid spine or cervical spine involvement are not common in children, especially in the early stage. The modified Schober test is a good tool for documenting thoracolumbar mobility. It is easily performed (Figure 7) and sequential measurements provide a useful parameter in the disease follow-up. With the child standing with the feet together, a line joining the iliac crests is used as a landmark for the lumbosacral junction. A mark is made 5 cm below (point A) and 10 cm above (point B) the lumbosacral joint. With the patient in maximal forward flexion with the knees straight, the increase in distance between points A and B is used as an indicator of lumbosacral joint mobility. In general, a distance less than 6 cm is regarded as abnormal. Measurement of the distance from the fingertips to the floor on maximal forward flexion is also used for quantification of spinal motion but it is poorly reproducible and does not correlate with Schober test. This measurement reflects hip flexion disturbances as well as back flexion. Nevertheless, because of lower height, measuring spine mobility with Schober test is potentially difficult in younger children.

Sequential measurements of thoracic excursions may be useful in documenting progressive loss of range. Since normal thoracic motion varies a lot depending on the age and sex of the patient, a single measurement is not useful. However, any chest excursion of less than 5 cm

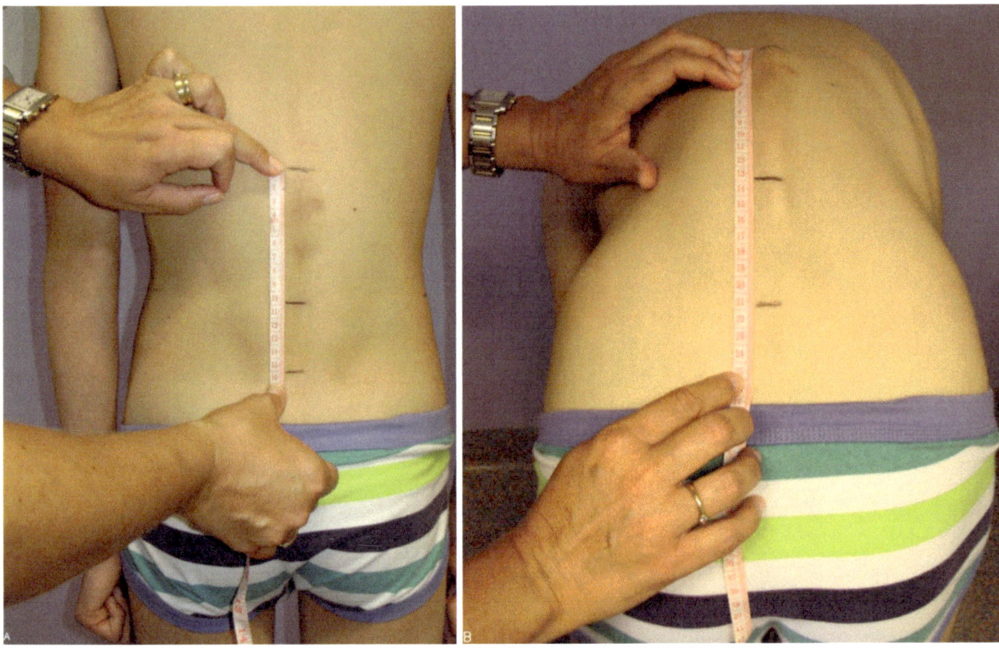

Fig. 7. Schober test. A, Measurement 10cm above and 5cm below the lumbosacral junction (the dimples of Venus) in the upright position. B, Measurement of the distance between the upper and the lower marks when the child is bending forward.

(maximum expiration and maximum inspiration measured at the fourth intercostal space) in the adolescent should be considered as abnormal (Burgos-Vargas, Castelazo-Duarte et al. 1993). In the late development of the disease it may be restricted to 1 or 2 cm, even in the absence of symptoms.

Pain and tenderness at costosternal and costovertebral joints, as well as sternoclavicular joints are often present, rarely at sternomanubrial junction and may be elicited by firm palpation.

Arthritis characteristics in the later course of jSpA are variable. Enteric bacteria may have a role in the exacerbation of disease in patients with ERA, implying that ERA could be a form of chronic reactive arthritis (Saxena, Misra et al. 2006). HLA-B27 negative patients usually have fewer episodes of arthritis and less symptoms of axial disease. HLA-B27 positive disease is associated with more severe and more frequent episodes of active oligoarthritis or polyarthritis, sacroillitis and axial involvement often. It also predicts evolvement to ankylosing spondylitis (AS) (Leirisalo, Skylv et al. 1982; Leirisalo-Repo 1998).

The long-term follow-up of children with HLA-B27 who have JIA reveals that between 18,5% and 75% develop spondyloarthritis (Burgos-Vargas, Pacheco-Tena et al. 2002).

7.3 Juvenile-onset ankylosing spondylitis (jAS)

Juvenile-onset ankylosing spondylitis (jAS) is a definite form of jSpA characterized by inflammation of the sacroiliac and vertebral joints leading to stiffening of the spine.

Back pain is common in young people with one year prevalence rates varying from 7% to 58% (Smith 2007). Low back pain (LBP) in childhood and adolescence is a significant risk factor for LBP in adulthood (Jones and Macfarlane 2005; Hestbaek, Leboeuf-Yde et al. 2006).

However, most cases of back pain are non-specific and self-limiting. A recent prospective study of 73 children under age 18 years, with back pain of greater than 3 months duration found only 21% of the patients with positive findings after diagnostic evaluation or a minimum of 2 years follow-up. Spondylolysis with or without spondylolisthesis was the most common diagnosis (Bhatia, Chow et al. 2008).

Children with jAS may present with back or buttock pain, but the typical history of morning stiffness, gradual resolution of pain with activity and clinical exam findings of limited lumbar mobility (Figure 7, Figure 8), sacroiliac joint tenderness and peripheral enthesitis or arthritis, usually allow the practitioner to make the correct diagnosis (Cassidy and Petty 2006).

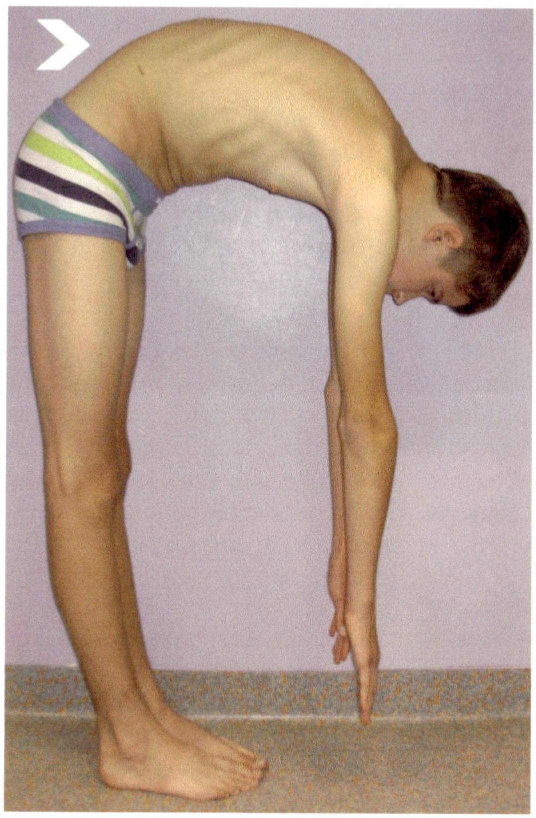

Fig. 8. Boy shown in the position of maximal forward flexion. Note the flattened back (arrow).

Inflammation in the caudal region of the sacroiliac joint is one of the earliest features of spinal disease in AS. Often this begins on the iliac side of the joint and then involves the sacral side as inflammation progresses (Bollow, Hermann et al. 2005). Frank erosions become evident, but may not appear for months to years after inflammation has begun. Sclerosis occurs and is often progressive, eventually resulting in fusion of the joint (Colbert 2010).

There is a less common subgroup of adult-like juvenile onset AS that is called genuine jAS, in which patients develop clinical and radiographic evidence of disease affecting the axial skeleton earlier than children progressing from SEA syndrome to AS. Seronegative enthesitis and arthritis (SEA) syndrome comprises the combination of enthesitis and arthritis, and probably represents the early stage of jAS or ERA. Most patients with persistent arthritis and enthesitis, who are HLA-B27 positive, develop ankylosing spondylitis five to ten years after initial symptoms. (Burgos-Vargas, Vazquez-Mellado et al. 1996).

jAS differs from adult-onset AS in clinical features at onset, presenting with higher prevalence of peripheral joint involvement and lower prevalence of axial disease. In contrast to adults, spinal pain in children does not seem to improve with movement. The prevalence of HLA-B27 is similar in both groups (Lin, Liang et al. 2009).

Although the pattern of peripheral arthritis and enthesitis is similar to that of other jSpA, jAS is characterized by persistent axial involvement. Enthesitis is usually more severe and episodes last for a longer period of time. During the initial period of six months most patients have oligoarthritis possibly evolving into polyarthritis by the end of the first year.

Axial symptoms first appear in the lumbar and thoracic spine, and less frequently in the cervical spine and sacroiliac joints.

Fever, weight loss, muscle weakness and atrophy, fatigue, lymphadenopathy, leukocytosis and anemia may be present in up to 10% of patients with JAS. Cardiovascular and nervous system manifestations are rare, although radiculopathy may be present in the late course of the disease. Interestingly, up to 80% of patients with jAS might have nonspecific intestinal bowel disease (Mielants, Veys et al. 1993).

7.4 Juvenile-onset psoriatic arthritis (jPsA)

According to the ILAR criteria, jPsA represents approximately 7% of patients with JIA. It is defined as arthritis with onset before the 16th birthday that lasts for at least 6 weeks, and is associated either with psoriasis or two of the following: dactylitis, nail pitting, onycholysis, or psoriasis in a first-degree relative (Cassidy and Petty 2001). ILAR criteria exclude the diagnosis of jPsA in patients with positive rheumatoid factor, HLA-B27 positive boys over the age of 6 years, or patients with a first-degree family history of HLA-B27 associated disease. In our opinion, the majority of jPsA patients fits under the jSpA umbrella and only a minority of patients will belong to other subtypes of PsA as seen in children or adults (Mease 2011; Stoll and Punaro 2011).

While the disease can have a variable presentation (especially in a younger child), in general, 50% of patients will have arthritis at disease onset, 40% will have psoriasis, and 10% of patients will have a coincidence of arthritis and skin changes. Dactylitis is common in both groups (20% to 40% of patients with jPsA), and refers to swelling within a digit that extends beyond the joints, giving the typical "sausage-like" appearance. Index finger and second toe are most commonly affected. Axial disease in jPsA is milder than in jAS, the cervical spine being involved more than other spinal segments, with a tendency for asymmetric sacroiliac joint involvement and a failure to progress to spinal ankylosis. The latter patients are frequently associated with HLA-B27 antigen. Enthesitis is prevalent in the older onset subgroup of patients with jPsA, which is similar to the patients with adult PsA. Severe skin and nail disease is rare in children with arthritis. Most children have mild psoriatic skin lesions in the capilitium, retroauricular, umbilical and intergluteal regions, extensor surfaces of the extremities, and slight nail pitting or onycholysis. Most patients with skin disease have psoriasis vulgaris (80%), 30% have guttata, and a minority of 2% have pustular psoriasis (Burgos-Vargas 2002). The severity of the skin lesions does not usually parallel the severity of arthritis. Systemic manifestations are rare and reflect chronic inflammation: fever, loss of appetite, anemia, growth retardation, and very rarely pericarditis, inflammatory bowel disease, or amyloidosis.

In contrast, patients with early-onset jPsA bear similarities to early-onset oligoarticular and polyarticular JIA patients, including female preponderance and antinuclear antibody (ANA) positivity. The majority of those patients will have oligoarthritis or polyarthritis of the upper and lower extremities (Stoll, Zurakowski et al. 2006; Stoll and Punaro 2011). Psoriasis and adult PsA are strongly associated with HLA-Cw*0602 HLA-B38, and non-MHC genes *psors 1* and *psors* 2, but HLA associations in jPsA are inconsistent, probably due to great variability within jPsA across the pediatric age spectrum (Stoll and Punaro 2011).
Other extra-articular manifestations include uveitis in about 15% of patients. The uveitis in psoriatic patients is heterogeneous in its aspect. Sometimes it resembles the acute anterior uveitis and is associated with the HLA B27 antigen, in other patients however it evolves as a chronic posterior and even panuveitis and needs regular ophthalmologic work out as well as preventive controls for relapse.

7.5 Inflammatory bowel disease-related arthritis (IBD)

Crohn's disease (CD) and ulcerative colitis (UC) are two major IBD associated with arthropathies. Peripheral or axial arthritis are the most common extraintestinal manifestations of these diseases, and are present in 7% to 21% of children with IBD, more frequently in UC than in CD (Burgos-Vargas 2002; Jose, Garnett et al. 2009). CD involves the mucosa and regional lymphatics of the colon, distal ileum and other segments of the intestinal tract, with characteristic noncaseating granulomas. UC is a diffuse inflammatory bowel disease with characteristic crypt abscesses in the colonic mucosa. Approximately one third of patients with CD and about 15% of those with UC have onset before the age of 20 years (Burbige, Huang et al. 1975; Hamilton, Bruce et al. 1979).
Initial gastrointestinal symptoms are cramping abdominal pain, often with localized tenderness, diarrhea, loss of appetite to anorexia, sometimes fever. Bloody diarrhea is more suggestive of UC, while perianal skin tags and fistulae are typical for CD. Gastrointestinal symptoms usually precede joint disease by months or even years and rarely they coincide.
Arthritis mostly affects peripheral joints with predomination on lower extremities (knees and ankles). Episodes of acute peripheral arthritis usually last not more than two weeks and rarely cause joint damage or functional loss. Axial disease and sacroillitis are rare, and association with HLA-B27 is common in the older age-onset patients with juvenile CD or juvenile UC.
Subclinical gut inflammation ("low-grade-IBD") is very common in jSpA and occurs in up to 80% of patients, and destructive arthritis of small joints is more common in biopsy proven "low-grade-IBD" children (Mielants, Veys et al. 1987). Peripheral arthritis (mono or oligo) improves with colectomy (disease control), but axial disease shows little improvement.
Erythema nodosum is commonly associated with IBD. Reddish, painful, nodular lesions usually occur in the pretibial region and persist for several weeks, recurring in crops sometimes for several months. Articular involvement often accompanies exacerbations of erythema nodosum.
Painful oral ulcerations could be a part of the initial clinical presentation, especially in CD, and should not be misdiagnosed as Behcet disease.
Children with IBD may also have asymptomatic uveitis.

7.6 Ankylosing tarsitis (AT)

Ankylosing tarsitis represents a set of clinical and radiological manifestations originally described in patients with HLA-B27 positive jSpA, and include inflammation from the ankle to the metatarsophalangeal joints (synovitis, enthesitis, tenosynovitis, bursitis), followed by proliferative changes that finally lead to the fusion of tarsal bones) (Burgos-Vargas, Pacheco-Tena et al. 2002; Alvarez-Madrid, Merino et al. 2009)

Clinical features are usually midfoot swelling, swelling around the malleoli, Achilles tendon and plantar region of the feet, with decreased mobility of tarsal, ankle and metatarsophalangeal joints. The condition has a variety of radiologic features, which include osteopenia of the tarsal bones at the beginning, with the progression to erosions, osseous proliferation at enthesis, bone cysts, joint space narrowing and finally ankylosis.

Ankylosing tarsitis may occur in patients with undifferentiated jSpA, but it can also be a part of the clinical manifestations in children with jAS. There are some differences between children diagnosed with jSpA initially affected with tarsitis and those without it. It can be often misdiagnosed as soft tissue infection at the beginning of disease (Alvarez-Madrid, Merino et al. 2009).

7.7 Clavicular cortical hyperostosis (CCH)

Clavicular cortical hyperostosis (CCH) is characterized by unilateral sterno-clavicular swelling (Figure 9). Some authors described it as a variant of chronic recurrent multifocal osteomyelitis (CRMO) (Girschick, Krauspe et al. 1998), and some as a sternoclavicular syndrome (Kalke, Perera et al. 2001). Histopathology is characterized by osteitis, hyperostosis and bone edema, without signs of microorganisms, or evidence of CRMO features. Some patients have jSpA features, and some are HLA-B27 positive. In adults, it is associated with spondyloarthritis, but the possible association to jSpA is not well established. Our preliminary data of the gene expression profiling study of patients with CCH and jSpA showed significant concordance in expression of genes linked to autoinflammatory (TLR-4, PTPN12) and autoimmune diseases (STAT3, CD36) (Harjacek, Lamot et al. 2011).

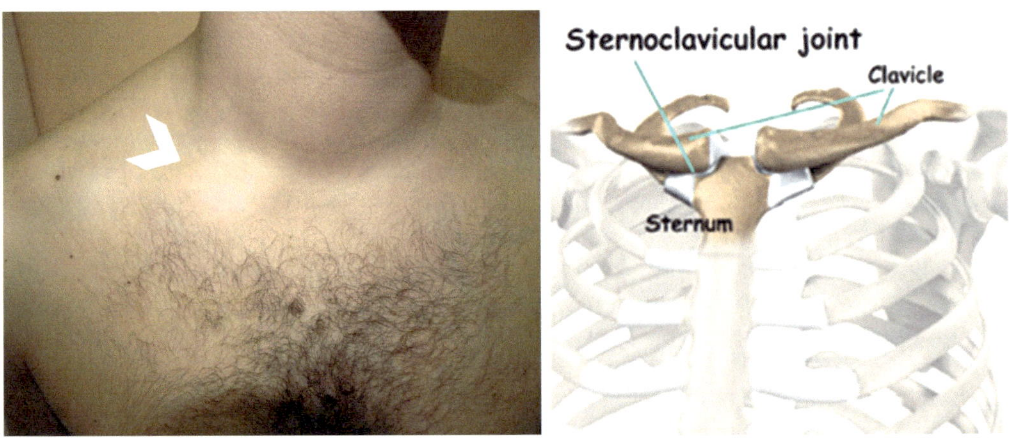

a) b)

Fig. 9. Seventeen-year-old male patient with CCH. Note the unilateral sternoclavicular swelling (A). Schematic representation of the sterno-clavicular joint (B).

Basic characteristics of juvenile spondyloarthritis are shown in Table 4.

	Reactive arthritis (Reiter's syndrome) (RA)	Undifferentiated jSpA (ERA)	Juvenile ankylosing spondylitis (jAS)	IBD-related arthritis (IBD)	Psoriatic arthritis (PsA)	Ankylosing tarsitis (AT)	Clavicular cortical hyperostosis (CCH)
Familial clustering	+	+	+	+	+	?	?
HLA B27 association	+	-/+	+	+	-/+	?	-/+
Enthesitis (fibro-cartilage entheses)	-	+	-/+	-/+	-/+	-	-
Synovitis (asymmetrical arthritis)	+	+	-/+	+	+	+	+
Axial involvement	-	-/+	+	-/+	+	-/+	-
Periositis	-	-	-	-	-	+	+
Colitis (asymptomatic and symptomatic)	+	-/+	-/+	+	-/+	-	-
Symptomatic uveitis	+	-/+	-/+	-/+	-/+	-	-
Bone marrow edema / subchondral edema	-/+	-/+	-	-/+	-/+	-/+	+
Ankylosis	-	-	+	-	-	-/+	-
Tarsitis ("midfoot disease")	-	-	-	-	-	+	-
Dactylitis	-	-	-	-	+	-	-
Nail pitting and psoriatic plaques	-	-	-	-	+	-	-
Other exraarticular manifestations	+	-/+	-/+	+	-	-	-

Table 4. The basic characteristics of jSpA

8. Laboratory yests

There are no pathognomonic blood tests for spondyloarthritis. Erythrocyte sedimentation rate might be elevated though it is nonspecific. The negative ANA and rheumatoid factor ("seronegativity"), in combination with positive HLA-B27 in a child with asymmetric arthritis and enthesitis, would be helpful. However, less than 5 percent of people who are HLA-B27 positive ever develop spondyloarthritis, so diagnosis should not rely solely on this finding.

9. Imaging in jSpA

Imaging studies usually reveal osteopenia mostly in the foot and hip area in the early stage, joint space narrowing and ankylosis in the later course of the disease. Erosions and destruction are rare, but enthesophytosis and bone bridging, particularly in the feet, are common. Subchondral sclerosis and irregularities of the articular surface in the lower third of the sacroiliac joints on the iliac side are usually seen, and this may progress to erosions, joint space narrowing, bone bridging and complete fusion of the sacroiliac bones. Long lasting disease activity leads also to syndesmophytosis and ligamentous calcification of the spine. Magnetic resonance (MR) and ultrasound (US) are useful methods for disease activity monitoring. MR may even reveal sacroiliac joint inflammation in children with neither symptoms nor radiographic changes (Braun and Baraliakos 2011).

9.1 Ultrasound

Musculoskeletal US assessment in general is safe, noninvasive, and comparably cheap, showing itself as a complimentary tool to clinical evaluation in Spa. Nevertheless, it is very user dependent (D'Agostino, Aegerter et al. 2011). US has an increasing and relevant role in the evaluation of SpA mainly for its ability to assess joint and periarticular soft tissue involvement and in particular for its capacity to detect enthesitis, the clinical hallmark feature of SpA. A number of ultrasound studies have also shown that clinically unrecognised enthesitis is common in the lower limbs including those insertions amenable to sonographic assessment adjacent to the knee joint in patients with jSpA (Riente, Delle Sedie et al. 2007; D'Agostino, Aegerter et al. 2011). Since most cases of enthesitis are subclinical, addition of gray-scale US and Power-Doppler US (PDUS) appears to be a valuable first-line diagnostic tool to confirm a diagnosis in a patient with suspected SpA (D'Agostino, Aegerter et al. 2011). Changes include thickening and edema of the insertions, increased vascularity, bone erosion, and new bone formation (Borman, Koparal et al. 2006). Also, in cases of dactylitis, US can accurately delineate the underlying pathology. US allow clinicians to guide needle positioning within inflamed joints, tendon sheaths and entheses in order to inject steroids or other drugs. The clinical application of US in SpA extends to the monitoring of therapy efficacy, particularly when coupled with power Doppler imaging. Very slight changes in vascularity are easily detected in joints, entheses or tendons, aiding the rheumatologist in the assessment of the effects of local or systemic therapies. Subclinical Achilles enthesitis, detected with gray-scale US, is described in a subset of AS patients and a significant improvement can be demonstrated after 2 months of TNF-alpha antagonist therapy (Aydin, Karadag et al. 2010). In addition, in children with JIA subclinical synovitis detected by US is common, and often missed clinically (Magni-Manzoni, Epis et al. 2009).

9.2 MRI

Diagnosing spondyloarthritis (SpA) early in young patients with inflammatory back pain and normal findings on radiographs of the sacroiliac joints (SIJ) remains a challenge in routine practice. Magnetic resonance imaging (MRI) is regarded as the most sensitive imaging modality for detecting early SpA before the radiographic appearance of structural lesions (Figure 10). Single MRI lesions suggestive of inflammation can be found in the SIJ and the spine in up to one quarter of healthy controls and young patients with mechanical back pain (Weber and Maksymowych 2011).

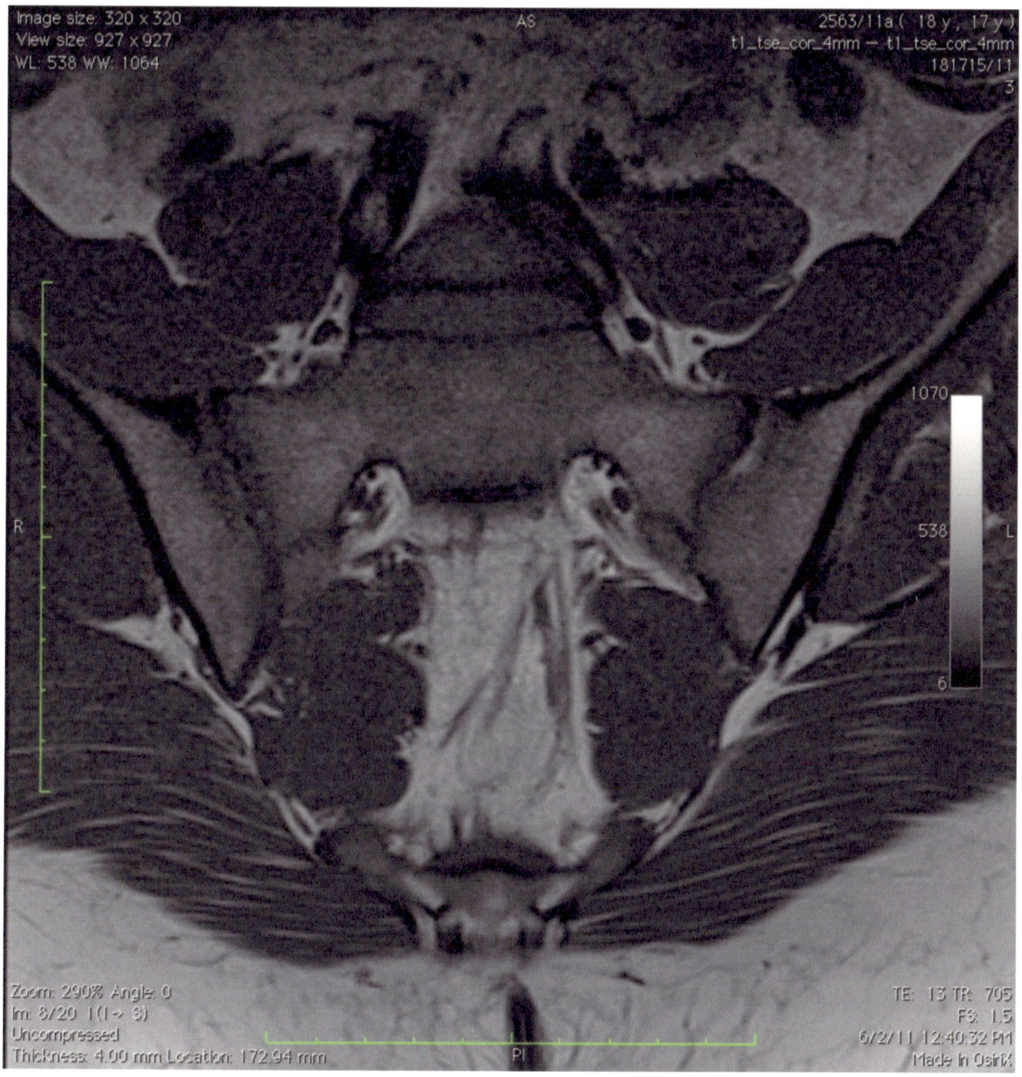

Fig. 10. MRI of the SI joints in a 12 year old boy with right-sided buttock pain. Coronal SE T1 WI shows erosive changes of articular facets of right sacroiliac joint with sclerotic subchondral bone.

MRI is highly sensitive for active enthesitis and depicts not only the enthesis itself but also associated findings such as soft-tissue involvement and bone marrow edema. Extensive and diffuse patterns of bone marrow edema are more closely related to inflammatory enthesitis, as shown in the hip. When soft-tissue involvement occurs in a synovial joint, synovitis may mask some, if not all, MRI features of enthesitis. Still, differentiation between the different causes of enthesitis (i.e., inflammatory, mechanical, metabolic) is only reliably possible in the context of the available clinical information. Despite these limitations, MRI represents a significant advance for the early diagnosis of ERA and for monitoring therapy that targets entheseal inflammation (Eshed, Bollow et al. 2007).

9.3 Conventional radiography

Imaging studies usually reveal osteopenia mostly in the foot and hip area in the early stage, joint space narrowing and ankylosis in the later course of the disease. Erosions and destruction are rare, but enthesophytosis and bone bridging, particularly in the feet, are common. Subchondral sclerosis and irregularities of the articular surface in the lower third of the sacroiliac joints on the iliac side are usually seen, and this may progress to erosions, joint space narrowing, bone bridging and complete fusion of the sacroiliac bones. Long lasting disease activity leads also to desmophytosis and ligamentous calcification of the spine. Plain radiography is insensitive to most of the early inflammatory changes in the sacroiliac joints in AS, yet to fulfill the modified New York criteria (van der Linden, Valkenburg et al. 1984), sacroillitis must be present as either grade 2 (erosion and sclerosis) or greater bilaterally, or grade 3–4 (erosion, sclerosis, and/or ankylosis) unilaterally (Figure 11). In one study, it took 5 years in 36%, and 10 years in 59% of patients with IBP and radiographically normal (or suspicious) sacroiliac joints to develop radiographic sacroillitis (Mau, Zeidler et al. 1988). Although conventional radiography is indicated in the initial evaluation of sacroiliac joints diseases, it is often insensitive for demonstrating the early changes of sacroillitis, so other imaging techniques typically are often necessary to clarify the pathology and for establishing the early diagnosis of seronegative SpA (Guglielmi, Scalzo et al. 2009).

We have to take into account that these New York criteria were designed for pathology in adult patients. In children the development of the skeleton does not allow us to interpret plain radiographs of the sacroiliac joints in a proper way until the Risser index reaches stage five. If that is not a case, sacroillitis may be misdiagnosed because of pseudowidening of the articular space and irregular margins.

10. Treatment of jSpA

In cases of juvenile-onset SpA, treatment decisions are based on clinical experience rather than on evidence from clinical trials (Burgos-Vargas, 2009). Medications and physical therapy are the mainstays of therapy. NSAIDs might be helpful to a degree, especially if there is inflammatory back pain or peripheral arthritis. Sulfasalazine can work well for peripheral arthritis, but it is not as effective for axial disease (Burgos-Vargas, Vazquez-Mellado et al. 2002). Methotrexate as second line agent is a good option in other forms of JIA, however its use in jSpA is limited. Steroids are used sparingly, mostly as intra-articular injections with triamcionolone hexacetonide. The combination of these conventional medications is often inadequate in controlling spondyloarthropathy.

The therapeutic value of low-energy lasers (LLLT) for enthesitis is controversial, and has not been systematically studied in children with spondyloarthritis. LLLT (Ga-Al-As laser) is a light source that generates extremely pure light, of a single wavelength. The effect is not thermal, but rather related to photochemical reactions in the cells (Brosseau, Robinson et al. 2005; Hawkins, Houreld et al. 2005). Laser therapy is used in many biomedical sciences to promote tissue regeneration (Mester, Mester et al. 1985; Karu 1999). Many studies involving the low-level laser therapy have shown that the healing process is enhanced by such therapy (Enwemeka 1988; Rochkind, Rousso et al. 1989; Nemeth 1993; Grossman, Schneid et al. 1998; O'Brien, Li et al. 1998; Lilge, Tierney et al. 2000; Maegawa, Itoh et al. 2000; Schlager, Kronberger et al. 2000; Sommer, Pinheiro et al. 2001; Wong-Riley, Bai et al. 2001; do Nascimento, Pinheiro et al. 2004; Eells, Wong-Riley et al. 2004; Pinheiro, Meireles et al. 2004; Hawkins, Houreld et al. 2005). In Table 5 we show the results of LLLT therapy in the pilot study of 38 children with jSpA diagnosed based on both ESSG and ILAR criteria, which we treated, in addition to standard NSAID therapy, with LLLT (Harjacek and Lamot 2008).

No. of patients	**38**
Cumulative dose	2.5 - 3 J/m^3
Treatment duration (days)	15,6 (10-40)
Enthesitis	
Infrapatelar	13
Achilles	20
AC	10
Inguinal	5
VAS before	5
VAS after	1,2

Table 5. LLLT (Ga-Al-As laser) treatment response.

In this pilot study we have shown that LLLT (Ga-Al-As laser) seems to be very effective in reducing pain in children with jSpA and enthesitis (76% VAS pain reduction). Visual analogue scales have become an acceptable measurement tool, and the use of a VAS to measure pain has been shown to have a high interclass correlation of 0.95. (Chow, Heller et al. 2006). This is in concordance with other studies that have found the lowering of VAS for the 2 points on a 10- point scale to be significant (Farrar, Portenoy et al. 2000; Farrar, Young et al. 2001; Chow, Heller et al. 2006; Van Breukelen 2006).

Currently, the best treatment for severe cases of juvenile-onset SpA is probably anti-TNF therapy. Anti-TNF alpha agents are also approved for use in Crohn's disease and psoriatic arthritis in children. Etanercept (Enbrel), infliximab (Remicade) and adalimumab (Humira) are in this group and work in the majority of patients. They have improved short-term outcomes in ankylosing spondylitis and psoriatic arthritis dramatically, and it seems they change the long-term disease course and outcome (Henrickson and Reiff 2004; Tse, Burgos-Vargas et al. 2005; Sulpice, Deslandre et al. 2009; Lamot, Bukovac et al. 2011). jSpA patients treated with TNF-blockers, such as infliximab and etanercept, have shown significant Improvements in the number of active joints and tender entheses, ESR, CRP levels, and CHAQ scores (Henrickson and Reiff 2004; Tse, Burgos-Vargas et al. 2005; Sulpice, Deslandre

et al. 2009; Lamot, Bukovac et al. 2011). In addition, the results of a 3-month, randomized, double-blind, placebo-controlled trial to assess the efficacy of infliximab showed that this treatment significantly improved most measures of disease activity compared to placebo, including the number of active joints and tender entheses, pain intensity, patient and/or parent assessment of well-being and physician assessments of disease activity, health status, CHAQ score and CRP level (Burgos-Vargas 2007). There was no difference between groups in the frequency of adverse events.Regular exercises for stretching the spine and physical therapy are important to keep spinal and joint mobility in patients with jSpA.
Basic principles in the treatment of jSpA are shown in Figure 12.

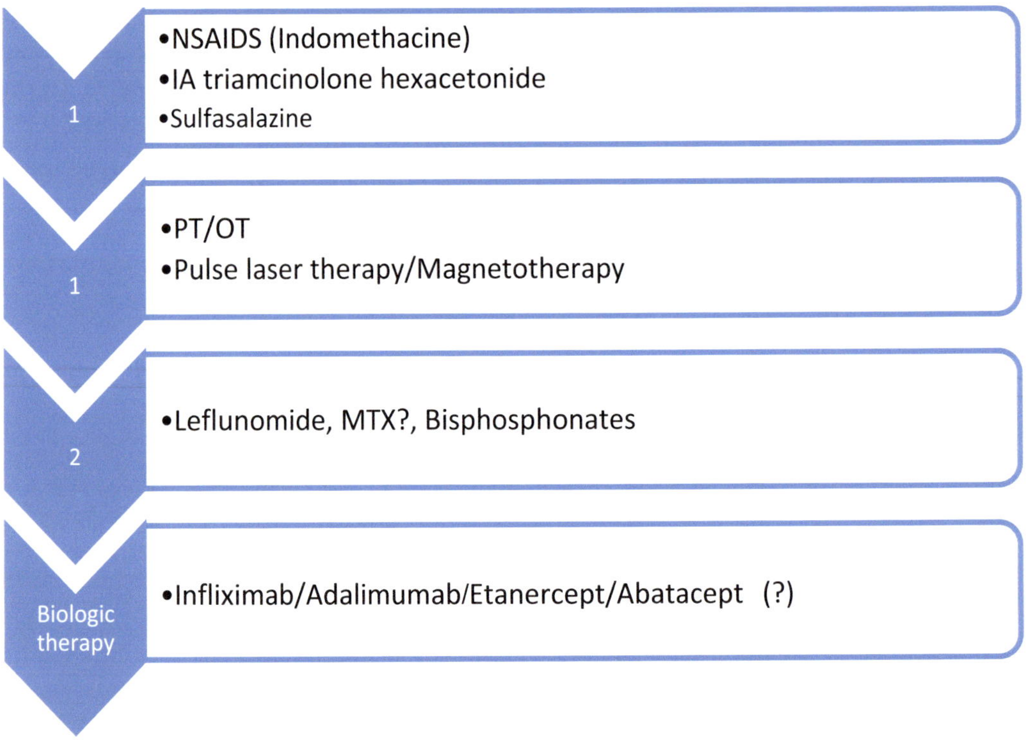

Fig. 12. Treatment of jSpA.

11. Prognosis

It is difficult to accurately estimate prognosis because the spectrum of jSpA is so broad. In comparison with other forms of juvenile arthritis, juvenile SpA tends to have a poorer outcome. While prognosis for ReA is clearly favorable, the majority of children who start out with undifferented jSpA (ERA), if not treated properly and early-enough, will eventually develop ankylosing spondylitis (Andersson Gare 1999; Burgos-Vargas 2002; Minden, Niewerth et al. 2002). In addition, patients might have long periods of remission, although "outgrowing" jSpA is not an expectation. In the pre-anti-TNF therapy reported remission rates of ERA following treatment and prior to adulthood range from 17% to 37%, and the risk of developing sacroillitis within the first 5 years after diagnosis ranges from 6% to approximately 50% across studies (Flato, Smerdel et al. 2002; Pagnini, Savelli et al. 2010;

Stoll, Bhore et al. 2010). Long term outcome is rather impaired as illustrated by a retrospective study by Flato *et al. (Flato, Hoffmann-Vold et al. 2006)* and by Minden *et al.* (Minden, Niewerth et al. 2002). Functional scores (measured by HAQ) are elevated and quality of life (measured by SF-36) is diminished. Remission rates varied from 18 % after 11 years (Minden, Niewerth et al. 2002) to 44 % after 15 years of disease (Flato, Hoffmann-Vold et al. 2006). In 35 % sacroillitis was found during the course of disease (Flato, Hoffmann-Vold et al. 2006) and in 39 % definite As developed (Minden, Niewerth et al. 2002). In older boys with JIA the positive HLA-B27 predicts increasingly extended disease within the first 3 years. It is also associated with involvement of small joints in the lower extremities (primarily subtalar and tarsal joints) in boys but not in girls, and with inflammatory back pain in both sexes (Berntson, Damgard et al. 2008). The new epidemiologic and outcome data in a "post-TNF-α" era are clearly warranted.

12. Conclusions

The juvenile spondyloarthritis is a group of seronegative, immune-mediated inflammatory pediatric disorders characterized by enthesitis and arthritis, and a variety of extra-articular symptoms. They must be distinguished from JIA, however the distinction may not always be obvious. While the reactive arthritis is by far the most common form, in many children, the specific chronic disorder remains "undifferentiated"; most of these children fulfill criteria for ERA . Other children might develop more differentiated forms: jAS, jPsA, as well as, IBD-related arthritis. Although these are distinctive diseases, they have a number of clinical, radiologic, and genetic characteristics in common, which permit them to be classified under the unifying term "spondyloarthritis. There is not a specific test to be used since HLA-B27 is neither necessary nor sufficient, but clearly involved in the pathogenesis of disease. Since plain radiograph is often difficult to interpret in a growing child, the US is becoming the primary and most important imaging modality for the assessment of these diseases. Children with jSpA are at risk for sacroillitis, which may be present in the absence of suggestive symptoms or physical examination findings. Therefore, a routine screening by MRI has been recently proposed. Axial involvement is usually a late finding. The treatment decisions are based on clinical experience rather than on evidence from clinical trials; NSAID's and physiotherapy (including LLLT) are frequently used to manage symptoms. Sulphasalazine seems to be more effective on peripheral arthritis then on axial disease. New biologic therapies appear to improve outcomes, but education, exercise, physical and occupational therapy for stretching and maintaining range of motion are still the key components of management. Despite significant advances in the treatment of jSpA over the past few years, a better understanding of pathogenesis is likely to improve outcome by identifying ways to provide greater and more sustained clinical responses.

13. Key points

1. Juvenile spondyloarthritis (jSpA) is a term that refers to group inflammatory disorders affecting children under the age of 16 years, characterized by enthesitis and arthritis affecting predominantly the joints of the lower extremities.
2. The jSpA often begins as 'undifferentiated' disease (ERA), the presentation of which differs in children and adults; most notably, spinal involvement is uncommon, while hip arthritis is frequently seen in juvenile-onset disease.

3. jSpA are multifactorial diseases in which a disturbed interplay occurs between the immune system and environmental factors on a predisposing genetic background. The jSpA are polygenic in nature, both MHC genes (e.g. HLA-B27, etc.), and non-MHC genes (e.g. TLR-4, etc.) play a significant role in the disease pathogenesis.
4. Subclinical gut inflammation has been demonstrated in patients with all forms of juvenile spondyloarthritis.
5. While classification of juvenile spondyloarthritis is a "work in progress" and clearly problematic, the Garmisch-Partenkirchen criteria are the major candidates for future research in identifying spondyloarthritis in juvenile patients.
6. There are no pathognomonic blood tests for spondyloarthritis.
7. Magnetic resonance (MR) and ultrasound (US) are useful methods for disease activity monitoring, even in the asymptomatic patient.
8. In cases of juvenile-onset SpA, treatment decisions are based on clinical experience rather than on evidence from clinical trials; in addition to NSAID's and sulfasalazine, anti-TNF therapy has become the best treatment for severe cases of jSpA.
9. Education, exercise, physical and occupational therapy for stretching and maintaining range of motion are still the key components of management
10. Prognosis in the post "anti-TNF-α" era is largely unknown but clearly more favorable than before. Better understanding of pathogenesis is likely to improve outcome by identifying ways to provide greater and more sustained clinical responses.

14. References

Aalto, K., A. Autio, et al. (2011). "Siglec-9 is a novel leukocyte ligand for vascular adhesion protein-1 and can be used in PET imaging of inflammation and cancer." Blood 118(13): 3725-3733.

Adarichev, V. A. and T. T. Glant (2006). "Experimental spondyloarthropathies: animal models of ankylosing spondylitis." Curr Rheumatol Rep 8(4): 267-274.

Agarwal, S., R. Misra, et al. (2009). "Synovial fluid RANKL and matrix metalloproteinase levels in enthesitis related arthritis subtype of juvenile idiopathic arthritis." Rheumatol Int 29(8): 907-911.

Alvarez-Madrid, C., R. Merino, et al. (2009). "Tarsitis as an initial manifestation of juvenile spondyloarthropathy." Clin Exp Rheumatol 27(4): 691-694.

Amor, B., M. Dougados, et al. (1991). "[Evaluation of the Amor criteria for spondylarthropathies and European Spondylarthropathy Study Group (ESSG). A cross-sectional analysis of 2,228 patients]." Ann Med Interne (Paris) 142(2): 85-89.

Amor, B., M. Dougados, et al. (1990). "[Criteria of the classification of spondylarthropathies]." Rev Rhum Mal Osteoartic 57(2): 85-89.

Andersson Gare, B. (1999). "Juvenile arthritis--who gets it, where and when? A review of current data on incidence and prevalence." Clin Exp Rheumatol 17(3): 367-374.

Appel, H., R. Maier, et al. (2011). "Analysis of IL-17+ cells in facet joints of patients with spondyloarthritis suggests that the innate immune pathway might be of greater relevance than the Th17-mediated adaptive immune response." Arthritis Res Ther 13(3): R95.

Arabshahi, B., K. M. Baskin, et al. (2007). "Reactive arthritis of the temporomandibular joints and cervical spine in a child." Pediatr Rheumatol Online J 5: 4.

Artamonov, V. A., S. Akhmadi, et al. (1991). "[The clinical and immunogenetic characteristics of reactive arthritis in children]." Ter Arkh 63(5): 22-24.

Assassi, S., J. D. Reveille, et al. (2011). "Whole-blood gene expression profiling in ankylosing spondylitis shows upregulation of toll-like receptor 4 and 5." J Rheumatol 38(1): 87-98.

Aydin, S. Z., O. Karadag, et al. (2010). "Monitoring Achilles enthesitis in ankylosing spondylitis during TNF-alpha antagonist therapy: an ultrasound study." Rheumatology (Oxford) 49(3): 578-582.

Barash, J., E. Mashiach, et al. (2008). "Differentiation of post-streptococcal reactive arthritis from acute rheumatic fever." J Pediatr 153(5): 696-699.

Barnes, M. G., B. J. Aronow, et al. (2004). "Gene expression in juvenile arthritis and spondyloarthropathy: pro-angiogenic ELR+ chemokine genes relate to course of arthritis." Rheumatology (Oxford) 43(8): 973-979.

Barnes, M. G., A. A. Grom, et al. (2009). "Subtype-specific peripheral blood gene expression profiles in recent-onset juvenile idiopathic arthritis." Arthritis Rheum 60(7): 2102-2112.

Benjamin, M. and D. McGonagle (2007). "Histopathologic changes at "synovio-entheseal complexes" suggesting a novel mechanism for synovitis in osteoarthritis and spondylarthritis." Arthritis Rheum 56(11): 3601-3609.

Berlin, C., R. F. Bargatze, et al. (1995). "alpha 4 integrins mediate lymphocyte attachment and rolling under physiologic flow." Cell 80(3): 413-422.

Berlin, C., E. L. Berg, et al. (1993). "Alpha 4 beta 7 integrin mediates lymphocyte binding to the mucosal vascular addressin MAdCAM-1." Cell 74(1): 185-195.

Berntson, L., M. Damgard, et al. (2008). "HLA-B27 predicts a more extended disease with increasing age at onset in boys with juvenile idiopathic arthritis." J Rheumatol 35(10): 2055-2061.

Bhatia, N. N., G. Chow, et al. (2008). "Diagnostic modalities for the evaluation of pediatric back pain: a prospective study." J Pediatr Orthop 28(2): 230-233.

Birnbaum, J., J. G. Bartlett, et al. (2008). "Clostridium difficile: an under-recognized cause of reactive arthritis?" Clin Rheumatol 27(2): 253-255.

Bollow, M., K. G. Hermann, et al. (2005). "Very early spondyloarthritis: where the inflammation in the sacroiliac joints starts." Ann Rheum Dis 64(11): 1644-1646.

Borman, P., S. Koparal, et al. (2006). "Ultrasound detection of entheseal insertions in the foot of patients with spondyloarthropathy." Clin Rheumatol 25(3): 373-377.

Bowyer, S. and P. Roettcher (1996). "Pediatric rheumatology clinic populations in the United States: results of a 3 year survey. Pediatric Rheumatology Database Research Group." J Rheumatol 23(11): 1968-1974.

Boyer, G. S., D. W. Templin, et al. (1993). "Evaluation of the European Spondylarthropathy Study Group preliminary classification criteria in Alaskan Eskimo populations." Arthritis Rheum 36(4): 534-538.

Braun, J. and X. Baraliakos (2011). "Imaging of axial spondyloarthritis including ankylosing spondylitis." Ann Rheum Dis 70 Suppl 1: i97-103.

Braun, J., M. Bollow, et al. (1998). "Prevalence of spondylarthropathies in HLA-B27 positive and negative blood donors." Arthritis Rheum 41(1): 58-67.

Braun, J., M. A. Khan, et al. (2000). "Enthesitis and ankylosis in spondyloarthropathy: what is the target of the immune response?" Ann Rheum Dis 59(12): 985-994.

Brophy, S., S. Hickey, et al. (2004). "Concordance of disease severity among family members with ankylosing spondylitis?" J Rheumatol 31(9): 1775-1778.

Brosseau, L., V. Robinson, et al. (2005). "Low level laser therapy (Classes I, II and III) for treating rheumatoid arthritis." Cochrane Database Syst Rev(4): CD002049.

Brown, M. A., S. Brophy, et al. (2003). "Identification of major loci controlling clinical manifestations of ankylosing spondylitis." Arthritis Rheum 48(8): 2234-2239.

Brown, M. A., K. D. Pile, et al. (1998). "A genome-wide screen for susceptibility loci in ankylosing spondylitis." Arthritis Rheum 41(4): 588-595.

Burbige, E. J., S. H. Huang, et al. (1975). "Clinical manifestations of Crohn's disease in children and adolescents." Pediatrics 55(6): 866-871.

Burgos-Vargas, R. (2002). "The juvenile-onset spondyloarthritides." Rheum Dis Clin North Am 28(3): 531-560, vi.

Burgos-Vargas, R. (2007). "Efficacy, safety, and tolerability of infliximab in juvenile-onset spondyloarthropathies (JO-SpA): results of the three-month, randomized, double-blind, placebo-controlled trial phase." Arthritis Rheum 56 (Suppl): S319.

Burgos-Vargas, R., G. Castelazo-Duarte, et al. (1993). "Chest expansion in healthy adolescents and patients with the seronegative enthesopathy and arthropathy syndrome or juvenile ankylosing spondylitis." J Rheumatol 20(11): 1957-1960.

Burgos-Vargas, R. and P. Clark (1989). "Axial involvement in the seronegative enthesopathy and arthropathy syndrome and its progression to ankylosing spondylitis." J Rheumatol 16(2): 192-197.

Burgos-Vargas, R., C. Pacheco-Tena, et al. (2002). "A short-term follow-up of enthesitis and arthritis in the active phase of juvenile onset spondyloarthropathies." Clin Exp Rheumatol 20(5): 727-731.

Burgos-Vargas, R., M. Rudwaleit, et al. (2002). "The place of juvenile onset spondyloarthropathies in the Durban 1997 ILAR classification criteria of juvenile idiopathic arthritis. International League of Associations for Rheumatology." J Rheumatol 29(5): 869-874.

Burgos-Vargas, R., J. Vazquez-Mellado, et al. (1996). "Genuine ankylosing spondylitis in children: a case-control study of patients with early definite disease according to adult onset criteria." J Rheumatol 23(12): 2140-2147.

Burgos-Vargas, R., J. Vazquez-Mellado, et al. (2002). "A 26 week randomised, double blind, placebo controlled exploratory study of sulfasalazine in juvenile onset spondyloarthropathies." Ann Rheum Dis 61(10): 941-942.

Campbell, D. J. and E. C. Butcher (2002). "Rapid acquisition of tissue-specific homing phenotypes by CD4(+) T cells activated in cutaneous or mucosal lymphoid tissues." J Exp Med 195(1): 135-141.

Carter, S. and R. J. Lories (2011). "Osteoporosis: A Paradox in Ankylosing Spondylitis." Curr Osteoporos Rep.

Cassidy, J. T. and R. E. Petty (2001). Textbook of pediatric rheumatology. Philadelphia, W.B. Saunders.

Cassidy, J. T. and R. E. Petty (2006). Textbook of pediatric rheumatology. Philadelphia, PA, Elsevier Saunders.

Cedoz, J. P., D. Wendling, et al. (1995). "The B7 cross reactive group and spondyloarthropathies: an epidemiological approach." J Rheumatol 22(10): 1884-1890.

Chow, R. T., G. Z. Heller, et al. (2006). "The effect of 300 mW, 830 nm laser on chronic neck pain: a double-blind, randomized, placebo-controlled study." Pain 124(1-2): 201-210.

Ciccia, F., A. Accardo-Palumbo, et al. (2010). "Expansion of intestinal CD4+CD25(high) Treg cells in patients with ankylosing spondylitis: a putative role for interleukin-10 in preventing intestinal Th17 response." Arthritis Rheum 62(12): 3625-3634.

Colbert, R. A. (2010). "Classification of juvenile spondyloarthritis: Enthesitis-related arthritis and beyond." Nat Rev Rheumatol 6(8): 477-485.

Colbert, R. A. (2010). "Early axial spondyloarthritis." Curr Opin Rheumatol 22(5): 603-607.

Colbert, R. A., M. L. DeLay, et al. (2010). "From HLA-B27 to spondyloarthritis: a journey through the ER." Immunol Rev 233(1): 181-202.

Conti, F., O. Borrelli, et al. (2005). "Chronic intestinal inflammation and seronegative spondyloarthropathy in children." Dig Liver Dis 37(10): 761-767.

Cury, S. E., M. J. Vilar, et al. (1997). "Evaluation of the European Spondylarthropathy Study Group (ESSG) preliminary classification criteria in Brazilian patients." Clin Exp Rheumatol 15(1): 79-82.

Cuttica, R. J., E. J. Scheines, et al. (1992). "Juvenile onset Reiter's syndrome. A retrospective study of 26 patients." Clin Exp Rheumatol 10(3): 285-288.

D'Agostino, M. A., P. Aegerter, et al. (2011). "How to diagnose spondyloarthritis early? Accuracy of peripheral enthesitis detection by power Doppler ultrasonography." Ann Rheum Dis 70(8): 1433-1440.

do Nascimento, P. M., A. L. Pinheiro, et al. (2004). "A preliminary report on the effect of laser therapy on the healing of cutaneous surgical wounds as a consequence of an inversely proportional relationship between wavelength and intensity: histological study in rats." Photomed Laser Surg 22(6): 513-518.

Dougados, M., S. van der Linden, et al. (1991). "The European Spondylarthropathy Study Group preliminary criteria for the classification of spondylarthropathy." Arthritis Rheum 34(10): 1218-1227.

Drexler, S. K. and B. M. Foxwell (2010). "The role of toll-like receptors in chronic inflammation." Int J Biochem Cell Biol 42(4): 506-518.

Duffy, C. M., R. A. Colbert, et al. (2005). "Nomenclature and classification in chronic childhood arthritis: time for a change?" Arthritis Rheum 52(2): 382-385.

Eells, J. T., M. T. Wong-Riley, et al. (2004). "Mitochondrial signal transduction in accelerated wound and retinal healing by near-infrared light therapy." Mitochondrion 4(5-6): 559-567.

el-Zaatari, F. A., K. C. Sams, et al. (1990). "In vitro mutagenesis of HLA-B27. Amino acid substitutions at position 67 disrupt anti-B27 monoclonal antibody binding in direct relation to the size of the substituted side chain." J Immunol 144(4): 1512-1517.

el-Zaatari, F. A. and J. D. Taurog (1992). "In vitro mutagenesis of HLA-B27: single and multiple amino acid substitutions at consensus B27 sites identify distinct monoclonal antibody-defined epitopes." Hum Immunol 33(4): 243-248.

Enwemeka, C. S. (1988). "Laser biostimulation of healing wounds: specific effects and mechanisms of action." J Orthop Sports Phys Ther 9(10): 333-338.

Eshed, I., M. Bollow, et al. (2007). "MRI of enthesitis of the appendicular skeleton in spondyloarthritis." Ann Rheum Dis 66(12): 1553-1559.

Evans, H. G., T. Suddason, et al. (2007). "Optimal induction of T helper 17 cells in humans requires T cell receptor ligation in the context of Toll-like receptor-activated monocytes." Proc Natl Acad Sci U S A 104(43): 17034-17039.

Fantini, F. (2001). "Classification of chronic arthritides of childhood (juvenile idiopathic arthritis): criticisms and suggestions to improve the efficacy of the Santiago-Durban criteria." J Rheumatol 28(2): 456-459.

Fantini, M. C., F. Pallone, et al. (2009). "Common immunologic mechanisms in inflammatory bowel disease and spondylarthropathies." World J Gastroenterol 15(20): 2472-2478.

Farrar, J. T., R. K. Portenoy, et al. (2000). "Defining the clinically important difference in pain outcome measures." Pain 88(3): 287-294.

Farrar, J. T., J. P. Young, Jr., et al. (2001). "Clinical importance of changes in chronic pain intensity measured on an 11-point numerical pain rating scale." Pain 94(2): 149-158.

Fendler, C., S. Laitko, et al. (2001). "Frequency of triggering bacteria in patients with reactive arthritis and undifferentiated oligoarthritis and the relative importance of the tests used for diagnosis." Ann Rheum Dis 60(4): 337-343.

Fernandez-Sueiro, J. L., C. Alonso, et al. (2004). "Prevalence of HLA-B27 and subtypes of HLA-B27 associated with ankylosing spondylitis in Galicia, Spain." Clin Exp Rheumatol 22(4): 465-468.

Fink, C. W. (1995). "Proposal for the development of classification criteria for idiopathic arthritides of childhood." J Rheumatol 22(8): 1566-1569.

Flato, B., A. M. Hoffmann-Vold, et al. (2006). "Long-term outcome and prognostic factors in enthesitis-related arthritis: a case-control study." Arthritis Rheum 54(11): 3573-3582.

Flato, B., A. Smerdel, et al. (2002). "The influence of patient characteristics, disease variables, and HLA alleles on the development of radiographically evident sacroiliitis in juvenile idiopathic arthritis." Arthritis Rheum 46(4): 986-994.

Gerard, H. C., J. A. Whittum-Hudson, et al. (2010). "The pathogenic role of Chlamydia in spondyloarthritis." Curr Opin Rheumatol 22(4): 363-367.

Girschick, H. J., R. Krauspe, et al. (1998). "Chronic recurrent osteomyelitis with clavicular involvement in children: diagnostic value of different imaging techniques and therapy with non-steroidal anti-inflammatory drugs." Eur J Pediatr 157(1): 28-33.

Gomez, K. S., K. Raza, et al. (1997). "Juvenile onset ankylosing spondylitis--more girls than we thought?" J Rheumatol 24(4): 735-737.

Grossman, N., N. Schneid, et al. (1998). "780 nm low power diode laser irradiation stimulates proliferation of keratinocyte cultures: involvement of reactive oxygen species." Lasers Surg Med 22(4): 212-218.

Gu, J., Y. L. Wei, et al. (2009). "Identification of RGS1 as a candidate biomarker for undifferentiated spondylarthritis by genome-wide expression profiling and real-time polymerase chain reaction." Arthritis Rheum 60(11): 3269-3279.

Guglielmi, G., G. Scalzo, et al. (2009). "Imaging of the sacroiliac joint involvement in seronegative spondylarthropathies." Clin Rheumatol 28(9): 1007-1019.

Hafner, R. (1987). "[Juvenile spondarthritis. Retrospective study of 71 patients]." Monatsschr Kinderheilkd 135(1): 41-46.

Hamilton, J. R., G. A. Bruce, et al. (1979). "Inflammatory bowel disease in children and adolescents." Adv Pediatr 26: 311-341.

Harjacek, M. and L. Lamot (2008). The therapeutic value of low-energy laser (LLLT) for enthesitis in children with juvenile spondyloarthropathies. 15th Paediatric Rheumatology European Society (PreS) Congress, London, UK, BioMed Central.

Harjacek, M., L. Lamot, et al. (2011). Clavicular cortical hyperostosis: new autoinflammatory entity or part of the juvenile spondyloarthropathies clnical picture? 18th European Pediatric Rheumatology Congress Bruges, Belgium

Harjacek, M., T. Margetic, et al. (2008). "HLA-B*27/HLA-B*07 in combination with D6S273-134 allele is associated with increased susceptibility to juvenile spondyloarthropathies." Clin Exp Rheumatol 26(3): 498-504.

Harjacek, M., J. Ostojic, et al. (2006). "Juvenile spondyloarthropathies associated with Mycoplasma pneumoniae infection." Clin Rheumatol 25(4): 470-475.

Harjacek M., L. L., Frleta M., Bukovac L.T., Borovecki F. (2010). Distinctive gene expression in patients with juvenile spondyloartropathy is related to autoinflammatory diseases. 17th Pediatric Rheumatology European Society Congress, Valencia, Spain.

Haroon, N. and R. D. Inman (2010). "Endoplasmic reticulum aminopeptidases: Biology and pathogenic potential." Nat Rev Rheumatol 6(8): 461-467.

Hawkins, D., N. Houreld, et al. (2005). "Low level laser therapy (LLLT) as an effective therapeutic modality for delayed wound healing." Ann N Y Acad Sci 1056: 486-493.

Henrickson, M. and A. Reiff (2004). "Prolonged efficacy of etanercept in refractory enthesitis-related arthritis." J Rheumatol 31(10): 2055-2061.

Hestbaek, L., C. Leboeuf-Yde, et al. (2006). "The course of low back pain from adolescence to adulthood: eight-year follow-up of 9600 twins." Spine (Phila Pa 1976) 31(4): 468-472.

Heuft-Dorenbosch, L., R. Landewe, et al. (2007). "Performance of various criteria sets in patients with inflammatory back pain of short duration; the Maastricht early spondyloarthritis clinic." Ann Rheum Dis 66(1): 92-98.

Hinks, A., P. Martin, et al. (2011). "Subtype specific genetic associations for juvenile idiopathic arthritis: ERAP1 with the enthesitis related arthritis subtype and IL23R with juvenile psoriatic arthritis." Arthritis Res Ther 13(1): R12.

Hofbauer, L. C. and M. Schoppet (2004). "Clinical implications of the osteoprotegerin/RANKL/RANK system for bone and vascular diseases." JAMA 292(4): 490-495.

Hofer, M. and T. R. Southwood (2002). "Classification of childhood arthritis." Best Pract Res Clin Rheumatol 16(3): 379-396.

Hussein, A. (1987). "[Spectrum of post-enteritic reactive arthritis in childhood]." Monatsschr Kinderheilkd 135(2): 93-98.

Hussein, A., H. Abdul-Khaliq, et al. (1989). "Atypical spondyloarthritis in children: proposed diagnostic criteria." Eur J Pediatr 148(6): 513-517.

Johansson-Lindbom, B., M. Svensson, et al. (2003). "Selective generation of gut tropic T cells in gut-associated lymphoid tissue (GALT): requirement for GALT dendritic cells and adjuvant." J Exp Med 198(6): 963-969.

Jones, G. T. and G. J. Macfarlane (2005). "Epidemiology of low back pain in children and adolescents." Arch Dis Child 90(3): 312-316.

Joos, R., J. Dehoorne, et al. (2009). "Sensitivity and specificity of criteria for spondyloarthritis in children with late onset pauciarticular juvenile chronic arthritis as well as their characteristics." Clin Exp Rheumatol 27(5): 870-876.

Jose, F. A., E. A. Garnett, et al. (2009). "Development of extraintestinal manifestations in pediatric patients with inflammatory bowel disease." Inflamm Bowel Dis 15(1): 63-68.

Kalke, S., S. D. Perera, et al. (2001). "The sternoclavicular syndrome: experience from a district general hospital and results of a national postal survey." Rheumatology (Oxford) 40(2): 170-177.

Karu, T. (1999). "Primary and secondary mechanisms of action of visible to near-IR radiation on cells." J Photochem Photobiol B 49(1): 1-17.

Kasapcopur, O., N. Demirli, et al. (2005). "Evaluation of classification criteria for juvenile-onset spondyloarthropathies." Rheumatol Int 25(6): 414-418.

Khare, S. D., M. J. Bull, et al. (1998). "Spontaneous inflammatory disease in HLA-B27 transgenic mice is independent of MHC class II molecules: a direct role for B27 heavy chains and not B27-derived peptides." J Immunol 160(1): 101-106.

Kivi, E., K. Elima, et al. (2009). "Human Siglec-10 can bind to vascular adhesion protein-1 and serves as its substrate." Blood 114(26): 5385-5392.

Kruithof, E., L. De Rycke, et al. (2006). "Identification of synovial biomarkers of response to experimental treatment in early-phase clinical trials in spondylarthritis." Arthritis Rheum 54(6): 1795-1804.

Kruithof, E., V. Van den Bossche, et al. (2006). "Distinct synovial immunopathologic characteristics of juvenile-onset spondylarthritis and other forms of juvenile idiopathic arthritis." Arthritis Rheum 54(8): 2594-2604.

Lamot, L., L. T. Bukovac, et al. (2011). "The 'head-to-head' comparison of etanercept and infliximab in treating children with juvenile idiopathic arthritis." Clin Exp Rheumatol 29(1): 131-139.

Laval, S. H., A. Timms, et al. (2001). "Whole-genome screening in ankylosing spondylitis: evidence of non-MHC genetic-susceptibility loci." Am J Hum Genet 68(4): 918-926.

Leirisalo-Repo, M. (1998). "Prognosis, course of disease, and treatment of the spondyloarthropathies." Rheum Dis Clin North Am 24(4): 737-751, viii.

Leirisalo-Repo, M., P. Helenius, et al. (1997). "Long-term prognosis of reactive salmonella arthritis." Ann Rheum Dis 56(9): 516-520.

Leirisalo, M., G. Skylv, et al. (1982). "Followup study on patients with Reiter's disease and reactive arthritis, with special reference to HLA-B27." Arthritis Rheum 25(3): 249-259.

Lilge, L., K. Tierney, et al. (2000). "Low-level laser therapy for wound healing: feasibility of wound dressing transillumination." J Clin Laser Med Surg 18(5): 235-240.

Lin, Y. C., T. H. Liang, et al. (2009). "Differences between juvenile-onset ankylosing spondylitis and adult-onset ankylosing spondylitis." J Chin Med Assoc 72(11): 573-580.

Lories, R. J., I. Derese, et al. (2005). "Modulation of bone morphogenetic protein signaling inhibits the onset and progression of ankylosing enthesitis." J Clin Invest 115(6): 1571-1579.

Lories, R. J., F. P. Luyten, et al. (2009). "Progress in spondylarthritis. Mechanisms of new bone formation in spondyloarthritis." Arthritis Res Ther 11(2): 221.

Mackie, S. L. and A. Keat (2004). "Poststreptococcal reactive arthritis: what is it and how do we know?" Rheumatology (Oxford) 43(8): 949-954.

Maegawa, Y., T. Itoh, et al. (2000). "Effects of near-infrared low-level laser irradiation on microcirculation." Lasers Surg Med 27(5): 427-437.

Magni-Manzoni, S., O. Epis, et al. (2009). "Comparison of clinical versus ultrasound-determined synovitis in juvenile idiopathic arthritis." Arthritis Rheum 61(11): 1497-1504.

Mahendra, A., R. Misra, et al. (2009). "Th1 and Th17 Predominance in the Enthesitis-related Arthritis Form of Juvenile Idiopathic Arthritis." J Rheumatol 36(8): 1730-1736.

Malleson, P. N., M. Y. Fung, et al. (1996). "The incidence of pediatric rheumatic diseases: results from the Canadian Pediatric Rheumatology Association Disease Registry." J Rheumatol 23(11): 1981-1987.

Manners, P., J. Lesslie, et al. (2003). "Classification of juvenile idiopathic arthritis: should family history be included in the criteria?" J Rheumatol 30(8): 1857-1863.

Manners, P. J. and C. Bower (2002). "Worldwide prevalence of juvenile arthritis why does it vary so much?" J Rheumatol 29(7): 1520-1530.

Mau, W., H. Zeidler, et al. (1988). "Clinical features and prognosis of patients with possible ankylosing spondylitis. Results of a 10-year followup." J Rheumatol 15(7): 1109-1114.

McGonagle, D. and M. Benjamin (2009). Entheses, Enthesitis and Enthesopathy. Reports on the Rheumatic Diseases Series 6, Arthritis Research UK. 4.

Mease, P. J. (2011). "Psoriatic arthritis: update on pathophysiology, assessment and management." Ann Rheum Dis 70 Suppl 1: i77-84.

Melis, L. and D. Elewaut (2009). "Progress in spondylarthritis. Immunopathogenesis of spondyloarthritis: which cells drive disease?" Arthritis Res Ther 11(3): 233.

Mester, E., A. F. Mester, et al. (1985). "The biomedical effects of laser application." Lasers Surg Med 5(1): 31-39.

Mielants, H., M. De Vos, et al. (1996). "The role of gut inflammation in the pathogenesis of spondyloarthropathies." Acta Clin Belg 51(5): 340-349.

Mielants, H., E. M. Veys, et al. (1993). "Gut inflammation in children with late onset pauciarticular juvenile chronic arthritis and evolution to adult spondyloarthropathy--a prospective study." J Rheumatol 20(9): 1567-1572.

Mielants, H., E. M. Veys, et al. (1987). "Late onset pauciarticular juvenile chronic arthritis: relation to gut inflammation." J Rheumatol 14(3): 459-465.

Minden, K., M. Niewerth, et al. (2002). "Long-term outcome in patients with juvenile idiopathic arthritis." Arthritis Rheum 46(9): 2392-2401.

Moorthy, L. N., S. Gaur, et al. (2009). "Poststreptococcal reactive arthritis in children: a retrospective study." Clin Pediatr (Phila) 48(2): 174-182.

Myles, A. and A. Aggarwal (2011). "Expression of Toll-like receptors 2 and 4 is increased in peripheral blood and synovial fluid monocytes of patients with enthesitis-related arthritis subtype of juvenile idiopathic arthritis." Rheumatology (Oxford) 50(3): 481-488.

Nemeth, A. J. (1993). "Lasers and wound healing." Dermatol Clin 11(4): 783-789.

Nistala, K. and L. R. Wedderburn (2009). "Th17 and regulatory T cells: rebalancing pro- and anti-inflammatory forces in autoimmune arthritis." Rheumatology (Oxford) 48(6): 602-606.

O'Brien, T. P., Q. Li, et al. (1998). "Inflammatory response in the early stages of wound healing after excimer laser keratectomy." Arch Ophthalmol 116(11): 1470-1474.

Pacheco-Tena, C., C. Alvarado De La Barrera, et al. (2001). "Bacterial DNA in synovial fluid cells of patients with juvenile onset spondyloarthropathies." Rheumatology (Oxford) 40(8): 920-927.

Packham, J. C. and M. A. Hall (2002). "Long-term follow-up of 246 adults with juvenile idiopathic arthritis: functional outcome." Rheumatology (Oxford) 41(12): 1428-1435.

Pagnini, I., S. Savelli, et al. (2010). "Early predictors of juvenile sacroiliitis in enthesitis-related arthritis." J Rheumatol 37(11): 2395-2401.

Petty, R. E., J. R. Smith, et al. (2003). "Arthritis and uveitis in children. A pediatric rheumatology perspective." Am J Ophthalmol 135(6): 879-884.

Petty, R. E., T. R. Southwood, et al. (1998). "Revision of the proposed classification criteria for juvenile idiopathic arthritis: Durban, 1997." J Rheumatol 25(10): 1991-1994.

Petty, R. E., T. R. Southwood, et al. (2004). "International League of Associations for Rheumatology classification of juvenile idiopathic arthritis: second revision, Edmonton, 2001." J Rheumatol 31(2): 390-392.

Pinheiro, A. L., G. C. Meireles, et al. (2004). "Phototherapy improves healing of cutaneous wounds in nourished and undernourished Wistar rats." Braz Dent J 15 Spec No: SI21-28.

Prieur, L. V., Dougados M, et al. (1990). "Evaluation of the ESSG and the Amor criteria for juvenile spondyloarthropathies (JSA). Study of 310 consecutive children referred to one pediatric rheumatology center." Arthritis Rheum 33 (Suppl 9): D195.

Prutki, M., L. Tambic Bukovac, et al. (2008). "Retrospective study of juvenile spondylarthropathies in Croatia over the last 11 years." Clin Exp Rheumatol 26(4): 693-699.

Reveille, J. D. and R. M. Maganti (2009). "Subtypes of HLA-B27: history and implications in the pathogenesis of ankylosing spondylitis." Adv Exp Med Biol 649: 159-176.

Reveille, J. D., A. M. Sims, et al. (2010). "Genome-wide association study of ankylosing spondylitis identifies non-MHC susceptibility loci." Nat Genet 42(2): 123-127.

Reynolds, T. L. and M. A. Khan (1988). "B7 crossreactive antigens in spondyloarthropathies." J Rheumatol 15(9): 1454.

Riente, L., A. Delle Sedie, et al. (2007). "Ultrasound imaging for the rheumatologist IX. Ultrasound imaging in spondyloarthritis." Clin Exp Rheumatol 25(3): 349-353.

Rochkind, S., M. Rousso, et al. (1989). "Systemic effects of low-power laser irradiation on the peripheral and central nervous system, cutaneous wounds, and burns." Lasers Surg Med 9(2): 174-182.

Rosenberg, A. M. and R. E. Petty (1982). "A syndrome of seronegative enthesopathy and arthropathy in children." Arthritis Rheum 25(9): 1041-1047.

Rudwaleit, M., R. Landewe, et al. (2009). "The development of Assessment of SpondyloArthritis international Society classification criteria for axial spondyloarthritis (part I): classification of paper patients by expert opinion including uncertainty appraisal." Ann Rheum Dis 68(6): 770-776.

Rudwaleit, M., D. van der Heijde, et al. (2009). "The development of Assessment of SpondyloArthritis international Society classification criteria for axial spondyloarthritis (part II): validation and final selection." Ann Rheum Dis 68(6): 777-783.

Rutkowska-Sak, L., I. Slowinska, et al. (2010). "[Juvenile spondyloarthropaties]." Ann Acad Med Stetin 56 Suppl 1: 29-33.

Salmi, M. and S. Jalkanen (1998). "Endothelial ligands and homing of mucosal leukocytes in extraintestinal manifestations of IBD." Inflamm Bowel Dis 4(2): 149-156.

Salmi, M. and S. Jalkanen (2001). "Human leukocyte subpopulations from inflamed gut bind to joint vasculature using distinct sets of adhesion molecules." J Immunol 166(7): 4650-4657.

Saraux, A., C. Guedes, et al. (1999). "Prevalence of rheumatoid arthritis and spondyloarthropathy in Brittany, France. Societe de Rhumatologie de l'Ouest." J Rheumatol 26(12): 2622-2627.

Saxena, N., A. Aggarwal, et al. (2005). "Elevated concentrations of monocyte derived cytokines in synovial fluid of children with enthesitis related arthritis and polyarticular types of juvenile idiopathic arthritis." J Rheumatol 32(7): 1349-1353.

Saxena, N., R. Misra, et al. (2006). "Is the enthesitis-related arthritis subtype of juvenile idiopathic arthritis a form of chronic reactive arthritis?" Rheumatology (Oxford) 45(9): 1129-1132.

Schett, G. (2009). "Bone formation versus bone resorption in ankylosing spondylitis." Adv Exp Med Biol 649: 114-121.

Schett, G. and M. Rudwaleit (2010). "Can we stop progression of ankylosing spondylitis?" Best Pract Res Clin Rheumatol 24(3): 363-371.

Schiellerup, P., K. A. Krogfelt, et al. (2008). "A comparison of self-reported joint symptoms following infection with different enteric pathogens: effect of HLA-B27." J Rheumatol 35(3): 480-487.

Schlager, A., P. Kronberger, et al. (2000). "Low-power laser light in the healing of burns: a comparison between two different wavelengths (635 nm and 690 nm) and a placebo group." Lasers Surg Med 27(1): 39-42.

Sharma, S. M., D. Choi, et al. (2009). "Insights in to the pathogenesis of axial spondyloarthropathy based on gene expression profiles." Arthritis Res Ther 11(6): R168.

Sieper, J., M. Rudwaleit, et al. (2002). "Diagnosing reactive arthritis: role of clinical setting in the value of serologic and microbiologic assays." Arthritis Rheum 46(2): 319-327.

Sieper, J., D. van der Heijde, et al. (2009). "New criteria for inflammatory back pain in patients with chronic back pain: a real patient exercise by experts from the Assessment of SpondyloArthritis international Society (ASAS)." Ann Rheum Dis 68(6): 784-788.

Simonet, W. S., D. L. Lacey, et al. (1997). "Osteoprotegerin: a novel secreted protein involved in the regulation of bone density." Cell 89(2): 309-319.

Singh, R., A. Aggarwal, et al. (2007). "Th1/Th17 cytokine profiles in patients with reactive arthritis/undifferentiated spondyloarthropathy." J Rheumatol 34(11): 2285-2290.

Smith, L. (2007). "Back pain in the young: a review of studies conducted among school children and university students." Current Pediatric Reviews 3: 69-77.

Sommer, A. P., A. L. Pinheiro, et al. (2001). "Biostimulatory windows in low-intensity laser activation: lasers, scanners, and NASA's light-emitting diode array system." J Clin Laser Med Surg 19(1): 29-33.

Souza, H. S., C. C. Elia, et al. (1999). "Expression of lymphocyte-endothelial receptor-ligand pairs, alpha4beta7/MAdCAM-1 and OX40/OX40 ligand in the colon and jejunum of patients with inflammatory bowel disease." Gut 45(6): 856-863.

Stenstad, H., A. Ericsson, et al. (2006). "Gut-associated lymphoid tissue-primed CD4+ T cells display CCR9-dependent and -independent homing to the small intestine." Blood 107(9): 3447-3454.

Stoll, M. L., R. Bhore, et al. (2010). "Spondyloarthritis in a pediatric population: risk factors for sacroiliitis." J Rheumatol 37(11): 2402-2408.

Stoll, M. L. and M. Punaro (2011). "Psoriatic juvenile idiopathic arthritis: a tale of two subgroups." Curr Opin Rheumatol 23(5): 437-443.

Stoll, M. L., D. Zurakowski, et al. (2006). "Patients with juvenile psoriatic arthritis comprise two distinct populations." Arthritis Rheum 54(11): 3564-3572.

Sulpice, M., C. J. Deslandre, et al. (2009). "Efficacy and safety of TNFalpha antagonist therapy in patients with juvenile spondyloarthropathies." Joint Bone Spine 76(1): 24-27.

Symmons, D. P., M. Jones, et al. (1996). "Pediatric rheumatology in the United Kingdom: data from the British Pediatric Rheumatology Group National Diagnostic Register." J Rheumatol 23(11): 1975-1980.

Tse, S. M., R. Burgos-Vargas, et al. (2005). "Anti-tumor necrosis factor alpha blockade in the treatment of juvenile spondylarthropathy." Arthritis Rheum 52(7): 2103-2108.

Tsuchiya, N., M. Shiota, et al. (1998). "MICA allele typing of HLA-B27 positive Japanese patients with seronegative spondylarthropathies and healthy individuals: differential linkage disequilibrium with HLA-B27 subtypes." Arthritis Rheum 41(1): 68-73.

Van Breukelen, G. J. (2006). "ANCOVA versus change from baseline: more power in randomized studies, more bias in nonrandomized studies [corrected]." J Clin Epidemiol 59(9): 920-925.

van der Heijde, D. and W. P. Maksymowych (2010). "Spondyloarthritis: state of the art and future perspectives." Ann Rheum Dis 69(6): 949-954.

van der Linden, S., H. A. Valkenburg, et al. (1984). "Evaluation of diagnostic criteria for ankylosing spondylitis. A proposal for modification of the New York criteria." Arthritis Rheum 27(4): 361-368.

Vegvari, A., Z. Szabo, et al. (2009). "The genetic background of ankylosing spondylitis." Joint Bone Spine 76(6): 623-628.

Weber, U. and W. P. Maksymowych (2011). "Sensitivity and specificity of magnetic resonance imaging for axial spondyloarthritis." Am J Med Sci 341(4): 272-277.

Wong-Riley, M. T., X. Bai, et al. (2001). "Light-emitting diode treatment reverses the effect of TTX on cytochrome oxidase in neurons." Neuroreport 12(14): 3033-3037.

Yang, Z. X., Y. Liang, et al. (2007). "Increased expression of Toll-like receptor 4 in peripheral blood leucocytes and serum levels of some cytokines in patients with ankylosing spondylitis." Clin Exp Immunol 149(1): 48-55.

Yli-Kerttula, T., R. Tertti, et al. (1995). "Ten-year follow up study of patients from a Yersinia pseudotuberculosis III outbreak." Clin Exp Rheumatol 13(3): 333-337.

7

Ultrasonography in Diagnosis and Follow-Up of Temporal Arteritis: An Update

Giovanni Ciancio, Marco Bruschi and Marcello Govoni
Rheumatology Unit Department of Clinical and Experimental Medicine- University of Ferrara Azienda Ospedaliero, Universitaria Sant'Anna, Ferrara Italy

1. Introduction

Giant cell arteritis (GCA), also known as temporal arteritis (TA) is a relatively frequent primary systemic vasculitis affecting large and medium-sized arteries, in particular aorta and its main branches (Hunder, 2000). It occurs, by definition, in patients older than fifty with a peak between 70 and 80 years. The disease primarily affects whites, specifically those of northern European descent, and the highest worldwide incidence is reported to be in southern Norway with 32.8 per 100.000 people over the age of 50 affected (Richards et al., 2010). GCA affects women 2–3 times more commonly than men (Richards et al., 2010).

The spectrum of clinical manifestations associated with TA includes a wide combination of symptoms and signs, ranging from tender and swollen temporal arteries, headache and jaw claudication to systemic and musculoskeletal symptoms such as fatigue, weight loss, low-grade fever, polymyalgia rheumatica, arthralgias and tenosynovitis (Hunder, 2000). Irreversible visual loss secondary to ischemic optic neuropathy is the most serious and dreaded complication, so prompt diagnosis and treatment are mandatory to prevent it (Gonzalez-Gay et al., 2005; Hunder, 2000).

1.1 Diagnosis of GCA: Current issues

Although a rapid and non-invasive diagnosis of TA would be desirable, it still remains a challenge for clinicians. History, typical clinical findings and elevation of acute phase reactants are usually sufficient to induce the suspicion for TA but they are insufficient to give diagnostic certainty. The American College of Rheumatology classification criteria (ACRC) for GCA (Hunder et al., 1990) help to distinguish TA from other primary vasculitides for research purposes, but they have significant limitations in clinical diagnosis (Rao et al., 1998). Therefore, temporal artery biopsy (TAB) is still considered the gold standard because of its high specificity and it is currently recommended in all suspected cases of TA (Drehmer et al., 2005). At present, segments of at least 2.5 cm are considered adequate to reduce - but not to completely avoid - the risk of skip lesions (Gonzalez-Gay, 2005). Since histology can be influenced by corticosteroids, TAB should be performed before starting therapy (Ray-Chaudhuri et al., 2002) but in most cases it is too hazardous to wait until biopsy is performed, thus steroids are usually started as soon as GCA is clinically suspected (Borg & Dasgupta, 2009). After starting high dose of corticosteroids, TAB can remain informative even for up to 4-6 weeks (Achkar et al., 1994; Ray-Chaudhuri et al., 2002) but it should be performed no later than two weeks (Borg & Dasgupta, 2009; Warrington & Matteson, 2007).

However TAB implies a number of problems. It is an invasive procedure that may lead to some complications (Bhatti & Goldstein, 2001; Haist, 1985; Siemssen, 1987; Slavin, 1986) and it is usually available much too late to influence therapeutic decision (Nesher et al., 2004). Moreover, TAB may result negative in up to 10%-44% of patients (Hall et al., 1983; Schmidt, 2006) and in these cases patients should undergo controlateral TAB if clinical suspicion of GCA is high (Gonzalez-Gay, 2005).

On this background, new non-invasive vascular diagnostic techniques, such as ultrasound (US) and vascular magnetic resonance imaging (MRI), have gained in the last years a growing interest and an increasing importance in clinical diagnosis (Schmidt, 2004). In particular US, whose resolution with regard to superficial anatomical structures is superior to that of MRI, can provide an excellent evaluation of vessel anatomy and inflammatory alterations (Gonzalez-Gay et al., 2006; Schmidt & Blockmans, 2005).

Regular use of these non invasive imaging modalities in the diagnosis of GCA instead of TAB is currently a debated issue.

2. Ultrasonography in TA

With the availability of high-resolution Color Doppler (CD) and the high-frequency transducers, ultrasonography has became an increasingly powerful tool also for rheumatologists (Grassi et al., 2004). High-frequency probes have a resolution of about 0.1 mm and provide an optimal examination of joints, muscles and tendons (Grassi et al., 2004; Schmidt, 2004). CD and Color Duplex US (CDUS) offer further benefits over conventional Doppler US. CD integrates Doppler effect in the greyscale image as a colour signal and allows an accurate study of both small vessels and large arteries (Romera-Villegas et al., 2004; Schmidt, 2004; Schmidt & Blockmans, 2005). The sensitivity of CD in detecting the small vessels is even more enhanced by the application of Power Doppler, which is extremely useful in highlighting the slow blood flow and, consequently, it allows to study articular, periarticular and peritendinous inflamed tissues more accurately (Grassi et al., 2004; Schmidt, 2004). In addition CD is able to depict the wall of large arteries and the associated inflammatory changes in detail, thus appearing very useful in the diagnostic assessment of vasculitis (Kissin & Merkel, 2004) compared to conventional continuous-wave Doppler, which cannot provide anatomical images (Dany et al., 1989; Kelley, 1978; Puechal et al., 1995; Vinckier et al., 1989). CDUS offers further benefits over CD. Through a combination of real-time imaging and Doppler sonography, it shows at the same time anatomical images with colour signals and pulsed-wave Doppler curves, allowing an evaluation of the velocity of blood flow by the integration of Doppler shift frequency in combination with an angle correction programme (Schmidt & Gromnica-Ihle, 2005). Thus alterations like stenosis and occlusions, that frequently occur in acute temporal arteritis, can be evaluated more easily (Schmidt & Gromnica-Ihle, 2005).

2.1 Sonographic features

The usefulness of CD and CDUS in the diagnosis of TA was demonstrated in 1995 by Schmidt and colleagues (Schmidt *et al.*, 1995). They first described in temporal arteries of patients affected by acute TA the 'halo' sign, ascribed to oedematous wall swelling and characterized by a hypoechoic and circumferential wall thickening localized around the perfused lumen with a diameter ranging between 0.3 and 2 mm (Schmidt et al., 1995) (Fig.1,2).

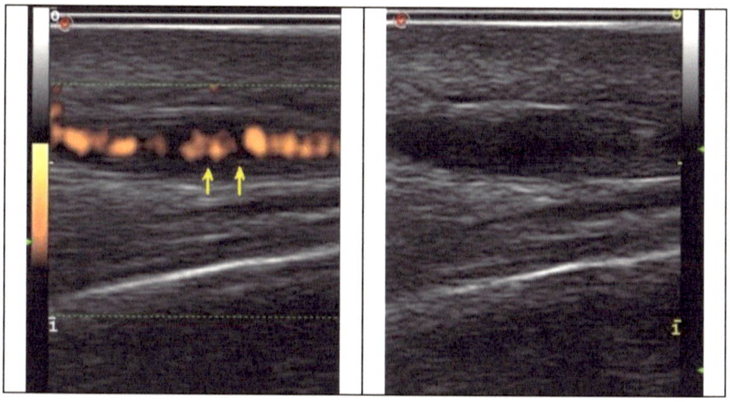

Fig. 1. US Color Doppler of the left parietal ramus in acute TA. Longitudinal plane. Very high-frequency transducer at 18MhZ (My Lab 70- Esaote). Hypoechoic dark area ("halo") is indicated by the yellow arrows (left side). On the right side: the same arterial segment in the greyscale.

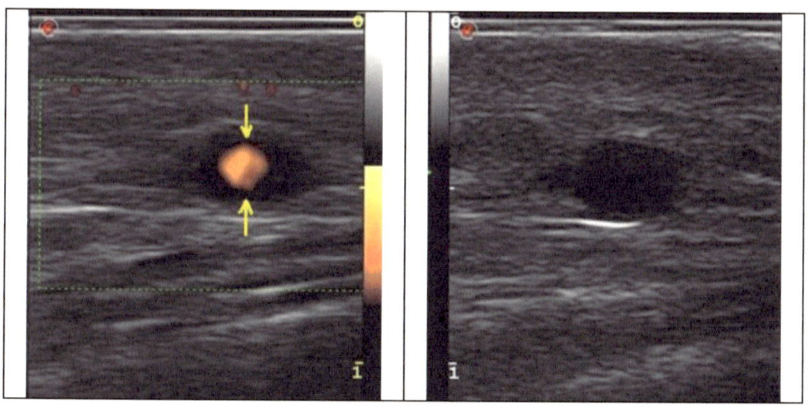

Fig. 2. US Color Doppler of the right distal third of the common superficial temporal artery in acute TA. Transverse plane. Very high-frequency transducer at 18MhZ (Esaote-My Lab 70). Hypoechoic dark area ("halo") is indicated by the yellow arrows (right side). On the right side: the same arterial segment in the greyscale.

The other two parameters considered relevant for the diagnosis of TA are stenosis and occlusion of the arteries. Stenosis, characterized by a narrowing of the vessel lumen, has been defined as a segmental increase in blood flow velocity and two time higher than in the area before the stenosis. Other ancillary US features are turbulence of the flow with reduced velocity behind the area of the stenosis and the persistence of the colour signal during diastole (Schmidt et al., 1995). Acute temporal artery occlusion is revealed by the complete absence of colour signals in a segment of temporal artery (Schmidt et al., 1995).

2.2 Sensitivity and specificity of CDUS in TA

In 1997, Schmidt and coll. published data on the sensitivity and specificity of CDUS in their series of 30 patients with active TA compared with 82 controls, with clinical diagnosis and biopsy as reference standard (Schmidt et al., 1997). Diagnosis of TA was confirmed by biopsy in 21 of the 30 patients. Hypoechoic halo was evidenced in 22/30 patients with TA; stenoses or occlusions in 24/30; stenoses, occlusions, or a halo in 28/30. On the contrary, no halo was evidenced in the 82 controls without TA but 6/82 had stenoses or occlusions. With regard to clinical diagnosis, sensitivity and specificity for the halo were 73% and 100%, whilst for stenosis and/or occlusion were 80% and 93%, respectively. With regard to histology, sensitivity and specificity for the halo resulted to be 76% and 92%, while for stenosis and/or occlusion were 86% and 88%, respectively. Noteworthy, if halo, stenosis and occlusion were considered together, sensitivity resulted higher both *vs* clinical diagnosis (93%) and *vs* histology (95%).

These results have been confirmed by the same authors in a larger study on 101 patients with acute TA vs 650 controls (Schmidt & Gromnica-Ihle, 2003). Sensitivity resulted low and specificity high vs clinical diagnosis and histology when the halo was considered alone, while sensitivity became significantly higher when halo, stenosis and occlusion were considered together (Schmidt & Gromnica-Ihle, 2003). Stenosis alone demonstrated a very low sensitivity in TA because it was commonly found even in elderly patients without TA, since they are usually affected by arteriosclerosis (Schmidt et al., 1997; Schmidt & Gromnica-Ihle, 2003, 2005). Conversely acute occlusions, although less frequent than stenosis, were more specific for TA being rarely found in patients without TA (Schmidt et al., 1997; Schmidt & Gromnica-Ihle, 2003, 2005)

Since the first description (Schmidt et al., 1997), several studies have been published on the diagnostic value of CDUS in TA with similar results (Aschwanden et al., 2010; Bley et al., 2008; Ghinoi et al., 2008; Houtman et al., 2008; Karahaliou et al., 2006; Lesar et al., 2002; Maldini et al., 2010; Morinobu et al., 2011; Murgatroyd et al., 2003; Nesher et al., 2002; Perez Lopez et al., 2009; Pfadenhauer & Weber, 2003; Reinhard et al., 2004; Romera-Villegas et al., 2004; Salvarani et al., 2002; Schmidt, 2000; Schmidt & Gromnica-Ihle, 2003; Suelves et al., 2010).

In the 2005, Karassa and coll. published a meta-analysis aimed to review the diagnostic value of CDUS in GCA (Karassa et al., 2005). The authors selected the most important studies published up to 2004. In all these reports, biopsy and the ACRC were used as the reference standard. The weighted sensitivity of halo sign resulted 69% (*vs* biopsy) and 55% (*vs* ACRC), while the specificity was 82% (*vs* biopsy) and 94% (*vs* ACRC criteria). Stenosis or occlusion showed quite a similar sensitivity (68% *vs* biopsy and 66% *vs* ACRC criteria). This analysis confirmed the utility of CDUS in diagnosing GCA and the high specificity of the halo sign, the detection of which strongly supports the diagnosis of TA. However most of the studies included in this meta-analysis were small, of modest quality and with a considerable degree of heterogeneity.

Two further meta-analysis were published more recently in 2010 (Arida et al., 2010; Ball et al., 2010). In the first one, the sensitivity and specificity of the halo sign versus the ACRC as a reference standard were examined. (Arida et al., 2010). Eight prospective studies, through December 2009, fulfilling technical quality criteria for ultrasound and involving 575 patients were finally selected. Compared with final diagnosis, sensitivity and specificity resulted of 68% and 91% for the presence of unilateral halo, and of 43% and 100% for bilateral halo, respectively.

In the second meta-analysis performed by Ball and coll., (Ball et al., 2010), all studies in english language published up to 2009 with a minimum of 5 patients and using TA biopsy and/or ACRC criteria as the reference standard were included. When the halo sign was compared with TA biopsy, the weighted sensitivity and specificity resulted 75% and 83% respectively. When the halo sign was compared with ACR criteria, the weighted sensitivity and specificity resulted 69% and 89% respectively. This study confirms the high specificity but also evidenced the higher sensitivity of the halo sign, that may reflect both the improvement of the duplex machines and the increased expertise of the ultrasonographers (Ball et al., 2010). Very interestingly, when halo, stenosis and occlusion were considered together, sensitivity further increased in comparison to TA biopsy and ACR criteria to 83% and 78%, respectively (Ball et al., 2010) (Table 1)

CDUS alterations	Reference standard	Karassa and coll.		Arida and coll.		Ball and coll.	
		Sens. (%)	Spec. (%)	Sens. (%)	Spec. (%)	Sens. (%)	Spec. (%)
H	TAB	69	82			75	83
S/O	TAB	68					
H + S + O	TAB					83	82
H	ACRC	55	94	68 (43 if bilat.)	91 (100 if bilat.)	69	89
S/O	ACRC	66					
H + S + O	ACRC					78	88

Table 1. CDUS signs vs references standard in the 3 meta-analysis. TA: temporal artery; ACRC: American College of Rheumatology Criteria. H: Halo; S: Stenosis; O: Occlusion. TAB: Temporal Artery Biopsy.

In summary, all these data confirm that the dark halo is the most specific CDUS sign in GCA, so its detection strongly supports a diagnosis of TA in patients with typical clinical signs. On the other hand, sensitivity of halo is lower than specificity, so the absence of a halo does not exclude TA. If halo, stenosis and occlusions are considered together, the sensitivity of CDUS is higher and comparable to histology.

Interestingly, in the study of Karahaliou (Karahaliou et al., 2006) it has been shown that the presence of a bilateral halo sign had a 100% specificity for the diagnosis of TA; this observation led the authors to conclude that bilateral "halo sign" may be substitutive of TA biopsy.

The results of a recent study by Maldini and coll. led to less enthusiastic conclusions about the real value of US in GCA (Maldini et al., 2010). Characteristics of US findings with continuous-wave Doppler or CDUS of temporal arteries was retrospectively evaluated and compared with biopsy and clinical diagnosis. Halo sign showed 100% specificity for GCA but only 10%-17% sensitivity; stenoses or occlusions appeared to have low diagnostic power. These data led the authors to conclude that US in GCA is neither an effective substitute for biopsy nor a reliable screening test to decide which patients can be safely spared from TAB.

2.3 US in follow-up of TA

In our experience, CDUS resulted very helpful in the diagnostic work-up, in identifying the best target segment to biopsy and in follow-up of patients with TA (Ciancio et al, 2009; Fotinidi et al, 2011).

We performed bilateral CDUS examination to check for the halo thickness, erythrocyte sedimentation rate (ESR) and C-reactive protein (CRP) in a group of 25 patients at baseline and after 2, 4 and 6 weeks. Both sensitivity and specificity for the halo resulted very high (100%) when compared to clinical diagnosis and biopsy. During follow-up, the halo thickness in all the 25 patients disappeared 2-weeks after starting corticosteroids (Fig. 3) and

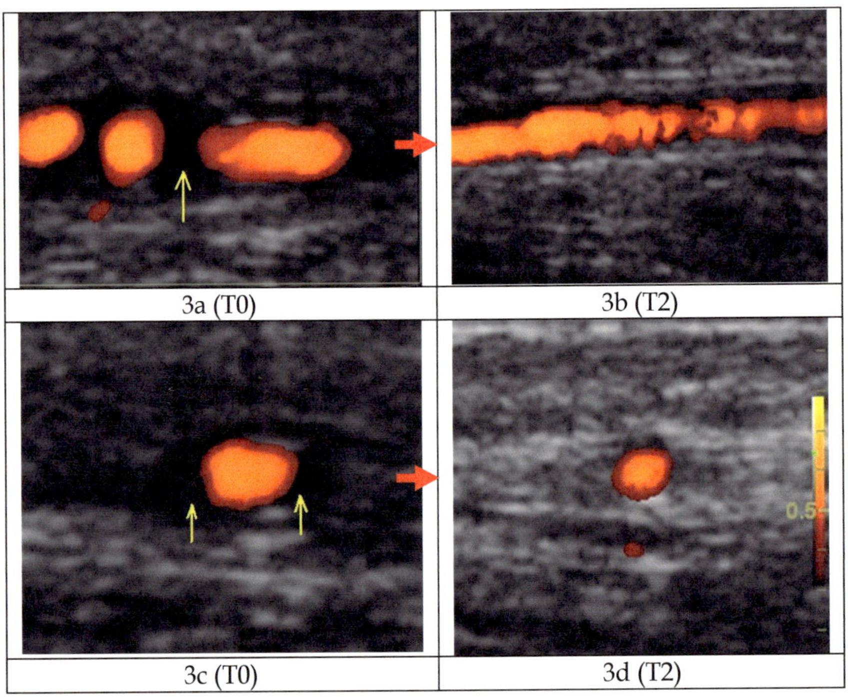

Fig. 3. Left parietal ramus of the superficial temporal artery in a patient with acute GCA at baseline (T0: on the left) and after two weeks of corticosteroid therapy (T2: on the right). High-frequency transducer at 12MhZ (*Logic 5 Pro*-GE)

3a. Longitudinal plane. Baseline (T0).The hypoechoic (black) area is indicated by the yellow arrows

3b.Longitudinal plane. Complete remission of the halo after two weeks (T2) of corticosteroids

3c. Transverse Plane of the same segment. Baseline (T0).The hypoechoic (black) area is indicated by the yellow arrows

3d. Transverse Plane. Complete remission of the halo after two weeks (T2) of corticosteroids this modification antedated the normalization of both ESR and CRP thus suggesting that CDUS may allow a better monitoring of clinical course and can guide a more careful tapering of glucocorticoid therapy (Chart 1). Obviously, this observation needs further confirmations in larger series since the role of CDUS in follow-up of TA is still currently considered rather doubtful and less useful for monitoring disease activity than the patient's history and/or ESR (Schmidt, 2004). Furthermore, in extracranial GCA the sonographic appearance of the arterial wall has not been validated yet as a reliable parameter for the assessment of disease activity (Tato & Hoffmann, 2008). Although the halo decreases during treatment, some degree of thickening of the arterial wall and stenosis can persist even in patients in complete remission, and complete recanalization of occluded arterial segments does not always occur (Schmidt & Blockmans, 2005; Tato e& Hoffmann, 2008).

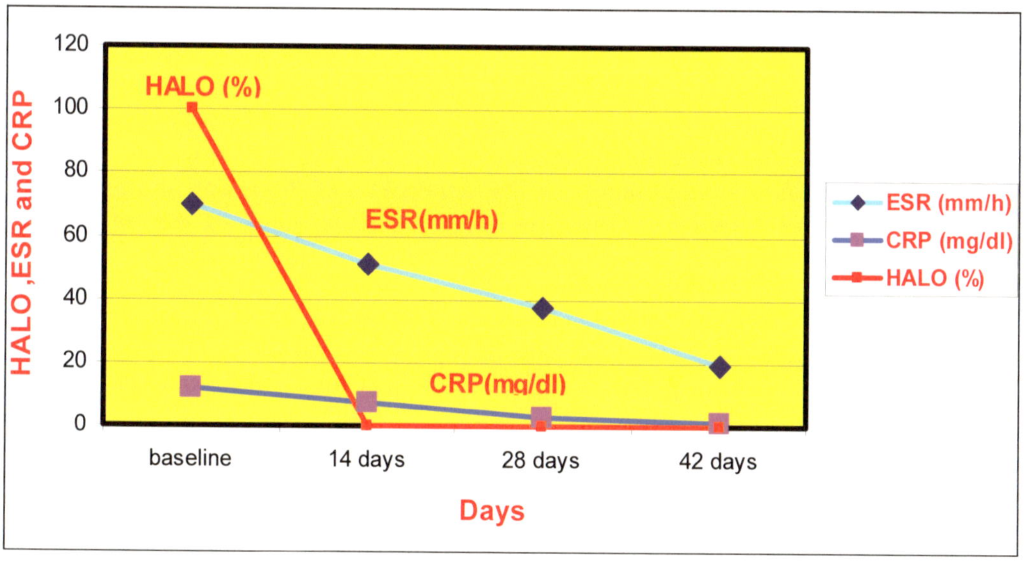

Chart 1. Variation of the monitored parameters (ESR and CRP *vs* HALO) in the 25 patients with GCA. ESR and CRP: mean value among the 25 patient at each time point.
ESR: erythrocyte sedimentation rate. CRP: C-reactive protein

2.4 Examination technique

Detailed technical aspects of the examination methodology have been described in an excellent review by Schmidt (Schmidt, 2004). Briefly, a high quality CD US equipment and standardised US machine adjustments, the use of linear probe with high frequency (>8 MHz) and a good experience of the operator are indispensable to adequately perform CDUS of temporal arteries.

2.4.1 US equipment

Excellent equipment is currently available and provided by different companies. However, even the best is likely to be ineffective for an adequate depiction of temporal arteries alterations if right machine settings are missing. A prerequisite to appropriately perform CD examination of temporal arteries is the availability of high frequency (>8 MHz) linear transducers. The availability of modern probes with frequencies of up to 15 MHz has greatly increased the resolution power for the evaluation of surface anatomical layers. Depending on the individual equipment, a too high frequency for the colour image may even reduce the sensitivity for the colour, and if grey scale and colour gains are too high or too low, it is possible to overlook hypoechoic areas or to generate false hypoechoic areas, respectively (Schmidt, 2004). Even the colour sample steering is important; it should have an angle of 20–30° when a branch parallel to the probe is examined, otherwise the colour signal would not be adequate (Schmidt, 2004). Again, pulse repetition frequency (PRF) should be carefully regulated to 2-2.5 KHz. Because of the high blood flow velocities, colour Doppler should be preferred to power Doppler since the latter may miss stenoses.

2.4.2 Experience of the sonographer

In order to properly examine temporal arteries, a good experience with vascular US should be warranted by a trained operator and a perfect knowledge of the US appearance of normal temporal arteries is mandatory. Artefacts may occur and the operator must be very familiar with them. It has been recommended that a minimum of 50 normal temporal arteries examination should be performed before starting to evaluate patients with suspected GCA (Schmidt, 2004). Recent experiences with standardized training programs to allow rheumatologists to learn the technique for US examination of the temporal arteries have shown encouraging results by proving effective and well accepted by the trainees (De Miguel et al., 2009)

2.5 Limits of CDUS in TA

False-positive and false-negative halos may be seen when performing CDUS. If the common superficial TA has an accompanying vein in which no flow is seen, this can be erroneously checked for a halo (Schmidt, 2000). False-positive halos are also seen in malignant and infectious diseases (Nesher et al., 2002).On the contrary, halo can be missed if a stronger colour intensity covering the inflamed wall is employed (Schmidt, 2000). Moreover, about 10 per cent of patients with a positive biopsy have normal duplex imaging as a result of very low inflammatory infiltrate possibly due both to mild disease or prolonged corticosteroid treatment (Schmidt, 2004; Weyand & Goronzy, 2003;). It has been demonstrated that CDUS findings in active TA do not correlate with occurrence and severity of ophthalmic complications (Schmidt et al., 2009). Furthermore, CDUS is not able to differentiate between GCA and other vasculitis that can involve temporal arteries, as it can occur in Wegener's granulomatosis, Churg-Strauss syndrome and microscopic polyangiitis (Schmidt & Gromnica-Ihle, 2005).

2.6 US findings in extracranial GCA

CDUS can also be very useful for diagnosis, assessment of severity and follow-up when extracranial large arteries are involved in GCA. (Aschwanden et al., 2010; Kolossvary et al., 2005; Reinhard et al., 2003; Schmidt et al., 2002; Schmidt et al., 2008;). In brachial, subclavian or axillary arteries, CDUS has been shown to be able to demonstrate the typical signs of vascular inflammation such as concentric and hypoechogenic wall thickening of arterial segments, the narrowing of the arterial lumen or a hypoechogenic occlusion. (Kolossvary et al., 2005; Schmidt et al., 2008). CDUS signs in association with clinical symptoms and elevated laboratory markers of systemic inflammation can be considered diagnostic for large-vessel vasculitis making it unnecessary to use of conventional angiography (Tato &

Hoffmann, 2008). With regard to the involvement of lower limbs in GCA, CDUS semeiology of femoropopliteal and crural arteries appears to be the same as in the vessels of the upper limbs (Aschwanden et al., 2010; Schmidt et al., 2002; Tato & Hoffmann, 2006;)

3. Other tools for the diagnosis of GCA

In recent years, other imaging techniques have been proved useful in the diagnosis of TA, such as magnetic resonance imaging (MRI), 18F-fluorodeoxyglucose positron emission tomography (FDG-PET), single-photon emission computed tomography (SPECT) and computed tomography (CT). High-resolution contrast-enhanced MRI and angio-MRI have proved useful in visualizing the involvement of temporal arteries and/or other large arteries such as aorta in extracranial GCA (Bley et al., 2005; Narvaez et al., 2005). MRI was also able to evidence isolate inflammation of the occipital arteries, with sparing of the temporal arteries (Bley et al., 2005).

The utility of FDG-PET in evaluating the active lesions of large arteries in patients with systemic vasculitis including GCA has recently been demonstrated(Schmidt e Blockmans, 2005). However, PET is not suitable for the assessment of temporal arteries (Schmidt & Blockmans, 2005) but it has proven useful in assessing disease activity during therapy in extracranial GCA (Walter et al., 2005).

In a pilot study, SPECT revealed positive findings in temporal arteries of nine patients with active temporal arteritis (Reitblat et al., 2003). In selected cases, angiography and CT may still have a role in investigating the involvement of large extracranial arteries in GCA (Stanson, 2000).

4. Conclusion

Although, to date, biopsy remains the gold standard for diagnosis of TA, CDUS may be considered a very useful tool. It is inexpensive, non-invasive, reproducible and easy-to-perform. Dark halo is the most specific CDUS sign in GCA, so its detection strongly supports a diagnosis of TA in patients with typical clinical signs. Sensitivity of halo is lower than specificity, so the absence of a halo does not exclude TA but if halo, stenosis and occlusions are simultaneously detected sensitivity of CDUS becomes high and comparable to histology. Finally, detection of the halo could allow a guided biopsy with an increased probability to avoid false negative results due to skip lesions. Therefore, CDUS should precede TA biopsy in all patients with suspected GCA. After initiating therapy, the disappearance of the halo has proved to be more sensitive than ESR and CRP. If confirmed by other studies, CDUS could be usefully employed also in follow-up allowing a better monitoring and tapering of glucocorticoid therapy. The contribution of CDUS is useful also for diagnosis, assessment of severity and follow-up in extracranial GCA.

Some limits of US evaluation should be well kept in mind, such as the possibility of false-positive and false-negative halos, the lack of correlations with ophthalmic complications and the inability to differentiate GCA by other vasculitis. The heavy dependence on operator expertise is another critical point to be considered.

Even if CDUS has gained an emerging role in the diagnostic workup of GCA, larger studies are needed in the near future to verify the possibility that this technique may really replace the TAB in the diagnostic work-up of TA and that it could be a reliable tool in the follow up evaluation.

5. Acknowledgments

We are very grateful to Prof. Francesco Trotta for his valuable advice in the preparation and review of the work.

6. References

Achkar, AA., Lie, JT., Hunder, GG., O'Fallon, WM. & Gabriel, SE. (1994). How does previous corticosteroid treatment affect the biopsy findings in giant cell (temporal) arteritis? Annals of Internal Medicine, Vol. 120, No 12, (June 1994), pp. 987-92, ISSN 0003-4819

Arida, A., Kyprianou, M., Kanakis, M. & Sfikakis, PP. (2010). The diagnostic value of ultrasonography-derived edema of the temporal artery wall in giant cell arteritis: a second meta-analysis. BMC Musculoskeletal Disorders, Vol. 11, (March 2010), p. 44, ISSN 1471-2474

Aschwanden, M., Kesten, F., Stern, M., Thalhammer, C., Walker, UA., Tyndall, A., Jaeger, KA., Hess, C. & Daikeler, T. (2010). Vascular involvement in patients with giant cell arteritis determined by duplex sonography of 2x11 arterial regions. Annals of the Rheumatic Diseases, Vol. 69, No. 7, (Jul 2010), pp. 1356-9, ISSN 1468-2060

Ball, EL., Walsh, SR., Tang, TY., Gohil, R. & Clarke, JM. (2010). Role of ultrasonography in the diagnosis of temporal arteritis. Br J Surg, Vol. 97, No. 12, (Dec 2010), pp. 1765-71, ISSN 1365-2168

Bhatti, MT. & Goldstein, MH. (2001). Facial nerve injury following superficial temporal artery biopsy. Dermatologic Surgery, Vol. 27, No.1, (Jan 2001), pp. 15-7, ISSN 1076-0512

Bley, TA., Wieben, O., Uhl, M., Thiel, J., Schmidt, D. & Langer, M. (2005). High-resolution MRI in giant cell arteritis: imaging of the wall of the superficial temporal artery. American Journal of Roentgenology, Vol. 184, No. 1 (Jan 2005), pp. 283-7, ISSN 0361-803X

Bley, TA., Reinhard, M., Hauenstein, C., Markl, M., Warnatz, K., Hetzel, A., Uhl, M., Vaith, P.& Langer M. (2008). Comparison of duplex sonography and high-resolution magnetic resonance imaging in the diagnosis of giant cell (temporal) arteritis. Arthritis and Rheumatism, Vol. 58, No. 8, (Aug 2008), pp. 2574-8, ISSN 0004-3591

Borg, FA.& Dasgupta, B. Treatment and outcomes of large vessel arteritis.(2009). Best Practice & Research Clinical Rheumatology, Vol. 23, No 3, (Jun 2009), pp. 325-37, ISSN 1532-1770

Ciancio, G., Colina, M., De Leonardis, F., Foschi, V., Govoni, M. & Trotta F. (2009). Colour duplex ultrasonography in the diagnosis and management of giant cell arteritis. Arthritis Rheumatism, Vol. 60, No. 10 (Supplement), (November 2009), p.672

Dany, F., Liozon, F., Chaumont, P., Chastang, A., Lacroix, P., Catanzano, R. & Christides C. (1989). Sensitivity and specificity of temporal Doppler in Horton's disease. Journal des maladies vasculaires, Vol. 14, Suppl. C, (1989), pp. 104-8, ISSN 0398-0499

De Miguel, E., Castillo, C., Rodriguez, A. & De Agustin, JJ. (2009). Learning and reliability of colour Doppler ultrasound in giant cell arteritis. Clinical and Experimental Rheumatology, Vol.. 27, No. 1, Suppl 52, (Jan-Feb 2009), pp. S53-8,. ISSN 0392-856X

Drehmer, TJ., Khanna, D., Markert, RJ. & Hawkins, RA. (2005). Diagnostic and management trends of giant cell arteritis: a physician survey. Journal of Rheumatology, Vol. 32, No. 7, (Jul 2005), pp. 1283-9, ISSN 0315-162X

Fotinidi, M., Farina, I., Bortoluzzi, A., Galuppi, E., Giacuzzo, S., Bruschi, M., Occhionorelli, S., Giusto, L., Vanini, A., Ciancio, G. & Govoni, M. (2011). Colour duplex ultrasonography in diagnostic assessment and follow-up of giant cell arteritis. Annals of the Rheumatic diseases. Abstract Book, European League Against Rheumatism (EULAR) Congress. London. Vol. 70, (Suppl 3), AB0976, (May 2011)

Ghinoi, A., Zuccoli, G., Nicolini, A., Pipitone, N., Macchioni, L., Bajocchi, GL., Nicoli, F., Silingardi, M., Catanoso, MG., Boiardi, L. & Salvarani C. (2008). 1T magnetic resonance imaging in the diagnosis of giant cell arteritis: comparison with ultrasonography and physical examination of temporal arteries. Clinical and experimental Rheumatology Vol. 26, No. 3, Suppl 49, (May-Jun 2008), pp. S76-80, ISSN 0392-856X

Gonzalez-Gay, MA. The diagnosis and management of patients with giant cell arteritis. (2005). Journal of Rheumatology, Vol. 32, No. 7, (Jul 2005), pp. 1186-8, ISSN 0315-162X

Gonzalez-Gay, MA., Barros, S., Lopez-Diaz, MJ., Garcia-Porrua, C., Sanchez-Andrade, A. & Llorca J. (2005). Giant cell arteritis: disease patterns of clinical presentation in a series of 240 patients. Medicine (Baltimore), Vol. 84, No. 5, (Sep 2005), pp. 269-76, ISSN 0025-7974

Gonzalez-Gay, MA., Garcia-Porrua, C. & Miranda-Filloy JA. (2006). Giant cell arteritis: diagnosis and therapeutic management. Current Rheumatology Reports, Vol. 8, No. 4, (Aug 2006), pp. 299-302, ISSN 1523-3774

Grassi, W., Filippucci, E. & Busilacchi P. (2004). Musculoskeletal ultrasound. Best Practice & Research Clinical Rheumatology, Vol. 18, No. 6, (Dec 2004), pp. 813-26, ISSN 1521-6942

Haist SA. Stroke after temporal artery biopsy. (1985). Mayo Clinic Proceedings, Vol. 60, No. 8, (Aug 1985), p. 538, ISSN 0025-6196

Hall, S., Persellin, S., Lie, JT., O'Brien, PC., Kurland, LT. & Hunder GG. (1983). The therapeutic impact of temporal artery biopsy. Lancet, Vol. 2, No. 8361, (Nov 1983), pp. 1217-20, ISSN 0140-6736

Houtman, P., Doorenbos, B., Dol, J. & Bruyn, G. (2008). Doppler ultrasonography to diagnose temporal arteritis in the setting of a large community hospital. Scandinavian Journal of Rheumatology, Vol. 37, No. 4, (Jul-Aug 2008), pp. 316-8, ISSN 0300-9742

Hunder, GG., Bloch, DA., Michel, BA., Stevens, MB., Arend, WP., Calabrese, LH., Edworthy, SM., Fauci, AS., Leavitt, RY., Lie, JT., Lightfoot, RW., Masi, AT., McShane, DJ., Mills, JA., Wallace, SL. & Zvaifler, NJ. (1990). The American College of Rheumatology 1990 criteria for the classification of giant cell arteritis. Arthritis and Rheumatism, Vol. 33, No. 8, (Aug 1990), pp. 1122-8, ISSN 0004-3591

Hunder, GG. Clinical features of GCA/PMR. (2000). Clinical and Experimental Rheumatology, Vol. 18, No. 4, Suppl 20, (Jul-Aug 2000), pp. S6-8, ISSN 0392-856X

Karahaliou, M., Vaiopoulos, G., Papaspyrou, S., Kanakis, MA., Revenas, K. & Sfikakis PP. (2006). Colour duplex sonography of temporal arteries before decision for biopsy: a prospective study in 55 patients with suspected giant cell arteritis. Arthritis Research & Therapy, Vol. 8, No. 4, (2006), R116, ISSN 1478-6362

Karassa, FB., Matsagas, MI., Schmidt, WA. & Ioannidis, JP. (2005). Meta-analysis: test performance of ultrasonography for giant-cell arteritis. Annals of Internal Medicine, Vol. 142, No. 5, (Mar 2005), pp. 359-69, ISSN 1539-3704

Kelley JS. (1978). Doppler ultrasound flow detector used in temporal artery biopsy. Archives of Ophthalmology, Vol. 96, No. 5, (May 1978), pp. 845-6, ISSN 0003-9950

Kissin, EY. & Merkel, PA.(2004). Diagnostic imaging in Takayasu arteritis. Current Opinion in Rheumatology, Vol. 16, No. 1, (Jan 2004), pp. 31-7, ISSN 1040-8711

Kolossvary, E., Kollar, A., Pinter, H., Erényi, E., Kiséry, I., Péter, H., Farkas, K., Mogán, L., Farsang, C. & Kiss I. (2005). Bilateral axillobrachial and external carotid artery manifestation of giant cell arteritis: important role of color duplex ultrasonography in the diagnosis. International Angiology, Vol. 24, No. 2, (Jun 2005), pp. 202-5, ISSN 0392-9590

LeSar, CJ., Meier, GH., DeMasi, RJ., Sood, J., Nelms, CR., Carter, KA., Gayle, RG., Parent, FN. & Marcinczyk MJ. (2002). The utility of color duplex ultrasonography in the diagnosis of temporal arteritis. Journal of Vascular Surgery, Vol. 36, No. 6, (Dec 2002), pp. 1154-60, ISSN 0741-5214

Maldini, C., Depinay-Dhellemmes, C., Tra, TT., Chauveau, M., Allanore, Y., Gossec, L., Terrasse, G., Guillevin, L., Coste, J. & Mahr A. (2010). Limited value of temporal artery ultrasonography examinations for diagnosis of giant cell arteritis: analysis of 77 subjects. Journal of Rheumatology, Vol. 37, No. 11, (November 2010), pp. 2326-30, ISSN 0315-162X

Morinobu, A., Tsuji, G., Kasagi, S., Saegusa, J., Hayashi, H., Nakazawa, T., Kogata, Y., Misaki, K., Nishimura, K., Sendo, S., Miura, N., Kawano, S. & Kumagai S. (2011). Role of imaging studies in the diagnosis and evaluation of giant cell arteritis in Japanese: report of eight cases. Modern Rheumatol, [Epub ahead of print], ISSN 1439-7609

Murgatroyd, H., Nimmo, M., Evans, A. & MacEwen, C. (2003) The use of ultrasound as an aid in the diagnosis of giant cell arteritis: a pilot study comparing histological features with ultrasound findings. Eye (Lond), Vol. 17, No. 3, (April 2003), pp. 415-9, ISSN 0950-222X

Narvaez, J., Narvaez, JA., Nolla, JM., Sirvent, E., Reina, D. & Valverde, J. (2005). Giant cell arteritis and polymyalgia rheumatica: usefulness of vascular magnetic resonance imaging studies in the diagnosis of aortitis. Rheumatology (Oxford), Vol. 44, No. 4, (April 2005), pp. 479-83, ISSN 1462-0324

Nesher, G., Shemesh, D., Mates, M., Sonnenblick, M. & Abramowitz, HB. (2002). The predictive value of the halo sign in color Doppler ultrasonography of the temporal arteries for diagnosing giant cell arteritis. Journal of Rheumatology, Vol. 29, No. 6, (June 2002), pp. 1224-6, ISSN 0315-162X

Nesher, G., Berkun, Y., Mates, M., Baras, M., Rubinow, A. &, Sonnenblick, M. (2004). Low-dose aspirin and prevention of cranial ischemic complications in giant cell arteritis. Arthritis & Rheumatism, Vol. 50, No. 4, (April 2004), pp. 1332-7, ISSN 0004-3591

Perez Lopez, J., Solans Laque, R., Bosch Gil, JA., Molina Cateriano, C., Huguet Redecilla, P. & Vilardell Tarres, M. (2009). Colour-duplex ultrasonography of the temporal and ophthalmic arteries in the diagnosis and follow-up of giant cell arteritis. Clinical and Experimental Rheumatology, Vol. 27, No. 1, Suppl. 52, (January-February 2009), pp. S77-82, ISSN 0392-856X

Pfadenhauer, K. & Weber, H. (2003). Duplex sonography of the temporal and occipital artery in the diagnosis of temporal arteritis. A prospective study. Journal of Rheumatology Vol. 30, No. 10, (October 2003), pp. 2177-81, ISSN 0315-162X

Puechal, X., Chauveau, M. & Menkes, CJ. (1995). Temporal Doppler-flow studies for suspected giant-cell arteritis. Lancet, Vol. 345, No. 8962, (June 1995), pp. 1437-8, ISSN 0140-6736

Rao,JK., Allen, NB. & Pincus, T. (1998). Limitations of the 1990 American College of Rheumatology classification criteria in the diagnosis of vasculitis. Annals of Internal Medicine, Vol. 129, No. 5, (September 1998), pp. 345-52, ISSN 0003-4819

Ray-Chaudhuri, N, Kine, DA., Tijani, SO., Parums, DV., Cartlidge, N., Strong, NP. & Dayan MR. (2002) Effect of prior steroid treatment on temporal artery biopsy findings in giant cell arteritis. British Journal of Ophthalmology, Vol. 86, No. 5, (May 2002), pp. 530-2, ISSN 0007-1161

Reinhard, M., Schmidt, D., Schumacher, M. & Hetzel, A. (2003). Involvement of the vertebral arteries in giant cell arteritis mimicking vertebral dissection. Journal of Neurology, Vol. 250, No. 8, (august 2003), pp. 1006-9, ISSN 0340-5354

Reinhard, M., Schmidt, D. & Hetzel A. (2004). Color-coded sonography in suspected temporal arteritis-experiences after 83 cases. Rheumatology International, Vol. 24, No 6, (November 2004), pp. 340-6, ISSN 0172-8172

Reitblat, T., Ben-Horin, CL & Reitblat, A. (2003). Gallium-67 SPECT scintigraphy may be useful in diagnosis of temporal arteritis. Annals of Rheumatic Diseases, Vol. 62, No. 3, (march 2003), pp. 257-60, ISSN 0003-4967

Richards, BL., March, L. & Gabriel, SE (2010). Epidemiology of large-vessel vasculidities. Best Practice & Research Clinical Rheumatology, Vol. 24, No. 6, (December 2010), pp. 871-83, ISSN 1532-1770

RRomera-Villegas, A., Vila-Coll, R., Poca-Dias, V. & Cairols-Castellote, MA. (2004). The role of color duplex sonography in the diagnosis of giant cell arteritis. Journal of Ultrasound in Medicine, Vol. 23, No. 11, (November 2004), pp. 1493-8, ISSN 0278-4297

Salvarani, C., Silingardi, M., Ghirarduzzi, A.., Lo Scocco, G., Macchioni, P., Bajocchi, G., Vinceti, M., Cantini, F., Iori, I. & Boiardi L. (2002). Is duplex ultrasonography useful for the diagnosis of giant-cell arteritis? Annals of Internal Medicine, Vol. 137, No. 4, (August 2002), pp. 232-8, ISSN 1539-3704

Schmidt, WA., Kraft, HE., Volker, L., Vorpahl, K. & Gromnica-Ihle, EJ. (1995). Colour Doppler sonography to diagnose temporal arteritis. Lancet, Vol. 345, No. 8953, (April 1995), p. 866, ISSN 0140-6736

Schmidt, WA., Kraft, HE., Vorpahl, K.., Volker, L.. & Gromnica-Ihle, EJ. (1997). Color duplex ultrasonography in the diagnosis of temporal arteritis. New England Journal of Medicine, Vol. 337, No. 19, (Novembre 1997), pp. 1336-42, ISSN 0028-4793

Schmidt, WA. (2000). Doppler ultrasonography in the diagnosis of giant cell arteritis. Clinical Experimental Rheumatology, Vo. 18, No. 4, Suppl 20, (July-August 2000), S40-2, ISSN 0392-856X

Schmidt, WA., Natusch, A., Moller, DE., Vorpahl, K. & Gromnica-Ihle, E. (2002). Involvement of peripheral arteries in giant cell arteritis: a color Doppler sonography study. Clinical Experimental Rheumatology, Vol. 20, No. 3, (May-June 2002), pp. 309-18, ISSN 0392-856X

Schmidt, WA. & Gromnica-Ihle, E. (2003). Duplex ultrasonography in temporal arteritis. Annals of Internal Medicine, Vol. 138, No. 7, (April 2003), p. 609; author reply 609-10, ISSN 1539-3704

Schmidt, WA. (2004). Doppler sonography in rheumatology. (2004). Best Practice & Research Clinical Rheumatology, Vol. 18, No. 6, (December 2004), pp. 827-46, ISSN 1521-6942

Schmidt, WA. & Blockmans, D. (2005). Use of ultrasonography and positron emission tomography in the diagnosis and assessment of large-vessel vasculitis, Vol. 17, No. 1, (January 2005), pp. 9-15, ISSN 1040-8711

Schmidt, WA, & Gromnica-Ihle, E. (2005). What is the best approach to diagnosing large-vessel vasculitis? Best Practice & Research Clinical Rheumatology, Vol. 19, No. 2, (April 2005), pp. 223-42, ISSN 1521-6942

Schmidt, WA. Current diagnosis and treatment of temporal arteritis. (2006), Current Treatment Options in Cardiovascular Medicine, Vol.8, No. 2, (April 2006), pp. 145-51, ISSN 1092-8464

Schmidt, WA., Seifert, A., Gromnica-Ihle, E., Krause, A. & Natusch, A (2008), Ultrasound of proximal upper extremity arteries to increase the diagnostic yield in large-vessel giant cell arteritis. Rheumatology (Oxford), Vol. 47, No. 1, (Jnuary 2008), SSN 1462-0332

Schmidt, WA., Krause, A., Schicke, B., Kuchenbecker, J, & Gromnica-Ihle, E. (2009). Do temporal artery duplex ultrasound findings correlate with ophthalmic complications in giant cell arteritis? Rheumatology (Oxford), Vol. 48, No. 4, (April 2009), pp. 383-5, ISSN 1462-0332

Siemssen SJ. (1987). On the occurrence of necrotising lesions in arteritis temporalis: review of the literature with a note on the potential risk of a biopsy. British Journal of Plastic Surgery, vol. 40, No. 1, (Jauary 1987), pp. 73-82, ISSN 0007-1226

Slavin, ML. (1986). Brow droop after superficial temporal artery biopsy. Archives of Ophthalmology, Vol. 104, No. 8, (Augut 1986), p. 1127, ISSN 0003-9950

Stanson, AW. (2000). Imaging findings in extracranial (giant cell) temporal arteritis. Clinical and Experimental Rheumatology, Vol. 18, No. 4 , Suppl 20, (Julyu-August 2000), pp. S43-8, ISSN 0392-856X

Suelves, AM., Espana-Gregori, E., Tembl, J., Rohrweck, S., Millan, JM. & Diaz-Llopis, M. (2010). Doppler ultrasound and giant cell arteritis.Clinical Ophthalmology, Vol. 25, No. 4,(November 2010), pp. 1383-4, ISSN 1177-5483

Tato, F.& Hoffmann U. (2006). Clinical presentation and vascular imaging in giant cell arteritis of the femoropopliteal and tibioperoneal arteries. Analysis of four cases. Journal of Vascular Surgery, Vol. 44, No 1, (July 2006), pp. 176-82, ISSN 0741-5214

Tato, F. & Hoffmann U. Giant cell arteritis: a systemic vascular disease. (2008). Vascular Medicine, Vol. 13, No. 2, (2008), pp. 127-40, ISSN 1358-863X

Vinckier, L., Hatron, PY., Gadenne, C.,, Catteau, MH., Gosset, D.& Devulder, B. (1989). Significance of arterial Doppler in Horton's disease. Prospective study of 59 case reports. Journal des Maladies Vasculaires, Vol. 14, Suppl C, (1989), ISSN 0398-0499

Walter, MA., Melzer, RA., Schindler, C., Muller-Brand, J., Tyndal,l A & Nitzsche EU (2005). The value of [18F]FDG-PET in the diagnosis of large-vessel vasculitis and the assessment of activity and extent of disease. European Journal of Nuclear Medicine and Molecular Imaging, Vol. 32, No. 6, (june 2005), pp. 674-81, ISSN 1619-7070

Warrington, KJ. & Matteson, EL. Management guidelines and outcome measures in giant cell arteritis (GCA). (2007). Clinical and Experimental Rheumatology, Vol. 25, No. 6, Suppl 47, (Novembre-December 2007), pp.137-41, 0392-856X

Weyand, CM. & Goronzy, JJ. (2003). Giant-cell arteritis and polymyalgia rheumatica. Annals of Internal Medicine, Vol.1 39, No. 6, (September 2003), pp. 505-15, ISSN 1539-3704

Part 4

Management and Therapy

8

Perioperative Management of Non-Biological and Biological Therapies in Rheumatic Patients Undergoing Orthopedic Surgery

Juan Salvatierra Ossorio, Magdalena Peregrina-Palomares, Francisco O´Valle Ravassa and Pedro Hernandez-Cortes
Department of Orthopedic Surgery, San Cecilio University Hospital
University of Granada, Granada
Spain

1. Introduction

Patients with rheumatoid arthritis (RA) or other inflammatory arthropathies often require orthopedic surgery, and the management of their medical treatments during the perioperative period is an important issue. The two main concerns during this period are the risk of infection and wound healing complications.

These patients receive multidisciplinary care from orthopedic surgeons, rehabilitators and rheumatologists (1). Before orthopedic surgery, the activity of the arthropathy and the non-biological and biological therapies of patients must be taken into consideration for an optimal outcome with no infectious or wound-healing complications. Good clinical and biological control of the disease must be obtained before the surgery, and effective coordination between surgeon and rheumatologist is essential (2).

The management of non-biological (immunosuppressive or immunomodulatory) and biological therapies in orthopedic surgery patients remains controversial. This chapter focuses on disease-modifying anti-rheumatic drugs (DMARDs) and biological therapies (see table 1). Although corticosteroids are immunosuppressants, protocols for their replacement or supplementation are well established in the literature and are not addressed here (3). DMARDs and especially biological therapies are the subject of multiple consultations between rheumatologists and orthopedists or anesthetists before surgery. The objective of this chapter is to discuss current protocols for the application of these treatments before and after orthopedic surgery, based on the best available scientific evidence or, in its absence, on accepted recommendations.

2. Disease-modifying anti-rheumatic drugs (DMARDS)

2.1 Methotrexate (MTX)

Until five years ago, there was a tendency to withdraw MTX at around two weeks before surgery, based on reports in various retrospective studies of a higher risk of postoperative complications, especially infections (4). However, a well-designed prospective study by Grennan et al. (5) in 388 patients concluded that the continuation of MTX treatment did not

MODIFYING DRUGS (DMARDS)	BIOLOGICAL THERAPIES
- METHOTREXATE	- INFLIXIMAB
- ANTI-MALARIALS	- ETANERCEPT
- LEFLUNOMIDE	- ADALIMUMAB (D2E7)
- SULFASALAZINE	- CERTOLIZUMAB
- CYCLOSPORINE A	- GOLIMUMAB
- GOLD COMPOUNDS	- ANAKINRA (rHuIL-1Ra)
- AZATHIOPRINE	- RITUXIMAB
	- ABATACEPT
	- TOCILIZUMAB

Table 1. Modifying drugs and biological therapies used in rheumatoid arthritis

increase infection risk or delay wound-healing. Furthermore, patients who had continued with their MTX treatment had fewer postoperative inflammatory outbreaks in comparison to those who had not, and the latter showed a non-significant tendency to a higher frequency of post-surgical complications. Nevertheless, although a rare complication, MTX-associated lymphoproliferative disorders consist of a heterogeneous group of lymphoid proliferations or lymphomas (mainly diffuse large B-cell lymphoma or Hodgkin lymphoma) that develop in patients with autoimmune diseases after prolonged MTX treatment. These lymphoproliferative disorders are often associated with Epstein-Barr virus infection and occasionally regress after the withdrawal of MTX therapy (6).

2.2 Anti-malarials

The anti-malarials used in RA patients are chloroquine and especially hydroxychloroquine, due to its lower ocular toxicity. After their prolonged administration, anti-malarials accumulate in multiple tissues (kidney, spleen, liver, etc). For this reason, despite the absence of well-designed studies, it does not appear appropriate or meaningful to interrupt their administration immediately before surgery. Nevertheless, it should be borne in mind that anti-malarials inhibit platelet aggregation and adhesion (7) and may therefore increase the risk of bleeding.

2.3 Leflunomide (LFN), sulfasalazine, and gold compounds

LFN inhibits pyrimidine synthesis and offers a similar effectiveness to that of MTX but with a greater selectivity, reversibly inhibiting the proliferation of activated autoimmune lymphocytes. Although a low risk of infection was reported in various clinical trials, there appear to be no studies that evaluate this risk or the effects on postoperative wound-healing. However, because LFN can potentiate anticoagulation, the dosage should be adjusted in patients receiving this drug as prophylaxis against deep vein thrombosis (7). With respect to sulfasalazine and gold compounds, no good scientific evidence is available on their perioperative administration. In general, however, the perioperative suspension of their administration is not recommended (8).

2.4 Cyclosporine A and azathioprine

Although there have been no well-designed studies, various publications (7,10) have reported that infections are more frequent after orthopedic surgery in patients receiving azathioprine or cyclosporine A. For this reason, it is recommended to withdraw these drugs one week before and reintroduce them two weeks after this surgery.

3. Biological therapies

Unlike the treatments reported above, biological therapies are designed to specifically block molecules with important pathophysiological roles in AR and other inflammatory arthropies. These molecules include various proinflammatory cytokines, such as tumor necrosis factor-alpha (TNF-a), interleukin 6 (IL-6), and interleukin 1 (IL-1), which are responsible for chronic synovitis, bone destruction, and systemic manifestations. Other biological drugs have been developed against cells that participate in the pathogenesis of RA, such as rituximab, directed against CD20 B cells, and abatacept, which prevents activation of T lymphocytes and has shown effectiveness in controlling the disease.

Biological drugs are proteins (monoclonal antibodies or soluble receptors against cytokines, receptors, or cell surface molecules) obtained by biotechnology that block the above-mentioned cytokines or modulate B or T cells in a specific manner. The following are currently available:

- Drugs directed against TNF-a, either monoclonal antibodies (infliximab, adalimumab, certolizumab, or golimumab) or soluble receptors (etanercept). Their administration form and dosage differ according to the pharmacokinetics of these products.
- Abatacept is a fusion protein that blocks the T lymphocyte co-stimulation signal mediated by CD28; it is administered intravenously every 4 weeks.
- Tocilizumab is a humanized monoclonal antibody against IL-6 receptor; it is administered intravenously at an initial dose of 4 mg/kg (USA) or 8 mg/kg (Europe, Japan) every 4 weeks.
- Rituximab is a chimeric monoclonal antibody against the CD20 marker for B lymphocytes; it is administered intravenously at a dose of 500 or 1000 mg on days 0 and 15 and repeated every 6-12 months according to the disease activity.
- Anakhinra is a recombinant human antagonist of IL-1 receptor; it is administered subcutaneously every day.

These drugs block cytokines or modulate cells involved in the cell immune response to infections. Hence, in theory, they should be withdrawn before surgery, despite the absence of clinical studies to support this decision. No clinical trial has addressed complications after orthopedic surgery in RA patients receiving biological treatments, but there have been some retrospective studies. Bibbo et al. (11) investigated the influence of infliximab and etanercept in orthopedic surgery and concluded that they could be administered safely in the perioperative period without increasing the risk of infectious or wound-healing complications. However, the pathologic study of the wounds is not reported, and the authors do not describe how they assessed wound-healing delay or bone-healing complications, two key variables in their study. A more recent retrospective study on clinical factors related to infliximab-treated RA patients undergoing orthopedic surgery (12) concludes that infliximab does not increase the risk of surgical or infectious complications at one year post-surgery. We did not observe any wound healing complications after hand surgery in fourteen rheumatoid patients treated with etanercept or infliximab (Fig. 1 and 2). Experimental results of TNF-a administration in murine models of wound-healing complications have not been consistent. Although TNF-a inhibition could theoretically have a negative impact on wound-healing (13), studies by our group and other authors suggest that it may improve collagenization of the wound (14), supporting its continuation during the perioperative period (Fig 3 and 4).

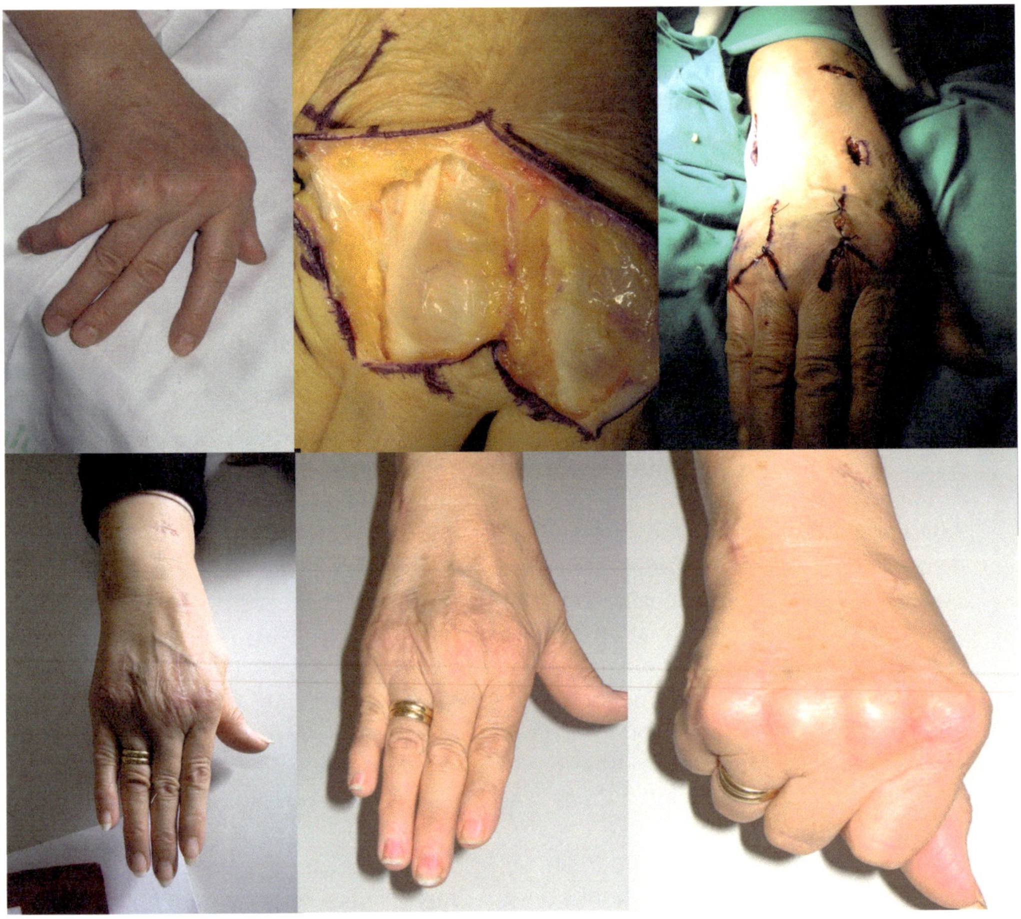

Fig. 1. Metacarpophalangeal deformity and arthritis in right hand of woman with rheumatoid arthritis and under treatment with etanercept. Surgical wound for implantation of metacarpophalangeal prosthesis. Treatment was not suspended during the perioperative period. Surgical wound healing was excellent.

No data are available on the effect of rituximab on surgical complications in RA patients. Its administration produces a prolonged (6 months–1 year) depletion of CD-19B lymphocytes and may therefore increase the risk of perioperative infection. Its effects on wound-healing are less clear. It therefore appears prudent to suspend treatment and delay surgery until the CD-19 lymphocyte B count of the patient is normalized (15). Nevertheless, experience with the administration of rituximab to lymphoma patients undergoing surgery suggests that it can be continued when surgery is essential and that its administration should not be a contraindication for surgery.

Tocilizumab blocks IL-6, inducing hepatic synthesis of C-reactive protein (CRP), which may mask signs and symptoms of post-surgical infectious complications, such as fever or elevated CRP (16, 17). The effects of IL-6 inhibition on wound-healing, by interfering with the initial inflammatory phase of the surgical wound, are not known.

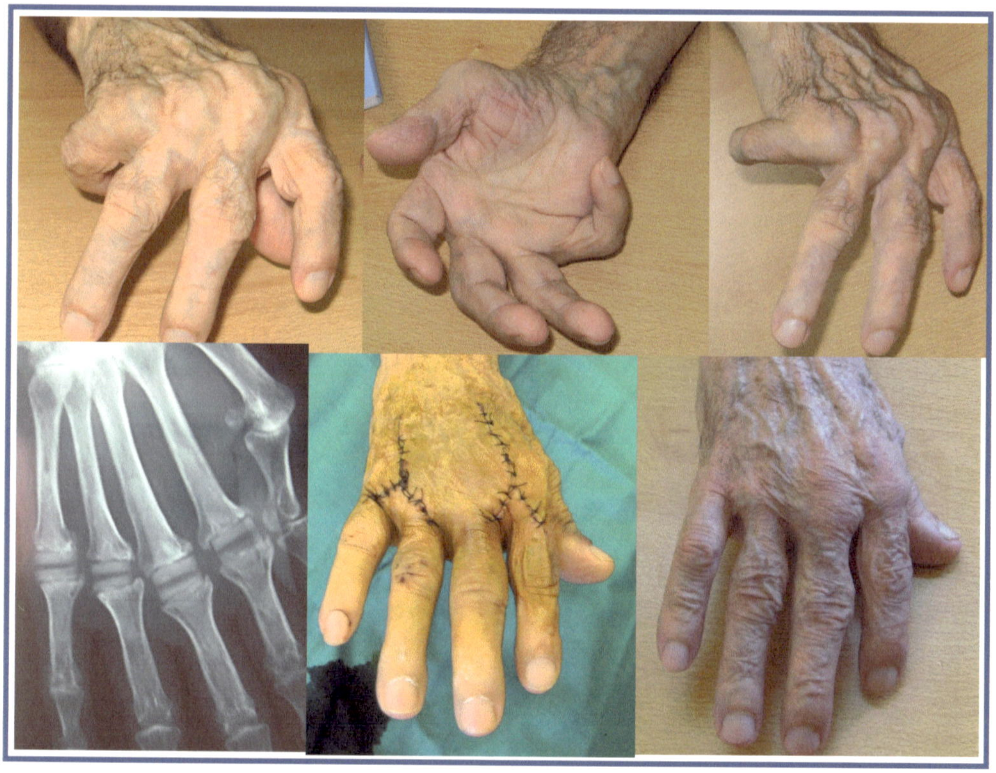

Fig. 2. Ulnar deformity and metacarpophalangeal arthritis in right hand of man with rheumatoid arthritis under treatment with infliximab and that underwent metacarpophalangeal prosthesis. Treatment was not suspended during the perioperative period. Wound-healing was satisfactory, with no complications.

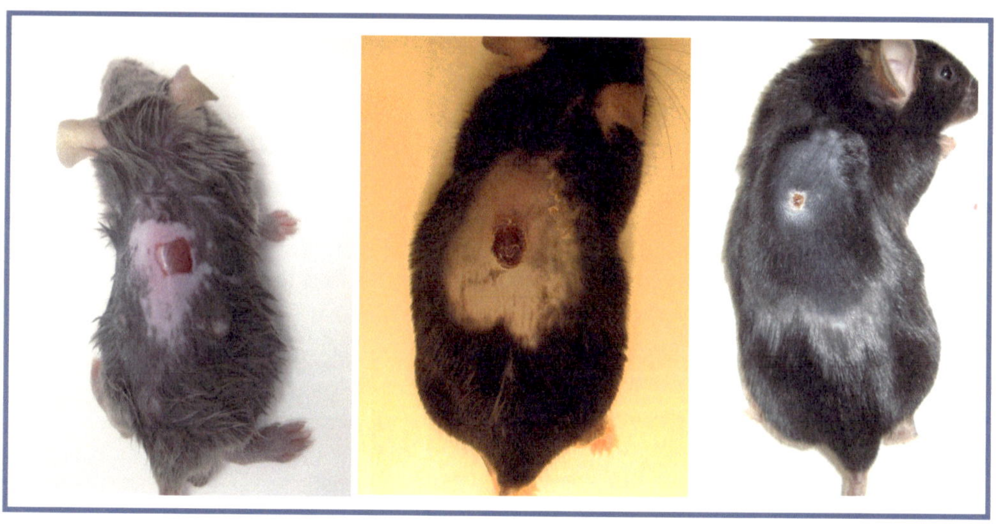

Fig. 3. Skin wound-healing during a 3-week period in etanercept-treated. DAB1J mice with collagen-induced arthritis

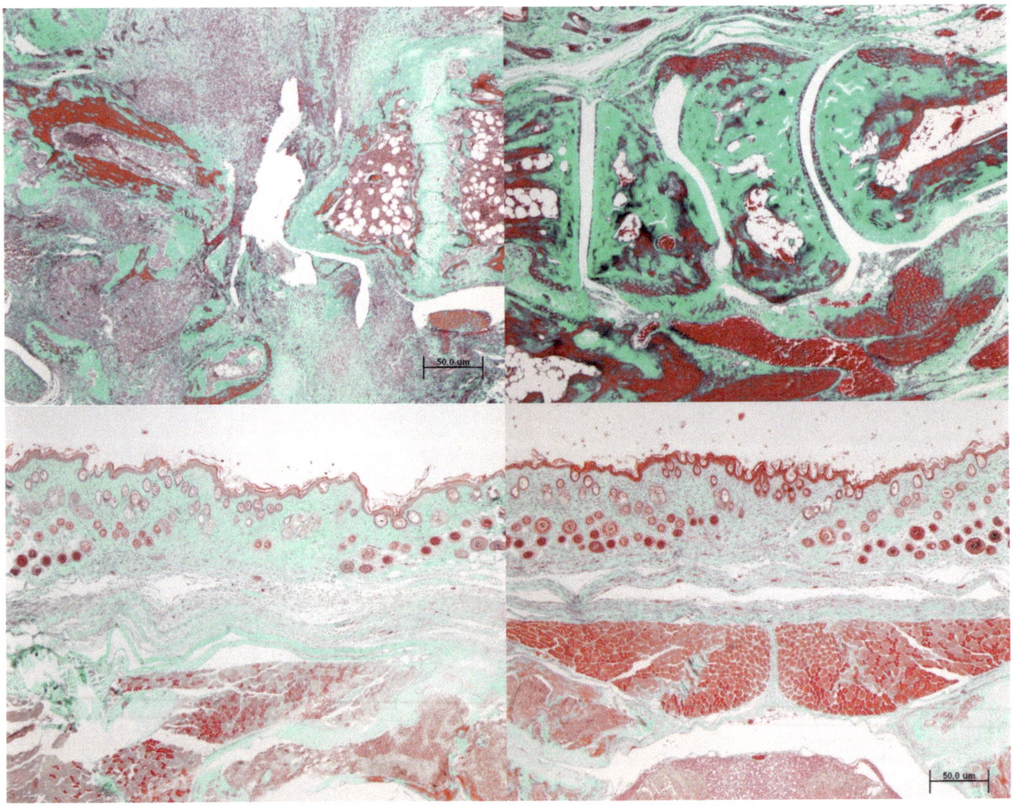

Fig. 4. Severe osteoarticular lesions in DAB1J mice with collagen-induced arthritis at day 15 (upper-left image). Absence of osteorticular lesions in etanercept-treated mice (upper-right image). Skin wound-healing in DAB1J mice with collagen-induced arthritis at day 15. Note complete re-epithelization and skin appendages recovery in control (lower left image) and etanercept-treated (lower right image) mice [original magnification 4x, Masson Trichrome stain].

We could find no study on the effect of abatacept on surgical complications or wound healing. However, no associated postoperative complications were described in case reports on infections in patients who underwent surgery while receiving this drug (18).

Given the above data, and until new scientific evidence becomes available, it appears sensible to suspend these treatments before surgery, determining the pre-surgical interval according to the drug's half-life, only reintroducing them when the wound has healed with no complications. We propose the following recommendations (summarized in Table 2) for each drug.

- Infliximab: suspend treatment 6 weeks before surgery.
- Adalimumab: suspend treatment 2 weeks before surgery.
- Golimumab/Certolizumab: suspend treatment 4 weeks before surgery.
- Etanercept: suspend treatment 1 week before surgery.
- Anakinra: suspend treatment 24-48 hours before surgery.
- Rituximab: suspend treatment and delay surgery until serum levels of CD-19 B lymphocytes normalize (usually 3-6 months after last dose). Nevertheless, if urgent

surgery is required or cannot be delayed due to the patient's condition, surgery can be performed without normalization of these serum levels.

- Tocilizumab: suspend treatment 4 weeks before surgery but take into account that patients with infectious complications may not present with elevated CRP levels or fever.
- Abatacept: suspend treatment 4 weeks before surgery.

BIOLOGICAL THERAPY	TIMING OF SUSPENSION BEFORE SURGERY
INFLIXIMAB	6 WEEKS
ETANERCEPT	1 WEEK
ADALIMUMAB (D2E7)	2 WEEKS
CERTOLIZUMAB	4 WEEKS
GOLIMUMAB	4 WEEKS
ANAKINRA (rHuIL-1Ra)	24-48 HOURS
RITUXIMAB	AFTER NORMALIZATION OF SERUM LEVELS OF CD-19 B LYMPHOCYTES (3-6 MONTHS)
ABATACEPT	4 WEEKS
TOCILIZUMAB	4 WEEKS

Table 2. Biological therapies and recommended timing of their suspension before surgery

Future therapies

Considerable clinical and experimental evidence suggests that various endogenous neuropeptides play a major role in educating our immune system to be self-tolerant. The fact that neuropeptides regulate various layers involved in the maintenance of tolerance, including regulation of the balance between pro-inflammatory and anti-inflammatory responses and between self-reactive Th1/Th17 cells and regulatory T cells, makes them attractive candidates for the development of novel therapies to treat autoimmune disorders such as RA. Vasoactive intestinal peptide is the paradigmatic immunomodulatory neuropeptide, but other neuropeptides possess similar properties, including melanocyte-stimulating hormone, urocortin, adrenomedullin, neuropeptide Y, cortistatin, and ghrelin (19). All have demonstrated marked beneficial effects in animal models of collagen-induced arthritis without affecting wound healing (20-23).

4. Conclusions

In the majority of cases, there are no well-designed studies to support clear recommendations on the perioperative management of patients with inflammatories arthropies receiving anti-rheumatic treatment, especially the new biological therapies. Available evidence suggests that methotrexate, anti-malarials, and gold compounds can be continued during surgery. However, leflunomide, sulfasalazine, azathioprine, and cyclosporine A should be withdrawn due to the increased risk of infection associated with their use. With regard to the new biological therapies, it should be borne in mind that they inhibit cytokines and modulate cells that participate in the physiological response against infections and in wound-healing. Until data from well-designed prospective studies become available, it therefore appears prudent to withdraw these drugs before surgery for a time interval based on their pharmacokinetics.

5. Key points

1. In patients with inflammatory arthropies requiring orthopedic surgery, good clinical and biological control of the disease must be obtained before the intervention; therefore, coordination between orthopedic surgeon and rheumatologist is essential.
2. We must know the biological and non-biological therapies received by our patients for their perioperative management, thereby reducing the risk of infection and surgical wound-healing complications.
3. Methotrexate can be maintained during the perioperative period, but leflunomide, sulfasalazine, azathioprine, and cyclosporine A should be suspended, because available studies suggest their association with a higher infection risk.
4. T and B cells and cytokines (tumor necrosis factor-alpha, interleukin 6, and interleukin 1) are involved in anti-infection defense and surgical wound-healing and are modulated or blocked by biological therapies administered to patients with inflammatory arthropaties.
5. There have been no clinical trials on surgical complications in patients with inflammatory arthropaties receiving biological therapies; therefore, recommendations are based on retrospective and animal studies.
6. Retrospective studies suggest that infliximab and etanercept can be safely administered during the perioperative period to patients undergoing orthopedic surgery without increasing their risk of infection or wound-healing complications.
7. Murine studies suggest that collagenization of the surgical wound is improved by the inhibition of tumor necrosis factor-alpha with etanercept.
8. In patients under treatment with rituximab, it is recommendable to program the surgery once the serum count of CD-19 B lymphocytes has normalized; however, if this is not possible, its administration should not be considered a contraindication for the surgery.
9. Tocilizumab blocks IL-6, inducing the hepatic synthesis of C-reactive protein (CRP), which can mask the signs and symptoms of infectious post-surgical complications such as fever or elevated CRP.
10. Given the absence of high-quality scientific evidence, we recommend suspending biological therapies before the surgery in accordance with their half-life and not reintroducing them until the surgical wound has healed.

6. References

[1] Carmona L, Ballina J, Gabriel R, Laffon A. The burden of musculoskeletal diseases in the general population of Spain: results from a national survey. Ann Rheum Dis 2001;60:1040-1045.

[2] Shaw M, Mandell BF. Perioperative management of selected problems in patients with rheumatic diseases. Rheum Dis Clin North Am 1999;25:623-638.

[3] Nicholson G, Burrin JM, Hall GM. Perioperative steroid supplementation. Anaesthesia 1998;53:1091-1104.

[4] Sany J, Anaya J, Canovas F, Combe B, Jorgensen C, Saker S, et al. Influence of methotrexate and the frequency of postoperative infections/complications in patients with rheumatoid arthritis. J Rheumatol 1993;20:1129-1132.

[5] Grennan DM, Gray J, Loudon J, Fear S. Methotrexate and early postoperative complications in patients with rheumatoid arthritis undergoing elective orthopaedic surgery. Ann Rheum Dis 2001; 60:214-217.

[6] Gaulard P, Swerdlow SH, Harris NL, Jaffe ES, Sundström C. Other iatrogenic immunodeficiency-associatedlymphoproliferative disorders. In: Swerdlow SH, Campo E, Harris NL, Jaffe ES, Pileri SA, Stein H, Thiele J, Vardiman JW, eds. WHO Classification of Tumours of Haematopoietic and Lymphoid Tissues. Sterling, VA: Stylus Publishing, LLC; 2008: 350-351.

[7] Lim V, Pande I. Leflunomide can potentiate the anticoagulant effect of warfarin. BMJ 2002; 325:1333.

[8] Jancinova V, Nosal R, Pretrikova M. On the inhibitory effect of chloroquine on blood platelet aggregation. Thromb Res 1994,74:495-504.

[9] Rothschild BM. Surgery and the patient with arthritis. Com Ther 2001;27:104-107.

[10] Sorokin R. Management of the patient with rheumatic diseases going to surgery. Med Clin North Am 1993; 77:453-464.

[11] Marchal L, D´Haens G, Van Assche G, Hiele M, D´Hoore Andre, Penninck F, Rutgeerts P. Infliximab does not increase postoperative complication rates in patients with Crohn´s disease. Gastroenterology suppl. Digestive Diseases Week, Orlando, FL; May 18-21, 2003. Abstract no. 100519.

[12] Brzezinski A, Armstrong L, Del Real GA, Parsi M, Lasher B, Achkar JP, Cleveland OH. Infliximab does not increase the risk of complications in the perioperative period in patients with Crohn´s disease. Gastroenterology suppl. Digestive Diseases Week, San Francisco, CA; May 19-22, 2002. Abstract no. 104783.

[13] Kawaguchi HH, Hizuta AA, Tanaka NN, Orita KK. Roles of endotoxin in wound healing impairment. Res Commun Mol Pathol Pharmacol 1995;89: 317-327.

[14] Iglesia E, O´Valle F, Salvatierra J, Aneiros-Fernández J, Cantero-Hinojosa J, Hernández-Cortés P. Effect of blockade of tumor necrosis factor-alpha with etanercept on surgical wound healing in SWISS-OF1 mice. J Rheumatol 2009;36:2144-48.

[15] Scanzello CR, Figgie MP, Nestor BJ, Goodman SM. Perioperative management of medications used in the treatment of Rheumatoid Arthritis. HSSJ 2006;2:141-147.

[16] Hirao M, Hashimoto J, Tsuboi H, Nampei A, Nakahara H, Yoshio N, et al. Laboratory and febrile feautures after joint surgery in patients with rheumatoid arthritis treated with tocilizumab. Ann Rheum Dis 2009;68:654-657.

[17] Hiroshima R, Kawakami K, Iwamoto T, Tokita A, Yano K, Sakuma Y, et al. Analysis of C-reactive protein levels and febrile tendency after joint surgery in rheumatoid arthritis patients treated with a perioperative 4-week interruption of tocilizumab. Mod Rheumatol 2011;21:109-111.

[18] Kakarala K, Durand ML, Emerick K. Retropharyngeal abscess in the setting of immune modulation for rheumatoid arthritis. Laryngoscope 2010:120 Suppl 4:S131.

[19] Gonzalez-Rey E, Delgado-Maroto V, Souza Moreira L, Delgado M. Neuropeptides as therapeutic approach to autoimmune diseases. Curr Pharm Des. 2010; 16(28): 3158-3172.

[20] Delgado M, Robledo G, Rueda B, Varela N, O'Valle F, Hernandez-Cortes P, Caro M, Orozco G, Gonzalez-Rey E, Martin J. Genetic association of vasoactive intestinal peptide receptor with rheumatoid arthritis: altered expression and signal in immune cells. Arthritis Rheum. 2008; 58(4): 1010-1019.

[21] Delgado M, Toscano MG, Benabdellah K, Cobo M, O'Valle F, Gonzalez-Rey E, Martín F. In vivo delivery of lentiviral vectors expressing vasoactive intestinal peptide complementary DNA as gene therapy for collagen-induced arthritis. Arthritis Rheum. 2008; 58(4): 1026-1037.

[22] Gonzalez-Rey E, Chorny A, Varela N, O'Valle F, Delgado M. Therapeutic effect of urocortin on collagen-induced arthritis by down-regulation of inflammatory and Th1 responses and induction of regulatory T cells. Arthritis Rheum. 2007; 56(2): 531-543.

[23] Gonzalez-Rey E, Chorny A, O'Valle F, Delgado M. Adrenomedullin protects from experimental arthritis by down-regulating inflammation and Th1 response and inducing regulatory T cells. Am J Pathol. 2007; 170(1):263-271.

9

Optimal Treatment Strategy for Amyloid A Amyloidosis in Rheumatic Diseases – Anti-Interleukin-6 Receptor Therapy

Yasuaki Okuda
Department of Internal Medicine,
Center for Rheumatic Diseases, Dohgo Spa Hospital
Japan

1. Introduction

Among the complications of inflammatory rheumatic diseases, amyloid A (AA) amyloidosis is one of the most severe because of its poor prognosis. AA amyloidosis commonly affects the kidney and the gastrointestinal tract, and is characterized by various clinical symptoms such as progressive proteinuria and renal dysfunction and failure. Control of the underlying disease, i.e. suppression of serum amyloid A (SAA) levels, is the most critical step in the treatment of AA amyloidosis. An immunosuppressant such as methotrexate, azathioprine, or cyclophosphamide, and moderate doses of prednisolone are commonly used to accomplish this. However, in some active cases, satisfactory suppression of SAA levels cannot be achieved, and the function of the affected organs deteriorates. The prognosis is usually poor for patients in advanced stages of AA amyloidosis. The major causes of death are renal failure and infection. Some retrospective studies and case reports have shown anti-tumor necrosis factor (TNF) therapies to be useful against AA amyloidosis (Elkayam et al., 2002; Fernándes-Nebro et al., 2010; Gottenberg et al., 2003; Kuroda et al., 2009; Nakamura et al., 2010). Although treatment with anti-TNF agents does reduce acute-phase reactants such as C-reactive protein (CRP) and SAA in chronic inflammatory diseases, unfortunately complete normalization of such acute-phase proteins is rarely observed.
On the other hand, several case reports and a retrospective comparative study have shown that tocilizumab, an anti-human interleukin-6 (IL-6) receptor monoclonal antibody, has an excellent ability to suppress SAA levels and improve clinical symptoms of AA amyloidosis with marked lasting regression of AA protein deposits (Inoue et al., 2010; Kishida et al., 2011; Nishida et al., 2009; Okuda & Takasugi, 2006; Okuda 2009; Sato et al., 2009; Ubara, 2009). Treatment with tocilizumab could, therefore, represent an important therapeutic strategy for AA amyloidosis secondary to rheumatic diseases.

2. Pathogenesis of AA amyloidosis in rheumatic diseases

AA amyloidosis resulting from deposition of AA protein in the extracellular matrices of various organs may lead to multiple organ dysfunction, and the prognosis is usually poor in patients with advanced AA amyloidosis.

Although formerly chronic infections such as tuberculosis were listed as the principal cause of AA amyloidosis, most cases of AA amyloidosis at present are closely associated with chronic inflammatory diseases such as rheumatoid arthritis (RA) (Sasatomi et al., 2007). SAA, the precursor of AA protein, is highly amplified in the liver under the stimulation of inflammation-associated cytokines such as IL-6, TNF, and IL-1 (Yamada, 1999). Prolonged elevation of SAA is the major inciting factor for AA amyloidosis developing in chronic inflammatory diseases. The extensive and persistent production of SAA under chronic active inflammatory conditions is the critical prerequisite for AA amyloidosis fibrillogenesis, and approximately 10–15% of Japanese RA patients have AA amyloidosis deposits in their gastroduodenal mucosa as shown by endoscopic biopsy (Kobayashi et al., 1996).

SAA is genetically polymorphic with four loci (SAA1, SAA2, SAA3, and SAA4) located on chromosome 11 (Yamada, 1999). The SAA gene products SAA1 and SAA2 are both elevated with acute inflammation and are therefore named acute-phase SAA. More than 90% of the precursor proteins of AA protein are derived from SAA1 (Liepnieks et al., 1995). SAA1 has several allelic variants, in which the exon 3 polymorphism generates three common isoforms in the Japanese population: *SAA1.1*:52Valine/57Alanine, *SAA1.3*:52Alanine/57Alanine, and *SAA1.5*:52Alanine/57Valine. It has been suggested that this polymorphism contributes to the susceptibility of the Japanese to RA-associated AA amyloidosis (Baba et al., 1995; Okuda et al., 1999; Moriguchi et al., 1999; Nakamura et al., 2006); *SAA1.3* may be a risk factor for AA amyloidosis, while *SAA1.1* acts as a defense. *SAA1.1*, however, has been reported to be a risk factor in Caucasians (Booth et al., 1998), suggesting a racial difference concerning the contribution of exon 3 polymorphism to the pathogenesis of AA amyloidosis in RA.

In animal model studies, elevated SAA was detected in ageing mice (Hsu et al., 1997), and organ extracts from aged mice had amyloid enhancing factor activity that accelerated experimental SAA production (Yokota et al., 1989). We examined the contributions of ageing to the induction of AA amyloidosis in RA in our large cohort (388 adult-onset RA patients with AA amyloidosis) including 144 patients who been analyzed for SAA1 polymorphism. We identified ageing as an independent risk factor for the formation of AA amyloidosis complicating RA (Okuda et al., 2011). Figure 1 shows the pathogenetic cascade of AA amyloidosis in rheumatic diseases.

3. Treatment of AA amyloidosis

The most rational treatment of AA amyloidosis is just to inhibit the production of SAA, the precursor of the AA proteins. As evidence of this, Gillmore et al. (2001) used serum amyloid P (SAP) scintigraphy to evaluate the level of amyloid deposits in organs in patients with AA amyloidosis associated with inflammatory diseases such as RA. They reported that when the SAA concentration in the blood was less than 10 mg/L, the level of amyloid deposits in the organs decreased and the 10 year survival rate was good at about 90%, whereas in patients with SAA levels of 10 mg/L or higher, the 10-year survival rate was about 40%. Maintenance of SAA concentrations within the normal range correlated significantly with reduced amyloid deposition and improved prognosis. The same group investigated 374 patients with AA amyloidosis and performed a more detailed analysis of the very close correlation between decreases in SAA concentration and improved survival prognosis. SAP scintigraphy revealed significant disappearance of AA protein in the low-concentration group compared with that in the high-concentration group. Control of the SAA

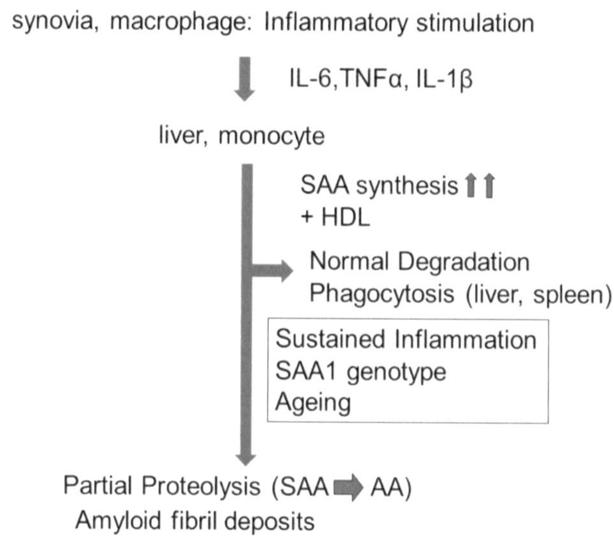

Fig. 1. SAA synthesis and pathogenesis of AA amyloidosis

concentration was stressed as the most important parameter in amyloidosis treatment (Lachmann et al., 2007). Therefore, it is very important to inhibit as much as possible the activity of the underlying disease itself. Rheumatic diseases are the most common underlying diseases of AA amyloidosis, and in the treatment of rheumatic disease patients, biologics show higher efficacy than do conventional treatments and can be used in current routine clinical practice. Anti-cytokine treatment is especially useful but there are certain characteristics and problems involved, which are discussed in detail in the next section. Among other treatments—when immunosuppressants and biologics are not adequate because of problems such as chronic infections or organ damage—there are often cases where moderate doses of corticosteroids (prednisolone 10–20 mg) are necessary. Because rheumatic diseases often affect elderly patients over the long term, complications can include onset of severe infections and thoracic and lumbar vertebral compression fractures due to osteoporosis.

For treatment of AA amyloidosis from a different standpoint, the organic solvent dimethyl sulfoxide (DMSO) is sometimes administered in an attempt to eliminate AA protein by increasing the degree of solubility of amyloid protein deposited in the tissues. Although not proven in controlled comparative studies, several case reports and case series reports suggesting its usefulness have appeared (Ravid et al., 1982, Gruys et al., 2005).

Eprodisate, a mimetic of glycosaminoglycan that serves as the extracellular scaffold for amyloid deposits in tissues, is expected to show therapeutic effects because it prevents accumulation of AA protein. A multicenter randomized double-blind placebo-controlled study was conducted mainly in Europe and the United States. It was reported that the risk of decline of renal function was lowered by 42%; however, no significant differences were found in the risk of decreases in the progression to end-stage renal failure and mortality (Dember et al., 2007). Applications were filed with the FDA, etc. as an orphan drug but they were not approved, and an additional international study is now in progress—International Randomized, Double-Blind, Placebo-Controlled, Phase 3 Study of the Efficacy and Safety of KIACTA™ in Preventing Renal Function Decline in Patients with AA Amyloidosis(Clinical Traials.gov Identifier:NCT01215747).

In the future we can expect to see the adjunctive or monotherapeutic use of biologics in patients who cannot undergo strong immunosuppressant treatment because of complications such as chronic infections.

Inhibition of SAA production

Immunosuppressive drugs
Biologics: IL-6 , TNF inhibitor
Corticosteroids

Inhibition of AA aggregation and deposition

Eprodisate (GAG mimic): GAG interaction

Amyloid fibril dissolution

Dimethyl sulfoxide

SAA: serum amyloid A; GAG: glycosaminoglycan

Fig. 2. Treatment strategies for AA amyloidosis

4. Treatment of AA amyloidosis with biologics

At present, reports of efficacy in the treatment of AA amyloidosis by biologics have stressed anti-TNF therapy and anti-IL-6 therapy, both of which are anti-cytokine therapies. First, anti-TNF therapy will be explained, and then anti-IL-6 therapy, which is the core topic of this overview, will be explained in detail.

4.1 Anti-TNF therapy

Elkayam et al. (2002) first reported that nephrotic syndrome was rapidly improved using the anti-TNF antibody drug infliximab in patients with AA amyloidosis associated with RA. Thereafter, a multicenter study was performed in France, and Gottenberg et al. (2003) evaluated anti-TNF therapy for renal disorders in 15 patients with AA amyloidosis associated with inflammatory arthritis (10 patients were given infliximab, four were given etanercept, and one was given both agents). They observed decreased proteinuria or elevated glomerular filtration rate in three patients, no progression of renal disorders in five, and worsening or progression of renal dysfunction in seven patients. Anti-TNF therapy was effective in more than half of the patients with renal disorders (Gottenberg et al., 2003). Case reports and case series reports from many facilities then appeared showing the efficacy of this therapy against AA amyloidosis associated with chronic inflammatory diseases such as rheumatic diseases (Bosca et al., 2006; Drewe et al., 2004;Kobak et al., 2007; Smith et al., 2004).

In Japan, the efficacy of anti-TNF therapy has been reported in many papers and reports given at academic society meetings. Kuroda et al. (2009) and Nakamura et al. (2010) reported efficacy in a large number of patients over a short time. Kuroda et al. analyzed therapeutic results in 14 RA patients complicated with AA amyloidosis in whom RA treatment was effective (four were given infliximab and 10 were given etanercept; mean observation period: 20.1 months). They found that 24-h creatinine clearance improved in three patients, was unchanged in five, and became worse in three. In a 24-h proteinuria assay, three patients showed decreased proteinuria, six were unchanged, and three became worse, indicating that progression of renal disorders was prevented in about 70% of patients. In nine patients subjected to serial gastroduoedenal biopsies, the level of amyloid deposits in the tissue was reported to decrease significantly (Kuroda et al., 2009). Nakamura et al. (2010) used etanercept to treat 14 Japanese patients who had the *SAA1.3* allele and high susceptibility to AA amyloidosis (mean observation period: 19 months) and analyzed their renal function profiles. Significant improvements were found in RA disease activity, SAA concentrations, 24-h proteinuria levels, and serum albumin levels. Creatinine was analyzed by grouping patients into those with creatinine levels of less than 2.0 mg/dL at introduction of etanercept and those with creatinine levels of 2.0 mg/dL or higher; no improvement in creatinine levels was reported in the 2.0 mg/dL or higher group. Nakamura et al. (2010) stressed the necessity of introducing etanercept treatment in the early stages of declining renal function.

Fernándes-Nebro et al. (2010) conducted a multicenter case-control study of the long-term treatment (mean observation period: 2.9 years) of many patients with an immune-mediated inflammatory disease complicated with AA amyloidosis. They evaluated 36 patients (29 given infliximab and seven given etanercept). A kidney response was observed in 12 of 22 patients (54.5%), kidney progression was observed in 6 of 36 patients (17%), and kidney amyloidosis remained stable in 16 of 36 patients (44%), which were considered good results. However, although proteinuria was significantly improved ($p < 0.001$), serum creatinine levels ($p = 0.783$) and creatinine clearance ($p = 0.721$) showed no significant differences before and after treatment. Significant improvement was found in inflammatory markers, but the normal range was not achieved. The four-year continuation rate of anti-TNF agents was 52%, and no differences from the control group were observed. Severe proteinuria was a risk factor for treatment response and continuation and for survival. The incidences of adverse drug reactions also showed no differences from the control group, but the frequencies of septicemia and severe infections were three times as high. Eight patients in the amyloid group and one in the control group of rheumatic disease patients without AA amyloidosis died, and an increased risk of infections was noted in the amyloid group in terms of safety (Fernándes-Nebro et al., 2010).

The above reports indicate that anti-TNF therapy is effective in patients with rheumatic diseases complicated with AA amyloidosis, but in patients with progressive renal dysfunction the possibility of irreversible changes is as high as in other chronic renal diseases and the risk of infections increases during the period up to multiple organ failure. Therefore, the utmost caution is necessary after introducing anti-TNF therapy and confirming the reduction in inflammatory markers, showing that the response to the underlying disease treatment is favorable.

4.2 Anti-IL-6 therapy

4.2.1 IL-6 and the mode of action of tocilizumab

IL-6 has a unique receptor system: although IL-6 receptor (IL-6R) specifically binds to IL-6, it is not directly involved in signal transduction. IL-6 forms a complex by binding to IL-6R on the cell membrane, which then combines with gp130, which also resides on the cell membrane, forming a homodimer and initiating intracellular signal transduction. Furthermore, IL-6R also exists in soluble form. After forming a complex with IL-6, soluble

IL-6R (sIL-6R) can also combine with gp130 on the cell membrane and enable signaling (Ward et al., 1994). sIL-6R is present in the blood of healthy individuals at a concentration of several tens of ng/mL, and if cells express gp130, IL-6 signaling can take place, even in the absence of IL-6R expression on the cell membrane. Reflecting this characteristic, the effects of IL-6 are diverse, and it is thought to have an extensive regulatory role, with involvement in the immune response, inflammation, bone metabolism, hematopoiesis, and the neuroendocrine system (Figure3).

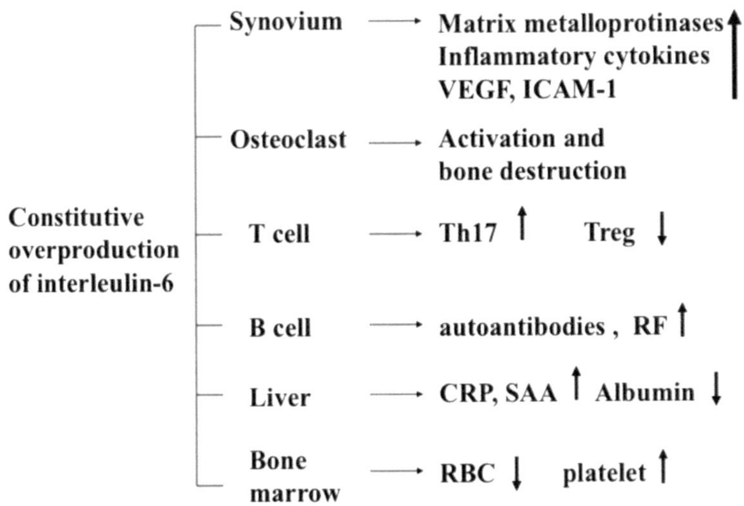

Constitutive overproduction of interleukin-6, a pleiotropic cytokine that regulates the immune system, inflammation, hematopoiesis, and bone metabolism, is thought to play pathologic roles in rheumatic diseases. VEGF: vascular endothelial growth factor; ICAM-1: intercellular adhesion molecule-1; T_h17: interleukin-17-producing $CD4^+$ T cell; T_{reg}: $CD4^+CD25^+$ regulatory T cell; RF: rheumatoid factor; CRP: C-reactive protein; SAA: serum amyloid A; RBC: red blood cell

Fig. 3. Pathological roles of interleukin-6 in rheumatic diseases

Tocilizumab is a recombinant monoclonal antibody that has been humanized by complementarity-determining region (CDR) grafting of a murine anti-human IL-6R antibody onto human IgG_1. Tocilizumab inhibits the induction of IL-6-mediated biological activity in cells that have expressed both membrane-bound IL-6R and gp130 molecules, and also inhibits the induction of biological activity mediated by IL-6/sIL-6R complex formation in cells that express gp130 alone. Furthermore, since tocilizumab has the capacity to dissociate IL-6/IL-6R complexes that have already formed (Mihara et al., 2005), it exhibits an extremely effective blocking action on IL-6 signal transduction (Figure 4).

4.2.2 Pivotal role of IL-6 in SAA synthesis

The signal transduction and transcription mechanisms of TNF-alpha, IL-1-beta, and IL-6 in the production of SAA have become clear. In a study using HepG2 cells, a cell line derived from hepatocytes, weak expression of SAA1 and SAA2 mRNA was induced by stimulation with IL-6 alone, but almost no expression was induced by stimulation with either IL-1-beta or TNF-alpha alone. However, synergistic induction of expression was observed by costimulation with IL-6 and IL-1-beta or with IL-6 and TNF-alpha (Hagihara et al., 2004).

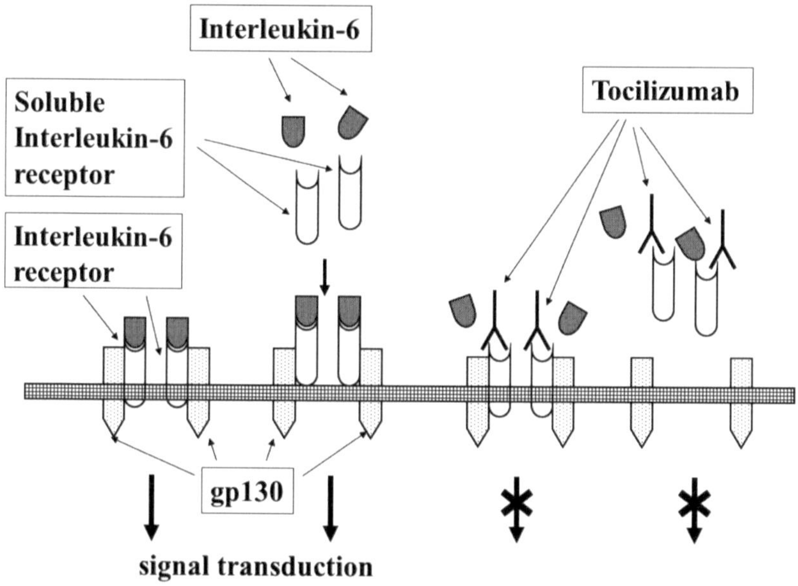

Fig. 4. Signal transduction of the interleukin-6/interleukin-6 receptor complex via gp130 and the mechanism of signal transduction blockade by tocilizumab.

Activation of STAT3 by IL-6 stimulation is essential in the production of SAA, and it is clear that SAA expression is strengthened by supplementation of NF-kappaBp65 activity by stimulation with TNF-alpha or IL-1-beta (Hagihara et al., 2005). Clinically, TNF inhibitors reduce SAA levels, but complete normalization is rare. However, tocilizumab can normalize SAA levels in almost all patients in whom a sufficient concentration of tocilizumab is maintained in the blood.

4.2.3 AA amyloidosis treatment by anti-IL-6 receptor therapy

Tocilizumab, a humanized anti-IL-6 receptor antibody drug, was approved in Japan in 2008 for RA, polyarticular juvenile idiopathic arthritis (JIA), and systemic JIA. At present, tocilizumab is the most effective agent against AA amyloidosis by the mechanism of action based on SAA reduction described above. Almost all patients undergoing anti-IL-6 therapy are those who can maintain tocilizumab blood concentrations, and SAA normalization is possible. In contrast, although it is already clear from routine clinical practice that anti-TNF therapy does decrease SAA, the percentage of patients undergoing anti-TNF therapy who achieve complete normalization is not high. And recently tocilizumab is reported to be very effective in many autoimmune and inflammatory diseases including auto-inflammatory diseases such as TNF receptor associated periodic syndrome which may cause AA amyloidosis (Tanaka, 2011).

Before its approval in 2008, we provided compassionate use of tocilizumab to a patient with life-threatening JIA complicated with rapidly progressing AA amyloidosis in whom many drugs were ineffective. SAA was completely normalized by early administration of tocilizumab, digestive tract symptoms (intractable diarrhea) disappeared, renal symptoms (proteinuria and renal dysfunction) were normalized, and AA protein showed marked disappearance from the tissues. The clinical course and usefulness in this case have been reported (Okuda & Takasugi, 2006) (Figures 5 & 6).

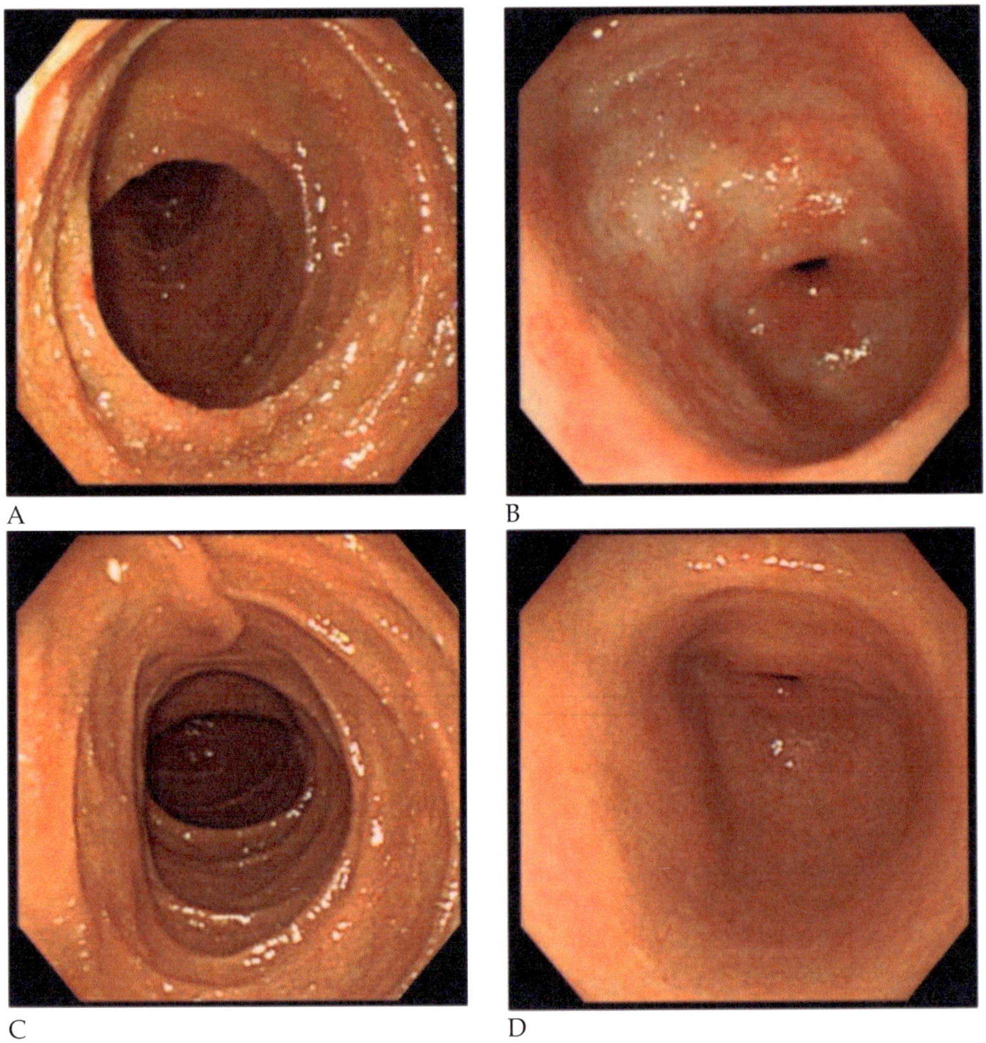

A: Before tocilizumab therapy was started, the appearance of the mucosa in the second portion of the duodenum was coarse, nodular, irregular, edematous, and reddish.
B: Before tocilizumab therapy, the appearance of the mucosa in the antrum of the stomach was coarse, with reddish and edematous changes.
C and D: After 18 months of tocilizumab therapy, no abnormality was observed in the second potion of the duodenum or in the antrum of the stomach, respectively
(Quoted from: Okuda Y, Takasugi K. (2006). Successful use of a humanized anti-interleukin-6 receptor antibody, tocilizumab, to treat amyloid A amyloidosis complicating juvenile idiopathic arthritis. *Arthritis Rheum.* Vol. 54, No. 9, pp. 2997–3000)

Fig. 5. Results of endoscopic examination before and after tocilizumab therapy (Case 1)

We have also reported that during a clinical study on tocilizumab, in a group of patients with RA complicated with AA amyloidosis, AA protein deposits disappeared from the digestive tract and renal function improved (Okuda, 2009). Figure 7 shows improved histological findings in a patient with RA complicated with AA amyloidosis obtained during the clinical study on tocilizumab. Many papers presented at meetings and case

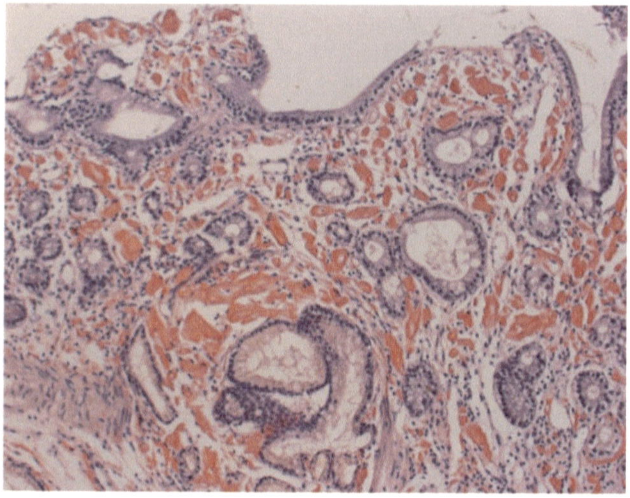

Massive amyloid A protein deposits were observed in duodenal mucosa and submucosa before the start of tocilizumab therapy.

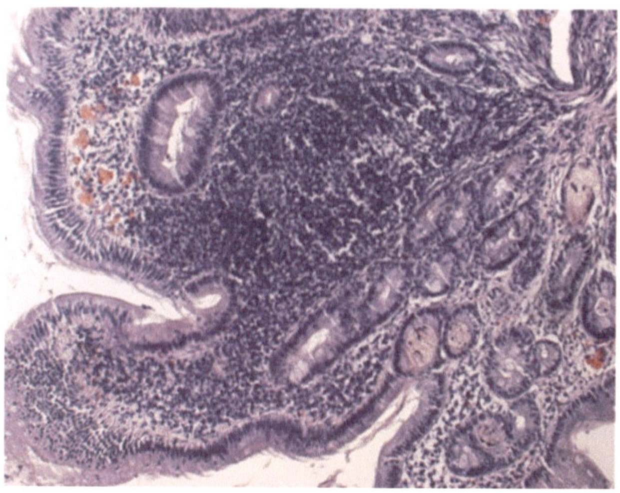

Lower: Marked regression of amyloid A protein deposits was seen in duodenal mucosa and submucosa after tocilizumab treatment. (Congo red stained; 200× magnification)
(Quoted from: Okuda Y, Takasugi K. (2006). Successful use of a humanized anti-interleukin-6 receptor antibody, tocilizumab, to treat amyloid A amyloidosis complicating juvenile idiopathic arthritis. *Arthritis Rheum.* Vol. 54, No. 9, pp. 2997–3000)

Fig. 6. Results of gastrointestinal biopsy before and after tocilizumab therapy (Case 1)

reports have since appeared suggesting the wide-ranging usefulness of tocilizumab in treating rheumatic diseases complicated with AA amyloidosis (Inoue et al., 2010; Kishida et al., 2011; Sato et al., 2009).

Even in patients that have switched to tocilizumab because of the insufficient effect or lack of effect of anti-TNF agents, it is reported that treatment with tocilizumab has marked effects on gastrointestinal disorders and histology (Nishida et al., 2009) and improves renal dysfunction (Ubara, 2009). Expectations related to the usefulness of tocilizumab are high.

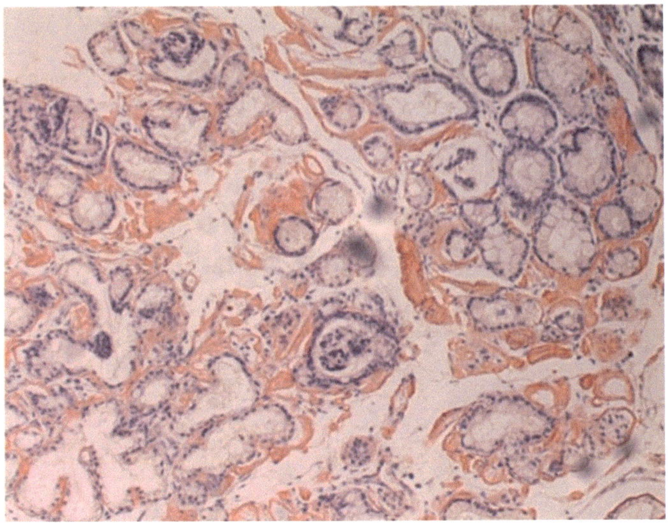

Massive amyloid A protein deposits were observed in duodenal mucosa and submucosa before the start of tocilizumab therapy. (Creatinine: 1.4 mg/dL)

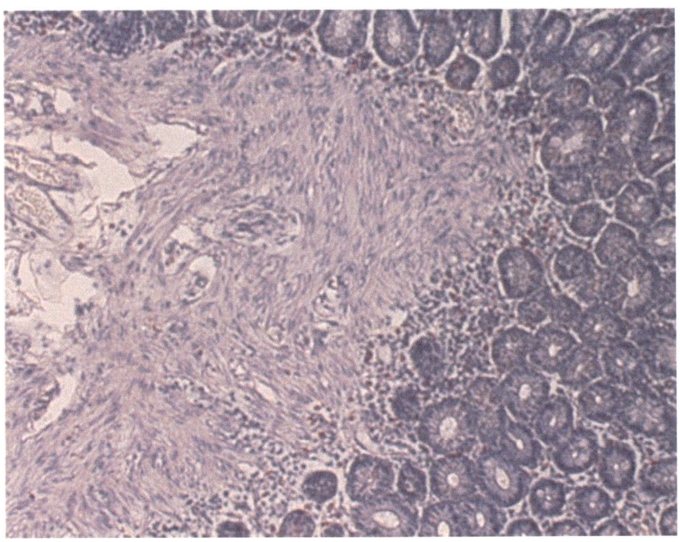

Complete regression of amyloid A protein deposits was seen in duodenal mucosa after 6.5 years of tocilizumab treatment. (Creatinine: 0.85 mg/dL) (Congo red stained; 200× magnification)

Fig. 7. Gastrointestinal biopsy before and after tocilizumab therapy (Case 2)

However, an all-case post-marketing survey for tocilizumab (Koike et al., 2010) found that, among patients with progressive renal disorders with multiple organ failure in whom tocilizumab was used for life-saving purposes, complications such as infections and deaths were reported. Therefore, considerable caution is required when tocilizumab is used. When considered from the standpoint of immunosuppression, it is desirable to use tocilizumab from an earlier stage when the risk of infections is lower, in the same way as anti-TNF therapy. At present, a multicenter investigator-initiated prospective clinical study comparing clinical and histological improvements in the tocilizumab group with a control group is underway in Japan, and evidence that proves more objectively the usefulness of tocilizumab exceeding that of other drugs is expected.

5. Conclusion

Tocilizumab has an excellent ability to suppress SAA levels and improve clinical symptoms of AA amyloidosis with marked lasting regression of AA protein deposits. Treatment with tocilizumab could, therefore, represent an important therapeutic strategy for AA amyloidosis secondary to rheumatic diseases.

6. Acknowledgements

This work was supported by a grant from the Amyloidosis Research Committee of the Intractable Disease Division of the Ministry of Health, Labour and Welfare of Japan.

7. Key points

AA amyloidosis, tocilizumab, a humanized anti-IL-6 receptor antibody, anti-cytokine therapy, rheumatic diseases, RA, IL- 6, TNF-alpha, SAA

8. References

Baba S, Masago SA, Takahashi T, Kasama T, Sugimura H, Tsugane S, et al. (1995). A novel allelic variant of serum amyloid A, SAA1γ: genomic evidence, evolution, frequency, and implication as a risk factor for reactive systemic AA-amyloidosis. *Hum Mol Genet.* Vol. 4, No. 6, pp. 1083–1087, ISSN 0964-6906

Booth DR, Booth SE, Gillmore JD, Hawkins PN, Pepys MB. (1998). SAA1 alleles as risk factors in reactive systemic AA amyloidosis. *Amyloid.* Vol. 5, No. 4, pp. 262–265, ISSN 1350-6129

Boscà MM, Pérez-Baylach CM, Solis MA, Antón R, Mayordomo E, Pons S, et al.. (2006). Secondary amyloidosis in Crohn's disease: treatment with tumor necrosis factor inhibitor. *Gut.* Vol. 55, No. 2, pp. 294–295, ISSN 1468-3288

Dember LM, Hawkins PN, Hazenberg BP, Gorevic PD, Merlini G, Butrimiene I, et al. (2007). Eprodisate for treatment of renal disease in AA amyloidosis. *N Engl J Med.* Vol. 356, No. 23, pp. 2349–2360, ISSN 0028-4793

Drewe E, Huggins ML, Morgan AG, Cassidy MJ, Powell RJ. (2004). Treatment of renal amyloidosis with etanercept in tumor necrosis factor receptor-associated periodic syndrome. *Rheumatology (Oxford).* Vol. 43, No. 11, pp. 1405–1408, ISSN 1462-0324

Elkayam O, Hawkins PN, Lachmann H, Yaron M, Caspi D. (2002). Rapid and complete resolution of proteinuria due to renal amyloidosis in a patient with rheumatoid arthritis treated with infliximab. *Arthritis Rheum.* Vol. 46, No. 10, pp. 2571–2573, ISSN 1529-0131

Fernándes-Nebro A, Olivé A, Castro MC, Varela AH, Riera E, Irigoyen MV, et al. (2010). Long-term TNF-alpha blockade in patients with amyloid A amyloidosis complicating rheumatic diseases. *Am J Med.* Vol. 123, No. 5, pp. 454–461, ISSN 0002-9343

Gillmore JD, Lovat LB, Persey MR, Pepys MB, Hawkins PN. (2001). Amyloid load and clinical outcome in AA amyloidosis in relation to circulating concentration of serum amyloid A protein. *Lancet.* Vol. 358, No. 9275, pp. 24–29, ISSN 0140-6736

Gottenberg JE, Merle-Vincent F, Bentaberry F, Allanore Y, Berenbaum F, Fautrel B, et al. (2003). Anti-tumor necrosis α therapy in fifteen patients with AA amyloidosis secondary to inflammatory arthritides: a followup report of tolerability and efficacy. *Arthritis Rheum.* Vol. 48, No. 7, pp. 2019–2024, ISSN 1529-0131

Gruys R, Sijens S, Biewenga J. (2005). Dubious effect of dimethlsulphoxide (DMSO) therapy on amyloid deposits and amyloidosis. VETRINARY RESEACH COMMUNICATIONS. Vol.5, No. 1, 21-32, ISSN 0165-7380

Hagihara K, Nishikawa T, Isobe T, Song J, Sugamata Y, Yoshizaki K. (2004). IL-6 plays a critical role in the synergistic induction of human serum amyloid A (SAA) gene when stimulated with proinflammatory cytokines as analyzed with an SAA isoform real-time quantitative RT-PCR assay system. *Biochem Biophys Res Commun.* Vol. 314, No. 2, pp. 363–369, ISSN 0006-291X

Hagihara K, Nishikawa T, Sugamata Y, Song J, Isobe T, Taga T, et al. (2005). Essential role of STAT3 in cytokine-driven NF-kappaB-mediated serum amyloid A gene expression. *Genes Cells.* Vol. 10, No. 11, pp. 1051–1063, ISSN 1365-2442

Hsu HC, Zhou T, Yang PA, Herrera GA, Mountz JD. (1997). Increased acute-phase response and renal amyloidosis in aged CD2-fas-transgenic mice. *J Immunol.* Vol. 158. No. 12, pp. 5988–5996, ISSN 0022-1767

Inoue D, Arima H, Kawanami C, Takiuchi Y, Nagano S, Kimura T, et al. (2010). Excellent therapeutic effect of tocilizumab on intestinal amyloid A deposition secondary to active rheumatoid arthritis. *Clin Rheumatol.* Vol. 29, No. 10, pp. 1195–1197, ISSN 0770-3198

Kishida D, Okuda Y, Onishi M, Takebayashi M, Matoba K, Jouyama K, et al. (2011). Successful tocilizumab treatment in a patient with adult-onset Still's disease complicated by chronic hepatitis B and amyloid A amyloidosis. *Mod Rheumatol.* Vol. 21, No. 2, pp. 215–218, ISSN 1439-7595

Koike T, Harigai M, Inokuma S, Ishiguro N, Ryu J, Takeuchi T, et al. (2010) Post-marketing surveillance program of tocilizumab for RA in Japan interim analyses of 3,881 patients. [abstract]. *Arthritis Rheum.* Vol. 62, Suppl. 10, pp. 399 DOI: 10.1002/art.28168

Kobak S, Oksel F, Kabasakal Y, Doganavsargil E. (2007). Ankylosing spondylitis-related secondary amyloidosis responded well to etanercept: a report of three patients. Clin Rheumatol. Vol. 26, No. 12, pp. 2191–2194, ISSN 0770-3198

Kobayashi H, Tada S, Fuchigami T, Okuda Y, Takasugi K, Matsumoto T, et al. (1996). Secondary amyloidosis in patients with rheumatoid arthritis. diagnostic and prognostic value of gastroduodenal biopsy. *Br J Rheumatol.* Vol. 35, No. 1, pp. 44–49, ISSN 1462-0324

Kuroda T, Wada Y, Kobayashi D, Murakami S, Sakai T, Hirose S, et al. (2009). Effective anti-TNF-α therapy can induce rapid resolution and sustained decrease of gastroduodenal mucosal amyloid deposits in reactive amyloidosis associated with rheumatoid arthritis. *J Rheumatol.* Vol. 36, No. 11, pp. 2409–2415, ISSN 0315-162X

Lachmann HJ, Goodman HJ, Gilbertson JA, Gallimore JR, Sabin CA, Gillmore JD, et al. (2007). Natural history and outcome in systemic AA amyloidosis. *N Engl J Med.* Vol. 356, No. 23, pp. 2361–2371, ISSN 0028-4793

Liepnieks JJ, Kluve-Beckerman B, Benson MD. (1995). Characterization of amyloid A protein in human secondary amyloidosis: the predominant deposition of serum amyloid A1. *Biochim Biophys Acta.* Vol. 1270, No. 1, pp. 81–86, ISSN 0925-4439

Mihara M, Katsutani K, Okazaki M, Nakamura A, Kawai S, Sugimoto M, et al(2005). Tocilizumab inhibits signal transduction mediated by both mIL-6R and sIL-6R, but the receptors of other members of IL-6 cytokine family. Int Immunophamacol Vol. 5, No 12, pp. 1731-1740, ISSN 1567-5769

Moriguchi M, Terai C, Koseki Y, Uesato M, Nakajima A, Inada S, et al. (1999). Influence of genotypes at SAA1 and SAA2 loci on the development and the length of latent period of secondary AA-amyloidosis in patients with rheumatoid arthritis. *Hum Genet.* Vol. 105, No. 4, pp. 360–366, ISSN 0340-6717

Nakamura T, Higashi S, Tomoda K, Tsukano M, Baba S, Shono M. (2006). Significance of SAA*1.3* allele genotype in Japanese patients with amyloidosis secondary to rheumatoid arthritis. *Rheumatology (Oxford).* Vol. 45, No. 1, pp. 43–49, ISSN 1462-0324

Nakamura T, Higashi S, Tomoda K, Tsukano M, Shono M. (2010). Etanercept can induce resolution of renal deterioration in patients with amyloid A amyloidosis secondary to rheumatoid arthritis. *Clin Rheumatol.* Vol. 29, No. 12, pp. 1395-1401, ISSN 0770-3198

Nishida S, Hagihara K, Shima Y, Kawai M, Kuwahara Y, Arimitsu J, et al. (2009). Rapid improvement of AA amyloidosis with humanized anti-interleukin 6 receptor antibody treatment. *Ann Rheum Dis.* Vol. 68, No. 7, pp. 1235–1236, ISSN 0003-4967

Okuda Y. (2009). Turnover and regression of amyloid A protein deposits in AA amyloidosis complicating rheumatoid arthritis. *Igaku no Ayumi.* Vol. 229. No. 5, pp. 337–340, ISSN 0039-2359 [Article in Japanese]

Okuda Y, Takasugi K. (2006). Successful use of a humanized anti-interleukin-6 receptor antibody, tocilizumab, to treat amyloid A amyloidosis complicating juvenile idiopathic arthritis. *Arthritis Rheum.* Vol. 54, No. 9, pp. 2997–3000, ISSN 1529-0131

Okuda Y, Yamada T, Takasugi K, Takeda M, Nanba S, Onishi M, et al. (1999). Serum amyloid A (SAA)1, SAA2 and apolipoprotein E isotype frequencies in rheumatoid arthritis patients with AA amyloidosis. *Ryumachi.* Vol. 39, No. 1, pp. 3–10, ISSN 0300-9157 [Article in Japanese]

Okuda Y, Yamada T, Matsuura M, Takasugi K, Goto M. (2011). Ageing: a risk factor for amyloid A amyloidosis in rheumatoid arthritis. *Amyloid.* Vol. 18, No. 3, pp. 108-111, ISSN 1350-6129

Ravid M, Shapira J, Lang R, Kedar I. (1982). Prolonged dimethylsulphoxide treatment in 13 patients with systemic amyloidosis. *Ann Rheum Dis.* Vol. 41, No. 6, pp. 587–592, ISSN 0003-4967

Sasatomi Y, Sato H, Chiba Y, Abe Y, Takeda S, Ogahara S, et al. (2007). Prognostic factors for renal amyloidosis: a clinicopathological study using cluster analysis. *Intern Med.* Vol. 46, No. 5, pp. 213–219, ISSN 0918-2918

Sato H, Sakai T, Sugaya T, Otaki Y, Aoki K, Ishii K, et al. (2009). Tocilizumab dramatically ameliorated life-threatening diarrhea due to secondary amyloidosis associated with rheumatoid arthritis. *Clin Rheumatol.* Vol. 28, No. 9, pp. 1113–1116, ISSN 0770-3198

Smith GR, Tymms KE, Falk M. (2004). Etanercept treatment of renal amyloidosis complicating rheumatoid arthritis. *Intern Med J.* Vol. 34, No. 9-10, pp. 570–572, ISSN 1445-5994

Tanaka T, Narazaki M, Kishimoto T. (2011). Anti-interleukin-6 receptor antibody, tocilizumab, for the treatment of autoimmune diseases. *FEBS Lett.* DOI: 10.1016/j.febslet.2011.03.023, ISSN 0014-5793

Ubara Y. (2009). Renal amyloidosis. *Medicina.* Vol. 13, No. 13, pp. 2009–2012, ISSN 0025-7699 [Article in Japanese]

Ward LD, Howlett GJ, Discolo G, Yasukawa K, Hammacher A, Moritz RL, et al. (1994). High affinity interleukin-6 receptor is a hexameric complex consisting of two molecules each of interleukin-6, interleukin-6 receptor, and gp-130. *J Biol Chem.* Vol. 269, No. 37, pp. 23286–23289, ISSN 0021-9258

Yamada T. (1999). Serum amyloid A (SAA): a concise review of biology, assay methods and clinical usefulness. *Clin Chem Lab Med.* Vol. 37, No. 4, pp. 381–388, ISSN 1434-6621

Yokota T, Ishihara T, Kawano H, Takahashi M, Fujinaga Y, Uchino F. (1989). Amyloid enhancing factor (AEF) in the aging mouse. *Virchows Arch A Pathol Anat Histopathol.* Vol. 414, No. 6, pp. 511–514, ISSN 0236-3636

10

Integral Treatment of Systemic Lupus Erythematosus

Raquel Ramírez Parrondo
Clínica, Universidad de Navarra, Madrid
Spain

1. Introduction

Systemic lupus erythematosus (SLE) is a chronic inflammatory autoimmune disease of unknown etiology. The prevalence of SLE is worldwide from 4 to 250 per 100,000. Statistics demonstrate that lupus is somewhat more frequent in Africans, Americans and people of Chinese and Japanese descent. It is a disease with predominance of the female sex, the ratio among SLE sufferers is about 9:1.

It is often discovered in their childbearing years. It affects heterogeneity multiple organs of the body and presents aberrant immunological findings and especially the presence of antinuclear antibodies. The clinical course and prognosis is unpredictable and may be characterized by periods of remissions and chronic or acute relapses. The mortality rate among patients with SLE is at least three times that of the general population. (Aberer, 2010; Ng & Chan, 2007; Ramírez, 2007)

2. Etiopathogenesis

The etiopathogenesis that causes lupus is not known. Interactions between susceptibility genes and environmental factors result in abnormal immune responses. The antigens, autoantibodies, and immune complexes persist for prolonged periods of time, allowing inflammation and contribute to irreversible tissue damage developing the disease.

The SLE is a multigenic disease. In most genetically susceptible individuals, if enough variations accumulate multiple genes they contribute to abnormal immune responses and disease results. Some genes influence clinical manifestations of disease in various ethnic groups. (Javierre & Richardson, 2011; Koike, 2011)

The SLE is more frequent in female sex. The females make higher antibody responses than the males. The estrogens favour a prolonged immune response increasing the risk of developing SLE.

Several environmental stimuli may influence in the development of the SLE. Exposure to ultraviolet light causes skin injures in approximately 70% of SLE patients. Some infections, for example Epstein-Barr virus (EBV), induce abnormal immune response. Occasionally, some drugs stimulate the immune system and can induce SLE. The extreme stress may trigger the illness. (Ng & Chan, 2007; Niller et al,2011; Nowicka-Sauer, 2007; Ramírez, 2007)

3. Clinical manifestations

The illness impacts in the patients with SLE, in three aspects: physical, psychological and social. (Ng & Chan, 2007; Ramírez, 2007)

3.1 Physical manifestations

The physical manifestations varies between different patients, and in a single patient the disease activity varies presenting exacerbations interspersed with periods of relative quiescence. SLE may involve one or several organ systems, but it is not usual for all systems to be affected simultaneously, and the severity varies from mild and intermittent to fulminant.

The general symptoms, particularly fatigue and fever, are present most of the time. The myalgias and or arthralgias are common. Most patients have intermittent polyarthritis most frequently in hands, wrists, and knees. The exercise capacity and muscular strength are reduced in these people.

Lupus dermatitis can be "butterfly" rash on the face, discoid lupus, photosensitivity, systemic rash, urticaria. About one-third of the patients have small, painful ulcerations on the oral or nasal mucosa.

The nephropathy in SLE varies from mild proteinuria and microscopical hematuria to end-stage renal failure.

The neuropsychiatric symptoms can be caused by a diffuse process or vascular occlusive disease. The manifestations of diffuse CNS lupus are cognitive dysfunction, depression and headache, myelopathy, peripheral neuropathy, seizures and psychosis. Many patients get a thromboembolic or haemorrhagic complication of the brain.

The pulmonary manifestations of SLE are pleuritis, acute pneumonitis and chronic fibrotising alveolitis.

The cardiac manifestations are pericarditis, myocarditis, fibrinous endocarditis of Libman-Sacks, heart failure, arrhythmia and myocardial infarctions.

The hematologic manifestations of SLE are anemia, usually normochromic normocytic, hemolysis, leukopenia lymphopenia, and thrombocytopenia.

The gastrointestinal manifestations are nausea, sometimes with vomiting, diarrhea or diffuse abdominal pain caused by peritonitis, intestinal vasculitis.

The ocular manifestations are sicca syndrome, nonspecific conjunctivitis, retinal vasculitis and optic neuritis.

Women with SLE have more risk of first and second trimester foetal losses and of premature birth. (Nakashima et al, 2011; Ng & Chan, 2007; Ramírez, 2007)

3.2 Psychological manifestations

Many persons with SLE experience high levels of emotional distress. The depression is the most common psychological symptom and the anxiety is another feeling quite frequently experienced.

The links between physical symptoms and psychological wellbeing have been studied in SLE relatively little research.

Studies have revealed that the physical symptoms from SLE affect psychologically to people which suffer.

The skin abnormalities and photosensitivity, disfiguring skin lesions and pleuritic pain are associated with depression, poor self-esteem and poor social functioning.

The sufferings from greater organ damage, such as the kidneys, experience greater psychological distress.
The disease-related changes to the direct central nervous system can result in depression or anxiety in SLE patients.
Levels of daily stress among patients with SLE are generally higher than those experienced by the general population. Such stress could cause depression and anxiety producing the worsening of physical and mental function in these people. (Ng & Chan, 2007; Ramírez, 2007; Zakeri et al, 2011).
The pharmacology treatment of physical symptoms of SLE can also contribute to feelings of desperation and helplessness among sufferers. The side effects of steroids, such as a "moon face" and weight gain have an additional negative impact on self-esteem. (Navarrete-Navarrete et al, 2010; Ng & Chan, 2007; Chaiamnuay et al, 2007)
The persons with SLE often have worries about their illness, their treatment plans, the level of pain caused by the illness, and the occurrence of the next "flare-up". These people often have a sense of helplessness that the illness is not yet curable even after appropriate treatment is adopted. These worries can be deleterious to their health and self-esteem. The researches associate abnormal illness-related behaviours, helplessness with increased levels of fatigue. (Burgos et al, 2009; Chuang et al, 2010; Ng & Chan,2007)
Few studies have pointed out that psychiatric symptomatology has been correlated significantly with family and social support. (Ng & Chan, 2007)

3.3 Social manifestations

The uncertainty of SLE affects the social life of these people.
Chronic fatigue and joint pains make it impossible for many with SLE to perform to the level expected by themselves and others. This loss of the ability to meet "normal" standards of performance can be very depressing.
Coupled with the side effects of drug treatment, this condition can lead to feelings of shame, isolation and worthlessness. To avoid the feeling of rejection, many may isolate themselves and refrain from interacting with friends and even family members.
The illness can also have an effect on major life decisions such as career development, wedding and pregnancy plans.
Some may have deep-seated fears of desertion and rejection by spouse and friends.
All these social problems are salient and tend to contribute to emotional and social disturbances (Baker & Pope, 2009; Ng & Chan, 2007)

4. Diagnosis

The integral diagnosis in the patients with SLE include the aspects: physical, psychological and social.

4.1 Physical diagnosis

4.1.1 Clinic and laboratory

The laboratory tests serve to establish the physical diagnosis, to follow the course of disease, and to identify adverse effects of therapies. These might include hemoglobin levels, platelet and leukocyte counts, erythrocyte sedimentation rate, urinalysis, and serum levels of creatinine or albumin, ANA, antibodies to double-stranded DNA (dsDNA), antibodies to Sm, antibodies antiphospholipid, anti-Ro, polyclonal gammaglobulinaemia, complement

Criterion	Definition
1. Malar Rash	Fixed erythema flat or raised, over the malar eminences, tending to spare the nasolabial folds
2. Discoid rash	Erythematous raised patches with adherent keratotic scaling and follicular plugging; atrophic scarring may occur in older lesion
3. Photosensitivity	Skin rash as a result of unusual reaction to sunlight, by patient history or physician observation
4. Oral ulcers	Oral or nasopharyngeal ulceration, usually painless, observed by physician
5. Nonerosive Arthritis	Involving 2 or more peripheral joints characterized by tenderness, swelling, or effusion
6. Pleuritis or Pericarditis	1 Pleuritis - convincing history of pleuritic pain or rubbing heard by a physician or evidence of pleural effusion 1. OR 2. Pericarditis - documented by electrocardiogram or rub or evidence of pericardial effusion
7. Renal Disorder	1. Persistent proteinuria > 0.5 grams per day or > than 3+ if quantitation not peformed 1. OR 2. Cellular casts –may be red cell, hemoglobin, granular, tubular, or mixed
8. Neurologic Disorder	1. Seizures - in the absence of offending drugs or known metabolic derangements; e.g., uremia, ketoacidosis, or electrolyte imbalance 1.OR 2. Psychosis - in the absence of offending drugs or known metabolic derangements, e.g., uremia, ketoacidosis, or electrolyte imbalance
9. Hematologic Disorder	1 Hemolytic anemia - with reticulocytosis 1. OR 2. Leukopenia -- < 4,000/mm3 on ≥ 2 occasions 1. OR 3. Lyphopenia --< 1,500/mm3 on ≥ 2 occaions 1. OR 4. Thrombocytopenia --< 100,000/mm3 in the absence of offending drugs
10. Immulogic Disorder	1. Anti- DNA: antibody to native DNA in abnormal titer 1. OR 2. Anti-Sm: presence of antibody to Sm nuclear antigen 1. OR 3. Positive finding of antiphospholipid anibodies on: 1.1-an abnormal serum level of IgG or anticardiolipin antibodies 2.2. a positive test result for lupus anticoagulant using a standard method, or 3.3.a false-positive test result for at least 6 months confimed by Treponema pallidum immobilization or fluorescent treponemal antibody absorption test
11. Positive Antinuclear Antibody	An abnormal titer of antinuclear antibody by immunofluorescence or an equivalent assay at any point in time an in the absence of drugs

Table 1. 1997 Update of the 1982 American College of Rheumatology Revised Criteria for Classification of Systemic Lupus Erythematosus Criterion.

values (C3 and C4), IFN-inducible genes, soluble IL-2, and urinary adiponectin or monocyte chemotactic protein 1.

In the diagnosis of SLE there is no single symptom or finding that is sufficient in itself, it is based on the clinical and the laboratory and on the American Rheumatism Association (ARA) classification criteria. Any combination of ≥4 of 11 criteria makes it likely that the patient has SLE. See TABLE 1.

Antinuclear antibodies (ANA) are positive in more 98% of patients during the course of disease; repeated negative tests suggest that the diagnosis is not SLE. The antibodies to double-stranded DNA and antibodies to the Sm antigen, specific for SLE, with compatible clinical favor the diagnosis. The presence in an individual of multiple autoantibodies without clinical symptoms should not be considered diagnostic for SLE, although such persons are at increased risk since clinical SLE begins in most patients years after autoantibodies appear.(Nakashima et al, 2011)

4.1.2 Disease activity and damage caused by SLE

4.1.2.1 Disease activity

The disease activity indices have been created at standardizing the SLE activity assessment. Some of such indices are: European Consensus Lupus Activity Measurement (ECLAM), Lupus Activity Index (LAI), British Isles Lupus Assessment Group (BILAG), Lupus symptom inventory (LSI) and Systemic Lupus Erythematosus Disease Activity Index (SLEDAI).

The ECLAM assesses disease activity over the last month, and comprises 15 clinical and laboratory parameters. Its scores ranges are from 0 to 10. (Griffiths et al, 2005)

The LAI comprises four scores to assess clinical activity: physician's global evaluation, opinion of the doctor about disease severity, laboratory findings and immunosuppressive treatment. Its scores ranges are from 0 to 3. (Griffiths et al, 2005)

The BILAG index measures SLE disease activity. It is composed of eight organ-based systems: general symptoms, mucocutaneous, respiratory, cardiovascular, neurological, musculoskeletal, renal and hematological. It is represented with alphabetical letters depending of the clinical characteristics present and their behavior during one month. BILAG "A" represents the presence of one or more severe SLE characteristics. BILAG "B" indicates more moderate characteristics of the disease. BILAG "C" includes mild symptomatic characteristics. BILAG "D" represents the previous activity. BILAG "E" indicates that a system has never been involved. (Isenberg et al, 2005)

The LSI measures clinical activity in the last month. It includes five main symptoms: flares, headaches, joint inflammation, muscles and weakness. Its score ranges are from 1 to 5. The higher score is the symptoms with more severity (Duvdevany et al, 2011)

The SLEDAI assesses disease activity in the previous ten days. It evaluates the organ affected, clinical and laboratory parameters. The scores greater than 8 indicates active disease. A three-point variation between medical visits indicates disease activation, and variations greater than or equal to 12 points mean severe activity. It was reviewed in the year 2000, originating SLEDAI-2K. The modifications included the persistence of rash, mucosal ulcers, alopecia, and proteinuria greater than 0.5 in 24h and had ability to differentiate clearly active patients from inactive ones or those with minimum activity. (Freire al, 2011)

4.1.2.2 Damage caused by SLE

The damage indices in organ-based systems can be used as a health measure in patients with chronic diseases. The damage caused by SLE has reference a symptom present at least six months that develops in tissue damage which produces irreversible organ damage. It detects damages in patients which can have resulted from disease activity or treatment or comorbidities.
The ACR published the Systemic Lupus International Collaborating Clinics/American College of Rheumatology - Damage Index (SLICC/ACR-DI), in 1996. This instrument approaches 12 organ-based systems. The damages caused by SLE affect to patients who result in physical or/and mental disabilities, worsening the patient's quality of life, which is an important indicator of the health status of patients with chronic diseases. (Freire al, 2011)

4.2 Psychological and social diagnosis

The committee on Outcome Measures in Rheumatology Clinical Trials (OMERACT) of the ACR has recognized the importance of measure function and wellbeing from the patient's view as a criterion to determine clinical improvement.
The psychological and social diagnosis can be obtain through data collection via a semi-structured interview performed by the same physician and measured about the illness perception of the own patient, experienced thought and behavior by chronic illness, the role of personality and coping with stressful life situations and social relationships. (Freire et al, 2011; Ramírez, 2007)

4.2.1 Illness perception

The model proposes by Leventhal support that self-regulatory patients are active problem-solvers who seek to make sense of illness and form illness perceptions that influence coping strategies.
These representations of illness are composed of cognitions about the name of the illness and its associated symptoms, timeline, causes, personal control and understanding, effectiveness of its treatment. These disease perceptions determine how individuals respond to illness in their emotions, behavior, health care, expectations, attitude to the illness, coping, functioning and cooperation with health professionals. (Kaptein & Broadbent, 2007; Nowicka-Sauer, 2007)
The methods used to assess illness perception are verbal and nonverbal tools. Among nonverbal are: Pictorial Representation of Illness and Self-Measure (PRISM) and drawing. Among verbal are the Brief-Illness Perception Questionnaire (B-IPQ). (Broadbent et al, 2006; Nowicka-Sauer, 2007).

Pictorial representation of illness and self-measure

Büchi et al have developed the Pictorial Representation of Illness and Self-Measure (PRISM). It is a measure of the "burden of suffering" due to illness from the patient's perspective that includes factors directly related to the disease, disease-related intrusion in relevant aspects of life, like family, work or friendship.
The burden of suffering is a subjective experience arising out of or identified by means of one´s awareness of his own states or processes, even clinician with great experience derived from direct observation (facial expression, body posture, signs of sorrow, etc) are unable to detect the inner feelings of their patient. PRISM is a measure, by simplicity of use, that is easily understood by patients and widely accepted by them.

A red disk , 5cm in diameter with magnet on the underside were given to the patient , this disk represents his/her illness and the patient is also presented with a metal board which has a fixed yellow disk 7cm in diameter at the bottom right hand corner, this yellow disk represents the patient "self". The patient is then asked "where in your life (board) would you put the (illness) disk at the moment?" The distance between the two disks, representing Illness and Self respectively, is inversely related to the burden of the illness. This distance, measured is called the Self- Illness Separation (SIS). The possible range of SIS is 0±27 cm.
PRISM can be used in people with SLE in everyday clinical practice as a quantitative assessment instrument of patient-focussed health. (Buchi et al, 1998; Buchi et al, 2000)

Drawing

The drawings allow to assess patients views on how are the heterogeneity of clinical presentations, variety of illness perception, understanding and experiences of the SLE patients. This method help to talk, it makes the patients open up to their emotions, views, and experiences. It improves understanding of these patients in a short amount of time. Together with questionnaire assessment, the drawings can be an important source of information on how the illness can be experienced and felt and how it influences patients emotions and behaviors. (Daleboudt et al, 2011; Nowicka-Sauer, 2007)

Brief-Illness Perception Questionnaire (B-IPQ)

The B-IPQ contains eight items to score on a scale from 0 to 10 and one open-ended question where the participants have to state the three most important causes for their disease. A mean score is calculated for every scale and the reported causes can be grouped into categories on the basis of common themes. The B-IPQ has been shown to be a valid and reliable measure to assess illness perceptions in ill populations, but no validation for patients with SLE has been done. (Broadbent et al, 2006).

4.2.2 Cognitive-behavioral analysis

The experience of chronic illness, one like SLE, could become for the patient the focus of all its daily attention, decreasing the time devoted to family, friends, work, or developing as a person. The ill could focus his time on trying to control or avoid his disease with its emotions, sensations, memories, or thoughts producing human suffering that restrict healthy behavior.
There are measures widely used for clinical outcomes, that assess human sufferers produced by chronic illness. These are: Beck Depression Inventory (BDI), Pain Anxiety Symptoms Scale (PASS), Sickness Impact Profile (SIP), Chronic Pain Acceptance Questionnaire (CPAQ), Mindful Attention Awareness Scale (MAAS), Chronic Pain Values Inventory (CPVI).

Beck Depression Inventory

The Beck Depression Inventory (BDI) is a measure of depression and general emotional distress. It has 21 items. Each scored goes from zero (neutral) to three (maximum severity). The BDI range is from zero to sixty three. The twenty is a cutoff for clinically significant symptoms. (Beck et al, 1988; McCracken et al, 2007)

Pain Anxiety Symptoms Scale

The Pain Anxiety Symptoms Scale (PASS) is a measure of anxiety responses and avoidance related to chronic pain. The original version is a 40-item measure. Patients indicate the frequency of anxiety from zero (never) to five (always). The total score ranges from zero to

two hundred. The PASS includes subscales: cognitive anxiety symptoms, escape and avoidance, fearful thinking and physiological anxiety responses.
The PASS-20 is a new version of PASS-40. It is a 20-item measure. It assesses of fear, avoidance, cognitive, and anxiety responses related to chronic pain. The rate each item goes from zero (never) to five (always) indicating how the patients do or experience each of the actions or thoughts described. (McCracken et al, 2004; McCracken & Yang, 2006; McCracken et al, 2007; Roelofs et al, 2004)

Sickness Impact Profile

The Sickness Impact Profile (SIP) is used to assess physical and psychosocial disability on daily functioning. It is a 136-item measure. It has three domains (physical, psychosocial and other aspects of disability) and twelve categories of daily functioning. The categories can be scored separately or combined with domains. The categories in the physical domain are ambulation, mobility, body care and movement. The categories in the psychosocial domain include social interaction, alertness behavior and emotional behavior. The categories in the other domain are sleep and rest, eating, home management, recreation and pastimes, work and communication. The patients, when answering the SIP, endorse statements that describe problems in relation to their health. All scores range from 0 to 1. Higher scores indicate greater disability. (McCracken & Yang, 2006; McCracken et al, 2007)

Chronic Pain Acceptance Questionnaire

The Chronic Pain Acceptance Questionnaire (CPAQ) is a measure of acceptance of chronic pain. It is a 20-item inventory. Each item has a scale of zero (never true) to six (always true). The total score ranges from zero to one hundred and twenty. It has two subscales: activity engagement (eleven items) and pain willingness (nine items). The activity engagement measures tendency to perform usual daily activities regardless of pain present. The pain willingness measures the relative absence of attempts to control or avoid pain present. (McCracken et al, 2004; McCracken & Yang, 2006; McCracken et al, 2007)

Mindful Attention Awareness Scale

The Mindful Attention Awareness Scale (MAAS) is a measure of mindfulness. It is a 15-item inventory. Each item is rated on a scale from one (almost always) to six (almost never). The items content reflects the opposite of mindfulness or mindlessness. The items of the lower frequency are taken to represent a higher level of mindfulness. The items greater than eighty correlate with measures of emotional distress and physical symptoms. (Brown and Ryan, 2003; McCracken et al, 2007)

Chronic Pain Values Inventory

The Chronic Pain Values Inventory (CPVI) is based on the acceptance and commitment therapy. It assesses two scores: success and the discrepancy between importance and success in six domains of patient values. The first set considers the values and rates the importance of these patients in each domain. The second set rates how these persons have lived according to their values in each domain. The values domains are: family, intimate relations, friends, work, health, and growth or learning. The rates of each item go from zero (not at all important/successful) to five (extremely important/successful). Low success in living in accord with an unimportant value produces less suffering than low success living in accord with important value. (McCracken & Yang, 2006)

4.2.3 Personality and coping variables

The capacities of patient to cope with stress to go off defence mechanisms that result in the psychological response to determine as these persons are living with the SLE. (Eriksson & Lindstrom, 2005)

4.2.3.1 Defence mechanisms

The defence mechanisms are defined by American Psychiatric Association as "automatic psychological processes that protect the individual against anxiety and from the awareness of internal or external dangers and stressors, mediating the individual's reactions to emotional conflicts and to internal or external stressors". (American Psychiatric Association. *Diagnostic and Statistical Manual of Mental Disorders DSM-IV-TR*, 1994)

The Defence Style Questionnaire (DSQ-88) estimate behaviour indicating four defence styles: namely maladaptive action, image-distorting, self-sacrificing and adaptive styles.

The Hostility and Direction of Hostility Questionnaire (HDHQ) provides a measure of hostility that reflects an attitudinal personality trait and shows the participant's reaction to frustrating occurrences. These questionnaires have been used with rheumatic patients. (Bai et al, 2009; Hyphantis et al,2006; Hyphantis, 2010)

4.2.3.2 Sense of coherence

The sense of coherence (SOC) introduced by Antonovsky, is defined as "a global life orientation that expresses the extent to which one has a pervasive, enduring though dynamic sense of confidence that the stimuli deriving from one's internal and external environments in the course of living are structural, predictable, and explicable; the resources are available to one to meet the demands posed by the stimuli; and these demands are worthy of investment and engagement".

The SOC scale assesses the three dimensions: comprehensibility, manageability, and meaningfulness. It is an instrument measuring of global orientation how people manage stressful situations, not to measure each of the three core components separately.

In patients with SLE, have been found correlations between SOC scores and physical and psychological quality of life components. The use of SOC scale detect those patients who are coping poorly with the illness because they have poor psychological resources, in order to promote psychotherapeutic interventions that improve patients' QOL. (Abu-Shakra et al, 2006; Hyphantis et al, 2011)

4.2.4 Quality of life

The quality of life (QOL) has been defined by WHO as "individuals perceptions of their position in life in the context of the culture and value systems in which they live and in relation to their goals, expectations, standards and concerns". (WHOQOL Group, 1995)

As health-related QOL scales are measures centered on the patient's opinion. It assessments the patient's health status throughout the disease and their satisfaction with treatment. These instruments are very used because these persons are the most interested in their own outcome. (Freire et al, 2011)

The instruments for QOL assessment can be self-administered or interview-administered. It can be generic or specific for a certain disease. Some generic instruments are the WHOQOL and Short Form 36-item Health Survey Questionnaire (SF-36). Other specific instruments are Systemic Lupus Erythematosus Symptom Checklist (SSC), Systemic Lupus Erythematosus Quality of Life Questionnaire (SLEQOL), Systemic Lupus Erythematosus Needs Questionnaire (SLENQ), Lupus Quality of Life (LupusQOL)

WHOQOL

The World Health Organization (WHO) has developed an international quality of life assessment. This measure shows physical, psychological and social well-being of patients connecting with the WHO's definition of quality of life. In clinical practice, the WHOQOL assessments help clinicians to discover the areas in which a patient is most affected by disease, and to decide about treatment.

The WHOQOL exists in twenty nine languages, contain hundred questions group by domains and sub-domains of quality of life. These are: I Physical Capacity (1 Pain and discomfort, 2 Energy and fatigue, 3 Sleep and rest), II Psychological (4 Positive feelings, 5 Thinking, learning, memory and concentration, 6 Self-esteem, 7 Bodily image and appearance, 8 Negative feelings), III Level of Independence (9 Mobility, 10 Activities of daily living, 11 Dependence on medication or treatments, 12 Work capacity), IV Social Relationships (13 Personal relationships, 14 Social support, 15 Sexual activity), V Environment (16 Physical safety and security, 17 Home environment, 18 Financial resources, 19 Health and social care: accessibility and quality, 20 Opportunities for acquiring new information and skills, 21 Participation in and opportunities for recreation/ leisure activities, 22 Physical environment (pollution/noise/traffic/climate), 23 Transport), VI Spirituality/Religion/ Personal Beliefs. (WHOQOL Group, 1995).

Short Form 36-item Health Survey Questionnaire

The Short Form 36-item Health Survey Questionnaire (SF-36) is a generic instrument for QOL assessment. It is a questionnaire with thirty-six items, grouped into the eight domains, which are: physical function, role limitations due to physical health, pain, general health perception, vitality, social function, role limitations due to emotional problems, and mental health. It summarize the results in two areas: physical and psychological. The score ranges are from zero to hundred and are directly proportional to the state of health.. There are validation studies in SLE patients, in a variety of socio-cultural contexts using many languages SF-36 versions. The SF-36 was recommended as the instrument of choice for measuring HRQOL in SLE. (Freire el al, 2011; Thumboo & Strand, 2007)

Systemic Lupus Erythematosus Symptom Checklist

The Systemic Lupus Erythematosus Symptom Checklist (SSC) measure the impact of the disease and its treatment on the individual. This questionnaire study 38 symptoms in a four-point scale, where zero is the best health status and four, the worst. (Freire et el, 2011; Sanchez et al, 2009; Thumboo & Strand, 2007)

Systemic Lupus Erythematosus Quality of Life Questionnaire

The Systemic Lupus Erythematosus Quality of Life Questionnaire (SLEQOL) has 40 items into the six domains: physical function, occupational activity, symptoms, treatment, mood and self-image. The scores vary from one to seven, and the lower (fourty) the score is the best the QOL and the higher (two hundred and eighty) the score is the worse QOL. This questionnaire showed to have more sensitivity to changes over time than SF-36. (Freire et el, 2011; Sanchez et al, 2009; Thumboo & Strand, 2007)

Systemic Lupus Erythematosus Needs Questionnaire

The Systemic Lupus Erythematosus Needs Questionnaire (SLENQ) has seven domains: that assess the following needs: psychological-spiritual-existential, health services, health information, physical, social support, daily living, and employment. This questionnaire showed moderate correlations with SF-36. (Moses et al, 2007; Freire et el, 2011).

Lupus Quality of Life

The Lupus Quality of Life (LupusQOL) contains thirty four items in eight domains: physical health, emotional health, body image, pain, planning, fatigue, intimate relationships and burden to others. (Freire et el, 2011; McElhone et al, 2007; Sanchez et al, 2009; Thumboo & Strand, 2007)

Cross-sectional studies and prospective studies have identified the age, the duration, the activity and damage disease, some specific manifestations of SLE as fatigue, pain or end-stage renal failure, the corticosteroids or cytotoxic, the knowledge of lupus, the illness related behaviours, the educational status, the self-efficacy, the learned helplessness, the ability to work, the home environment and the social support as factors associated may influence health-related quality of life (HRQOL) in SLE patients. (McElhone K et al, 2006; Navarrete-Navarrete et al, 2010; Thumboo & Strand, 2007)

5. Treatment

The SLE is no curable and complete remissions are rare, sometimes is cyclical and sometimes is progressive, is heterogeneous in manifestations and has significant mortality risk. It is a disease that requires lifelong treatment.

SLE may have a higher impact on patients' life than other chronic illnesses, and the level of impact may be influenced by type of treatment. SLE is a disease that can significantly impact physiological, psychological and social functioning, influencing in health-related quality of life of the patients. The pharmacologic and non-pharmacologic therapies may have an additive or synergistic effect on improving on these patients HRQOL (Daleboudt et al, 2011; Thumboo & Strand, 2007).

5.1 Patient-centred care

The treatment of SLE's people should be patient-centred ensuring that the patients are treated with dignity and respect. Good communication between doctors and patients is essential. These ills and their families and carers need a high-quality communication, supported by evidence-based information that provides treatment and care based on best practice. Patients should have the opportunity to be involved in the decisions about their treatment and care. The physician should take into account needs and preferences of the patients. Families and carers should have the information and support they need. Information, treatment and care should be given at patients, families and carers by culturally appropriate written information tailored to their needs. (Michalski & Kodner , 2010; van der Giesen et al, 2007; Villanueva, 2009)

5.2 Multidisciplinary treatment

SLE is a complex disease. Healthcare professionals of these patients must pay careful attention to all items of illness (physical, psychological, family and social) in multidisciplinary cooperation. It is the most frequent that patient comes at primary care physicians. The American College of Rheumatology Ad Hoc Committee on SLE guidelines recommends that primary care physicians should refer SLE patients to rheumatologists to establish SLE definitive diagnosis, activity and severity disease and treatment of general disease and some medication side effects. Rheumatologists should work with a multidisciplinary team allowing coordinated care of patient. This includes family physicians, other specialist physicians, psychotherapies, rehabilitations, nurses and social workers. Family Medicine is a specialty focused person-centred care. Competent and polyvalent family physicians may be allowed to attend the patient in his/her whole life. From primary care should monitored ill a long time and treated when presents other pathologies or some medication side effects (infection, cardiovascular disease, osteoporosis,) or mild symptom SLE. From other specialist physicians should treat damaged major organ. From psychotherapy should teach coping strategies to favor psychosocial adjustment. (Aberer, 2010; Beckerman et al, 2011; Michalski & Kodner , 2010; Ramírez, 2007; Taylor & McMurray, 2011; van der Giesen et al, 2007; Villanueva, 2009)

5.3 Physical treatment

Medical treatment and a recommended lifestyle are necessary for optimal functioning in life SLE patients.

The pharmacological treatment is always individual. It depends if it is to control acute, severe flares or to develop maintenance strategies that suppress symptoms and prevent organ damage. This therapy also depends on adverse effects of medications, whether disease manifestations are life-threatening or to cause organ damage, whether manifestations are potentially reversible and the best approaches to preventing complications of disease. (Michalski & Kodner , 2010; Taylor & McMurray, 2011; Yildirim-Torner C & Diamond B, 2011.)

The most important drugs are: nonsteroidal anti-inflammatory drugs, hydroxychloroquine corticosteroids, immunosuppressive drugs (azathioprine, cyclophosphamide, methotrexate, mycophenolate). Almost all patients should take hydroxychloroquine and most corticosteroids with immunosuppressive drugs. With better management, patients with lupus live longer but are at increased risk of disease and treatment-related complications, including infection, cardiovascular disease, and osteoporosis. (Michalski & Kodner , 2010; Taylor & McMurray, 2011; Yildiri-Toruner C & Diamond B, 2011.)

Pharmacologic and biologic therapies reducing disease activity and/or levels of anti-dsDNA antibodies improving HRQOL for SLE patients.(Thumboo & Strand, 2007; Dall'era & Chakravarty, 2011)

The damages disease in skin or alopecia can be improved with treatment of these lesions and/or use of cosmetics to camouflage these lesions.

The use of a highly protective broad-spectrum (UVB and UVA) sunscreen can effectively prevent skin photosensitive lesions in patients's SLE. (Kuhn et al, 2011; Obermoser & Zelger B, 2008 ; Thumboo & Strand, 2007)

5.4 Psychological and social treatment

The psychotherapy programs should help to equip the SLE's patients with knowledge and skills of coping for managing the illness and to build up familiar and social support.

The patients with rheumatic illness experience significant restrictions into their daily life. There are researches that prove that the cognitive behavioral therapy (coping methods and contextual methods) improves on these persons their experience of physical symptom (pain, fatigue), daily activity, psychology and social functioning.

Although there are few researches on SLE's patients, the cognitive behavioral therapy (CBT) (coping methods and contextual methods) reaches above average levels in physical functioning, psychic functioning and social functioning obtaining a significant improvement in the HRQOL, independent of the activity level of the disease. (McCracken & Vowles, 2008; Navarrete-Navarrete et al, 2010; Ramírez, 2007)

5.4.1 Psychotherapy methods

The behavioral therapy is in a state of development. Actually, there are three generations. They are based on chosen strategies the two firsts direct change, coping methods, and the third indirect change, contextual methods. The coping methods are focused on control or change in the content of psychological experiences and the contextual methods include acceptance, mindfulness and values. These therapies are characterized: the first by behavioral change, the second by cognitive models and the third by processes of acceptance and values-based action. They are integrative and not exclusive, they encompass each other. In these therapies the problems are rationalized and contextualized and the sensations produced by them can improve experience and acceptance.

The psychotherapy that use coping methods includes: understanding SLE providing information, understanding one's rights as a patient, controlling pain and fatigue oneself, teaching stress management through concept of stress and relaxation techniques (diaphragm breathing and deep muscle relaxation), alternative thought control strategies that help to manage frustration and emotion (self-instructional training and thought stopping), humour and optimism as coping strategies, cognitive restructuring (identifying and discussing the consequences of main errors in thinking, main core beliefs, challenging thoughts), demonstrating problem-solving skills, developing personal strengths, training in social skills (assertiveness techniques, how to say no without feeling bad, asking another person to change their behavior) locating community resources for rehabilitation. (Navarrete-Navarrete et al, 2010; Ng P & Chan, 2007; Ramírez, 2007; Robles-Ortega & Peralta-Ramírez, 2006; Sheldon,1995)

The psychotherapy that includes contextual methods is acceptance and commitment therapy (ACT) and mindfulness.

The ACT centers on building positive and flexible behavior patterns rather than removing symptoms carrying up processes of acceptance, contact with the present moment and values-based action. This model includes: acceptance, cognitive defusion, contact with the present moment, self-as-context, values and committed action (Hayes et al, 2006). The studies with this treatment on patient's rheumatic illness are very up to date. (McCracken & Vowles, 2008)

Mindfulness is a technique and a component of the acceptance and commitment therapy. It can be understood as attention, awareness and reflection of present moment non-judgmental. This model include: nonconceptual, focused on the present, non-judgmental, intentional, participatory observation, emotional, exploratory and liberating. The researches with this technique on patient's rheumatic are also very up to date. (Germer et al, 2005)

5.4.2 Psychotherapy in SLE

The patients with SLE live with fears about the illness because they have nothing or little knowledge about the clinic, treatment and prognosis of the illness. The researches have shown that to improve the understanding of these persons with accurate information of the mechanisms of SLE contribute to a better adjustment to live with their illness because their negative beliefs about it are reduced influencing on their self-esteem. (Ng P & Chan, 2007)

5.4.2.1 Chronic pain

The chronic pain is a great suffering for SLE's patient.
The medical and surgical treatments may produce variable results and adverse events and iatrogenic complications on any patient with chronic pain. The use of other means for pain reduction, as the programs of physical activity may reduce pain improving HRQOL in these ills.
The subjective nature of pain makes complicated this problem. The pain is a response to nociception on the patient influenced by genetic, personal history, physiologic state and psychological and social context. And the pain influences on physical, psychological and social functioning.
The patients with chronic pain may be influenced by distressing thoughts and emotions and ineffective behaviors focusing on their pain. The increasing attempts to control pain may be associated with increasing the limits of their functioning interfering with healthy living. An alternative approach, are personal's choice of adaptive responses adjusted to chronic pain. The research has shown the utility of ACT. The experienced pain, with control, allows more healthy activities.
The acceptance-oriented responses to chronic pain may improve physical (disability), psychological (suffering) and social (working) functioning over time. The positive purposes of families and friends, with more patient attitude about behavior pattern, may make easier the processes of acceptance.
The mindfulness-based treatment methods are addressed to these patients suffering chronic pain. The mindfulness is based: present-focused, realistic contact with pain, neutral awareness of pain, change experience pain and effective behavioral. Mindfulness is observation and commitment. The researches show mindfulness may get better well-being of patients with chronic pain. It gives them more realistic experiences and more effective flexible behavioral. (McCracken et al, 2007; Thumboo & Strand, 2007)

5.4.2.2 Fatigue

Fatigue is lack of energy, physical and mental tiredness. On SLE's patients, it compromises quality of life, reducing psychological well-being, because these difficulties on daily activities affect personal and social life.
Fatigue is present on many chronic ills, for example: multiple sclerosis, cancer, chronic fatigue syndrome, rheumatoid arthritis, SLE.
The physiopathology of fatigue in SLE have been difficult to identify but likely to be multi-factorial.
Fatigue may be associated with SLE disease process and with pain, lack of physical exertion, sleep disturbance, depression, anxiety, stressful life events, infection, medication side effects and characteristics of the local environment (lighting and temperature). (Bakshi 2003; Dittner et al, 2004 ; Godaert et al, 2002 ; Neill, 2005 ; Zifko, 2004).
Researches for reducing fatigue in people with SLE are few and show strategies not completely effective in the long-term. The treatment of chronic illnesses fatigue usually combines pharmacological and nonpharmacological therapy. Pharmacological therapy efficacy is questioned in fatigue of SLE's patients and nonpharmacological therapy is essential for her management. This therapy include exercise, rehabilitation programmes and cognitive behavioral therapy. (Godaert et al, 2002)
Studies suggest aerobic exercise is effective for reducing fatigue in some people with SLE. This exercise includes low-impact aerobics, walking, cycling, and jogging. It should be

appropriate for each ill and take into account individual fluctuations in fatigue intensity, if feasible, it might be executed home-based or in supervised classes. This exercise should begin early in the disease course or following the disease, start with low intensity activities and avoid provoking symptoms, gradually increasing in intensity, duration and frequency, combine aerobic and resistance training where possible. It is recommended to carry out between fifteen and thirty minutes at least three times weekly if it is tolerated. This exercise type appears to be effective in reducing fatigue in patient with cancer and chronic fatigue syndrome. (Mancuso et al, 2010; Stricker et al. 2004 ; Watson & Mock, 2004).

Fatigue is a variable and subjective experience that may decline inactive life-style disproportionally affecting physical activity, psychological and societal participation. In this case, it might be required to promote interventions of self-management of fatigue and better illness cognitions and coping styles by means of CBT.

Cognitive behavioural therapy helps to identify and to challenge perpetuating factors. These are: insufficient coping with the disease and dysfunctional cognitions about fatigue such as lack of control and catastrophizing (negative thoughts are put into reality perspective), deregulation of sleep (to adhere biologic rhythm and to fixed bedtimes and wake-up times during the day), deregulation of activity (a base level activity and alternating rest and activity should be established), low social interactions (to favor realistic expectations toward the participation in social relations).

Studies show that cognitive behavioural therapy with/without exercise is effective in reducing fatigue in chronic fatigue syndrome, multiple sclerosis, cancer-related fatigue and SLE because it improves self-efficacy, increasing their quality of life. (Edmonds et al, 2004; Navarrete-Navarrete et al, 2010; Neill et al, 2006; Wagner & Cella, 2004)

5.4.2.3 Neuropsychiatric manifestations

Cognitive dysfunction, anxiety and depression are frequent in patient's SLE. The consequences of SLE living may impact personal life, including interpersonal relationships and professional rol. The majority of SLE patients present depression and emotional distress. These affective disturbances are very rarely attributed to disease activity alone, and may influence psychosocial factors. Cognitive dysfunction may coexists with psychiatric disorders. Their association in SLE is not clear. Some study shows the psychological state of the ill may influence self-reporting of cognitive problems (Farrin et al, 2003; Kozora et al, 2006; Kozora et al, 2007; Nowicka-Sauer et al, 2011; Panopalis et al, 2007; Vogel et al, 2011; Zakeri et al, 2011.)

Neuropsychiatric manifestations should be diagnosed and treated in these patients first as if they had not SLE, and secondarily as if they had it. (Bertsias et al, 2010)

Clinical guideline about care of patients with depression and a chronic physical health problem recommend physical activity programme and cognitive behavioural therapy. (NICE, 2009)

Cognitive behavioural therapy sets up role cognitive representations or perceptions and emotional responses of patient's SLE that can influence individual's ability to manage his illness by selecting coping strategies. The ill may organize an individual's response around five cognitives. These include: representation of their illness, perceived duration, unpredictability, control, perceived of severity and cause. There are researches that show better depressive symptoms and cognitive dysfunction in patient SLE following cognitive behavioural therapy.(Bertsias & Boumpas, 2010 ; Bertsias et al, 2010; Greco et al, 2004; Philip et al, 2009)

6. Conclusion

Systemic lupus erythematosus (SLE) is a chronic inflammatory autoimmune disease of unknown etiology, with predominance of the female sex in their childbearing years.
SLE affects heterogeneity multiple organs of the body and presents aberrant immunological findings. The clinical course and prognosis is unpredictable. It can affect socio-psychologically to patients experiencing high levels of emotional distress by affecting physical, pharmacology treatment, their own worries about illness, abnormal illness-related behaviours and affecting social life.
The integral diagnosis in the patients with SLE include the aspects: physical, psychological and social. The physical diagnosis of SLE is based on the clinical and the laboratory and on the American Rheumatism Association (ARA) classification criteria. The psychological and social diagnosis can be obtain through data collection via a semi-structured interview performed by the same physician and measure about the illness perception of the own patient, experienced thought and behavior by chronic illness, the role of personality and coping with stressful life situations and social relationships.
The integral treatment of patient's SLE include pharmacological and non-pharmacological therapies that may have an additive or synergistic effect on these patients. These treatment should be patient-centred favouring high-quality communication between doctors and patients with their families and carers supported by evidence-based information that provides treatment and care based on best practice. These patients should be treatment by multidisciplinary team that include family physicians, rheumatologists, other specialist physicians, psychotherapies, rehabilitations, nurses and social workers. Pharmacological treatment and recommended lifestyle are always individual and necessary for optimal functioning in life SLE patients. The psychotherapy should help to equip the SLE's patients, that experience significant restrictions into their daily life, with knowledge and skills of coping for managing the illness and to build up familiar and social support. The cognitive behavioural therapy (coping methods: behavioural change and cognitive models, and contextual methods: acceptance and commitment therapy and mindfulness) improves on these persons their experience of physical symptom (pain, fatigue,…), daily activity, psychology and social functioning.

7. Key points

1. The SLE is a chronic inflammatory autoimmune disease of unknown etiology with predominance on the female sex in their childbearing years.
2. The SLE affects heterogeneity multiple organs of the body and presents aberrant immunological findings.
3. The clinical course and prognosis of SLE is unpredictable, it is a disease no cure.
4. The SLE affect patient's bio-psycho-social unit.
5. The integral diagnosis in patients with SLE includes : physical, psychological and social aspects.
6. The treatment of SLE patients should be physical, psychological and social.
7. The treatment of SLE's people should be patient-centred.
8. Healthcare to SLE patients should be multidisciplinary including rheumatologists, family physicians, other specialist physicians, psychotherapies, rehabilitations, nurses and social workers.

9. Medical treatment and a recommended lifestyle are necessary for optimal functioning in the life of SLE patients.
10. The psychotherapy programs should help to equip the SLE's patients with knowledge and skills of coping for managing the illness and to build up familiar and social support.
11. The cognitive behavioural therapy (coping methods and contextual methods) improves on the persons' SLE their experience of physical symptom (pain, fatigue, neuropsychiatric manifestations), daily activity, psychology and social functioning.

8. References

Aberer E. (2010). Epidemiologic, socioeconomic and psychosocial aspects in lupus erythematosus Lupus (2010) 19, 1118–1124

Abu-Shakra M, Keren A, Livshitz I. (2006). Sense of coherence and its impact on quality of life of patients with systemic lupus erythematosus. Lupus 2006; 15: 32–37.

American Psychiatric Association. Diagnostic and Statistical Manual of Mental Disorders DSM-IV-TR (4th ed.,text rev.). Washington, American Psychiatric Press, 1994.

Bai M, Tomenson B, Creed F.(2009). The role of psychological distress and personality variables in the disablement process in rheumatoid arthritis. Scand J Rheumatol 2009; 38: 419–430.

Baker K & Pope J. (2009). Employment and work disability in systemic lupus erythematosus: a systematic review. Rheumatology (Oxford).2009 Mar;48(3):281-4. Epub 2009 Jan 19.

Bakshi R. (2003) Fatigue associated with multiple sclerosis: diagnosis, impact and management. Multiple Sclerosis 9(3), 219–227.

Beck AT, Steer RA, Garbin MG. (1988). Psychometric properties of the Beck Depression Inventory: twenty-five years of evaluation. Clin Psychol Rev 1988;8:77–100.

Beckerman N. L., Auerbach Ch., Blanco I. (2011). Psychosocial dimensions of SLE: implications for the health care team. Journal of Multidisciplinary Healthcare 2011:4 63–72

Bertsias GK, Boumpas DT. (2010). Pathogenesis, diagnosis and management of neuropsychiatric SLE manifestations. Nat Rev Rheumatol. Jun 6(6):358-67.

Bertsias GK, J P A Ioannidis, M Aringer, E Bollen, S Bombardieri, I N Bruce, R Cervera, M Dalakas, A Doria, J G Hanly, T W J Huizinga, D Isenberg, C Kallenberg, J C Piette, M Schneider, N Scolding, J Smolen, A Stara,I Tassiulas, M Tektonidou, A Tincani, M A van Buchem, R van Vollenhoven, M Ward, C Gordon, D T Boumpas (2010). EULAR recommendations for the management of systemic lupus erythematosus with neuropsychiatric manifestations: report of a task force of the EULAR standing committee for clinical affairs. Ann Rheum Dis 69:2074–2082. doi:10.1136/ard.2010.130476

Broadbent E, Petrie KJ, Main J, Weinman J. (2006). The brief illness perception questionnaire. J Psychosom Res 2006; 60: 631–637.

Brown KW, Ryan RM. (2003). The benefits of being present: mindfulness and its role in psychological well-being. J Pers Soc Psychol 2003; 84:822–48.

Büchi S, Villiger P, Kauer Y, Klaghofer R, Sensky T & Stoll T. (2000). PRISM (Pictorial Representation of Illness and Self Measure) a novel visual method to assess the global burden of illness in patients with systemic lupus erythematosus. Lupus (2000) 9, 368±373.

Büchi S, Sensky T, Sharpe L, Timberlake N. (1998). Graphic representation of illness: a novel method of measuring patients' perceptions of the impact of illness. Psychother Psychosom 1998; 67: 222± 225.

Burgos PI, Alarcón GS, McGwin G Jr, Crews KQ, Reveille JD, Vilá LM. (2009). Disease activity and damage are not associated with increased levels of fatigue in systemic lupus erythematosus patients from a multiethnic cohort: LXVII. Arthritis Rheum.2009 Sep 15;61(9):1179-86.

Chaiamnuay S, Bertoli AM, Fernández M Apte M, Vilá LM, Reveille JD, Alarcón GS. (2007). The impact of increased body mass index on systemic lupus erythematosus: data from LUMINA, a multiethnic cohort. J Clin Rheumatol. 2007 Jun;13(3):128-33.

Chuang TH, Lin KC, Gau ML. (2010). Validation of the braden self-help model in women with systemic lupus erythematosus. J Nurs Res.2010 Sep;18(3):206-14.

Dalléra M, Chakravarty EF. (2011). Treatment of Mild, Moderate, and Severe Lupus Erythematosus: Focus on New Therapies. urr Rheumatol Rep. 2011 May 17.

Daleboudt GMN, Broadbent E, Berger SP & Kaptein AA. (2011). Illness perceptions in patients with systemic lupus erythematosus and proliferative lupus nephritis. Lupus (2011) 20, 290–298

Dittner A., Wessley S. & Brown R. (2004) The assessment of fatigue – a practical guide for clinicians and researchers. Journal of Psychosomatic Research 56(2), 157–170.

Duvdevany I, Cohen M, Minsker-Valtzer A & Lorber M. (2011). Psychological correlates of adherence to self-care, disease activity and functioning in persons with systemic lupus erythematosus. Lupus (2011) 20, 14–22

Edmonds M., McGuire H. & Price J. (2004) Exercise therapy for chronic fatigue syndrome. The Cochrane Database of Systematic Reviews, issue 3, art no.: CD003200.pub2.

Errol J. Philip, M.A, Helen Lindner, Ph.D., Leah Lederman, B.B.Sc. (2009). Relationship of illness perceptions with depression among individuals diagnosed with lupus depression and anxiety. 2009, 26:575–582

Farrin L, Hull L, Unwin C, Wykes T, David A. (2003). Effects of depressed mood on objective and subjective measures of attention. J Neuropsychiatry Clin Neurosci 15: 98–104.

Freire, Souto, Ciconelli3. (2011). Assessment measures in systemic lupus erythematosus. Rev Bras Reumatol 2011;51(1):70-80

Germer, C.K., Siegel, R.D., & Fulton, P.R. (2005). Mindfulness and psychotherapy. New York: GuilfordPress.

Giesen van der, Nelissen, Rozing, Arendzen, de Jong, Wolterbeek, Vliet Vlieland. (2007). A Multidisciplinary Hand Clinic for Patients with Rheumatic Diseases: a Pilot Study Journal of Hand Therapy. July-September 2007

Griffiths B, Mosca M, Gordon C. (2005). Assessment of patients with systemic lupus erythematosus and the use of lupus disease activity indices. Best Pract Res Clin Rheumatol 2005; 19(5):685-708.

Hyphantis T. (2010). The Greek version of the Defense Style Questionnaire: psychometric properties in three different samples. Compr Psychiatry 2010; 51: 618–629.

Hyphantis T, Bai L, Siafaka V. (2006). Psychological distress and personality traits in early rheumatoid arthritis: a preliminary survey. Rheum Int 2006; 26: 828–836.

Hyphantis T, Palieraki K, Voulgari PV, Tsifetaki N & Drosos AA (2011). Coping with health-stressors and defence styles associated with health-related quality of life in patients with systemic lupus erythematosus. Lupus (2011) 0, 1–11

Isenberg DA, Rahman A, Allen E, Farewell V, Akil M, Bruce IN. (2005). Development and initial validation of an updated version of the British Isles Lupus Assessment Groups disease activity index for patients with systemic lupus erythematosus. Rheumatology (Oxford) 2005.

Javierre BM, Richardson B. (2011). A new epigenetic challenge: systemic lupus erythematosus. Adv Exp Med Biol. 2011;711:117-36.

Jong Z.de, Wolterbeek R., Vliet Vlieland T.P.M., (2007). A Multidisciplinary Hand Clinic for Patients with Rheumatic Diseases: a Pilot Study. Journal of Hand Therapy (July-September 2007) doi:10.1197/j.jht.2007.04.004

Godaert G.L., Hartkamp A., Geenen R., Garssen A., Kruize A.A., Bijlsma J.W. & Derksen R.H. (2002) Fatigue in daily life in patients with primary Sjogren's syndrome and systemic lupus erythematosus. Annals of the New York Academy of Sciences 966, 320–326.

Greco CM, Rudy TE, Manzi S. (2004) Effects of a stress-reduction program on psychological function, pain, and physical function of systemic lupus erythematosus patients: a randomized controlled trial. Arthritis Rheum 51 : 625 - 34 .

Hayes, S. C., Luoma, J. B., Bond, F. W., Masuda, A., Lillis, J. (2006). Acceptance and Commitment Therapy: Model, processes and outcomes. Behaviour Research and Therapy, 44, 1–25.

Jarpa E, Babul M, Calderón J, González M, Martínez ME, Bravo-Zehnder M, Henríquez C, Jacobelli S, González A, Massardo L (2011). Common mental disorders and psychological distress in systemic lupus erythematosus are not associated with disease activity. Lupus. 2011 Jan;20(1):58-66. Epub 2010 Nov 15.

Kaptein AA, Broadbent E. (2007). Illness cognition assessment. In: Ayers S, Baum A, McManus C, et al. Handbook of Psychology, Health and Medicine, 2nd ed. Cambridge: Cambridge University Press; 2007. p. 268–273.

Koike T. (2011). The new era of autoimmune disease research. Arthritis Res Ther. 2011 May 31;13(3):113.

Kozora E, Arciniegas DB, Zhang L, West S. (2007). Neuropsychological patterns in systemic lupus erythematosus patients with depression. Arthritis Res Ther; 9: R48

Kozora E, Ellison MC, West S. (2006). Depression, fatigue, and pain in systemic lupus erythematosus (SLE): relationship to the American College of Rheumatology SLE neuropsychological battery. Arthritis Rheum 55: 628–635.

Kuhn A., Gensch K., Haust M., Meuth AM., Boyer F., Dupuy P, Lehmann P., Metze D, Ruzicka T. (2011). Photoprotective effects of a broad-spectrum sunscreen in ultraviolet-induced cutaneous lupus erythematosus: A randomized, vehicle-controlled, double-blind study. J Am Acad Dermatol Vol.64, No.1 (January 2011) ; 64:37-48.

Lance M. McCracken. (2007) Jeremy Gauntlett-Gilbert, Kevin E. Vowles (2007). The role of mindfulness in a contextual cognitive-behavioral analysis of chronic pain-related suffering and disability. Pain 131 (2007) 63–69

Eriksson M, Lindstrom B. (2005). Validity of Antonovsky's sense of coherence scale: a systematic review. J Epidemiol Community. Health 2005; 59: 460–466.

Mancuso CA, Perna M, Sargent AB & Salmon JE. (2010). Perceptions and measurements of physical activity in patients with systemic lupus erythematosus .Lupus (February 2010) 0, 1–12

McCracken L.M., Vowles K. E., Gauntlett-Gilbert J. (2007). A Prospective Investigation of Acceptance and Control-Oriented Coping with Chronic Pain. J Behav Med 30:339–349

McCracken L.M. & Vowles K.E. (2008) A Prospective Analysis of Acceptance of Pain and Values-Based Action in Patients With Chronic Pain. Health Psychology Vol. 27, No. 2, 215–220

McCracken L M., MacKichan F, Eccleston C. (2007). Contextual cognitive-behavioral therapy for severely disabled chronic pain sufferers: Effectiveness and clinically significant change. European Journal of Pain 11 (2007) 314–322

McCracken LM, Gauntlett-Gilbert J, Vowles KE. (2007). The role of mindfulness in a contextual cognitive-behavioral analysis of chronic pain-related suffering and disability. Pain 131 (2007) 63–69

McCracken LM, Yang S. (2006) The role of values in a contextual cognitive-behavioral approach to chronic pain. Pain 123 (2006) 137–145

McCracken LM, Vowels KE, Eccleston C. (2004). Acceptance of chronic pain: component analysis and a revised assessment method. Pain 2004;107:159–66.

McElhone K, Abbott J, Shelmerdine J, Bruce IN, Ahmad Y, Gordon C. (2007). Development and validation of a disease-specific healthy-related quality of life measure, the LupusQOL, for adults with systemic lupus erythematosus. Arthritis Rheum 2007; 57(6):972-9.

McElhone K, Abbott J, Teh LS. (2006). A review of health related quality of life in systemic lupus erythematosus. Lupus 2006; 15: 633–643.

Michalski JP & Kodner C. (2010) Systemic lupus erythematosus: safe and effective management in primary care. rim Care. (Dec 2010) 37(4):767-78, vii.

Moses N, Wiggers J, Nicholas C, Cockburn J. (2007). Development and psychometric analysis of the systemic lupus erythematosus questionnaire (SLENQ). Qual Life Res 2007; 16(3):461-6.

Nakashima CA, Galhardo AP, Silva JF, Fiorenzano GR, Santos AB Leite MF, Nogueira MA, Menolli PV, Menolli RA. (2011). Incidence and clinical-laboratory aspects of systemic lupus erythematosus in a Southern brazilian city. Rev Bras Reumatol. 2011 Jun;51(3):235-239.

National Collaborating Centre for Mental Health. National Institute for Health and Clinical Excellence [NICE] (2009) Depression in adults with a chronic physical health problem. Treatment and management. www.nice.org.uk/CG91

Ng P. & Chan W. (2007). Group psychosocial program for enhancing psychological well-being of people with systemic lupus erythematosus. J Soc Work Disabil Rehabil. 2007;6(3):75-87.

N Navarrete-Navarrete, MI Peralta-Ramírez, JM Sabio, I Martínez-Egea, A Santos-Ruiz, J Jiménez-Alonso. (2010). Quality-of-life predictor factors in patients with SLE and their modification after cognitive behavioural therapy. Lupus 19, 1632–1639.

Niller HH, Wolf H Ay E, Minarovits J. (2011). Minarovits J Epigenetic dysregulation of epstein-barr virus latency and development of autoimmune disease. Adv Exp Med Biol. 2011;711:82-102.

Neill J. (2005) Exploring underlying life patterns of women with multiple sclerosis or rheumatoid arthritis: comparison with NANDA dimensions. Nursing Science Quarterly 18(4), 344–352.

Neill J . , Belan I . & Ried K. (2006) Effectiveness of non-pharmacological interventions for fatigue in adults with multiple sclerosis, rheumatoid arthritis, or systemic lupus erythematosus: a systematic review. Journal of Advanced Nursing 56(6),617–635

Nowicka-Sauer K. (2007). Patients' perspective: lupus in patients' drawings. Assessing drawing as a diagnostic and therapeutic method. Clin Rheumatol. 2007 Sep;26(9):1523-5. Epub 2007 Apr 20

Nowicka-Sauer K, Czuszynska Z, Smolenska Z, Siebert J (2011) Neuropsychological assessment in systemic lupus erythematosus patients: clinical Clin Exp Rheumatol. Mar-Apr;29(2):299-306. Epub 2011 Apr 19.

Obermoser G, Zelger B. (2008). Triple need for photoprotection in lupus erythematosus. Lupus 17:525-7.

Panopalis P, Julian L, Yazdany J. (2007). Impact of memory impairment on employment status in persons with systemic lupus erythematosus. Arthritis Rheum; 57 : 1453 – 60.

Ramírez R. (2007). Depresión, primera manifestación de Lupus Eritematoso Sistémico. Semergen 2007; 33:438-40. Vol.33, No. 8.

Robles-Ortega H, Peralta-Ramıírez MI. (2006). Programa para el control del estrés, (ed). Pirámide; 2006.

Roelofs J, McCracken L, Peters ML, Crombez G, van Breukelen G. (2004). Vlaeyen JWS. Psychometric evaluation of the Pain Anxiety Symptoms Scale (PASS) in chronic pain patients. J Behav Med 2004;27:167–83.

Sanchez ML, McGwin G Jr, Durán S, Fernández M, Reveille JD, Vilá LM, Alarcón GS. (2009). Factors predictive of overall health over the course of the disease in patients with systemic lupus erythematosus from the LUMINA cohort (LXII): use of the SF-6D. Clin Exp Rheumatol.2009 Jan-Feb;27(1):67-71.

Sheldon, B. (1995) Cognitive-Behavioural Therapy. Research, practice and philosophy. Routledge, London.

Stricker C.T., Drake D., Hoyer K.A. & Mock V. (2004) Evidencebased practice for fatigue management in adults with cancer: exercise as an intervention. Oncology Nursing Forum 31(5), 963–974.

Taylor JK. & McMurray RV. (2011). Medical therapy for systemic lupus erythematosus. J Miss State Med Assoc..2011 Feb;52(2):39-43.

Thumboo J, Strand V. (2007) Health-related Quality of Life in Patients with Systemic Lupus Erythematosus: An Update. Ann Acad Med Singapore February 2007;36 (2):115-22

Villanueva T. (2009). Family Medicine, the specialty of the future: the Portuguese situation within the European context. International Archives of Medicine 2009, 2:36

Vogel A, Bhattacharya S, Larsen JL & Jacobsen S (2011). Do subjective cognitive complaints correlate with cognitive impairment in systemic lupus erythematosus? A Danish outpatient study. Lupus (2011) 20, 35-43

WHOQOL Group. The World Health Organization quality of life assessment (WHOQOL): position paper from the World Health organization. Soc Sci Med 1995; 41: 1403-1409.

Wagner L.I. & Cella D. (2004) Fatigue and cancer: causes, prevalence and treatment approaches. British Journal of Cancer 91(5), 822-828.

Watson T. & Mock V. (2004) Exercise as an intervention for cancerrelated fatigue. Physical Therapy 84(8), 736-743.

Yildirim-Toruner C. & Diamond B. (2011). Current and novel therapeutics in the treatment of systemic lupus erythematosus. J Allergy Clin Immunol February 2011, Vol. 127, No.2

Zakeri Z, Shakiba M, Narouie B, Mladkova N, Ghasemi-Rad M, Khosravi A. (2011). Prevalence of depression and depressive symptoms in patients with systemic lupus erythematosus: Iranian experience. Rheumatol Int.2011 Jan 21.

Zifko U. (2004) Management of fatigue in patients with multiple sclerosis. Drugs 64(12), 1295-1304.